Pheromones and Reproduction in Mammals

Contributors

F. H. Bronson

M. K. Izard

Robert E. Johnston

Eric B. Keverne

Michael Leon

Martha K. McClintock

Bruce Macmillan

Anna Marchlewska-Koj

Michael Meredith

John G. Vandenbergh

Pheromones and Reproduction in Mammals

Edited by

John G. Vandenbergh

Department of Zoology
School of Agriculture and Life Sciences
North Carolina State University
Raleigh, North Carolina

1983

ACADEMIC PRESS

A Subsidiary of Harcourt Brace Jovanovich, Publishers

New York   London
Paris   San Diego   San Francisco   São Paulo   Sydney   Tokyo   Toronto

COPYRIGHT © 1983, BY ACADEMIC PRESS, INC.
ALL RIGHTS RESERVED.
NO PART OF THIS PUBLICATION MAY BE REPRODUCED OR
TRANSMITTED IN ANY FORM OR BY ANY MEANS, ELECTRONIC
OR MECHANICAL, INCLUDING PHOTOCOPY, RECORDING, OR ANY
INFORMATION STORAGE AND RETRIEVAL SYSTEM, WITHOUT
PERMISSION IN WRITING FROM THE PUBLISHER.

ACADEMIC PRESS, INC.
111 Fifth Avenue, New York, New York 10003

United Kingdom Edition published by
ACADEMIC PRESS, INC. (LONDON) LTD.
24/28 Oval Road, London NW1 7DX

Library of Congress Cataloging in Publication Data
Main entry under title:

Pheromones and reproduction in mammals.

   Includes bibliographical references and index.
   1. Mammals--Reproduction.   2. Pheromones.
I. Vandenbergh, John G.
QL739.2.P48   1983   599'.016   82-22776
ISBN 0-12-710780-0

PRINTED IN THE UNITED STATES OF AMERICA

83 84 85 86   9 8 7 6 5 4 3 2 1

591.51
P529

This volume is dedicated to Wesley K. Whitten and to the memory of Hilda M. Bruce. Their original discoveries of estrus synchronization and pregnancy blockage in mice stimulated much of the work reported here.

Contents

I   Signalling Pheromones

1   Chemical Signals and Reproductive Behavior

Robert E. Johnston

2   Chemical Communication in Mother–Young Interactions

Michael Leon

6 Pregnancy Blocking by Pheromones

Anna Marchlewska-Koj

7 Hormonal Responses to Primer Pheromones

F. H. Bronson and Bruce Macmillan

8 Sensory Physiology of Pheromone Communication

Michael Meredith

9   Pheromones and Reproduction in Domestic Animals

M. K. Izard

Contributors

Numbers in parentheses indicate the pages on which the authors' contributions begin.

F. H. Bronson (175), Department of Zoology, Institute of Reproductive Biology, University of Texas, Austin, Texas 78712

M. K. Izard (253)* Department of Zoology, North Carolina State University, Raleigh, North Carolina 27650

Robert E. Johnston (3), Department of Psychology, Cornell University, Ithaca, New York 14850

Eric B. Keverne (79), Department of Anatomy, Cambridge University, Cambridge CB2 3DY, England

Michael Leon (39), Department of Psychobiology, University of California, Irvine, California 92717

Martha K. McClintock (113), Department of Behavioral Sciences, The University of Chicago, Chicago, Illinois 60637

Bruce Macmillan (175), Department of Zoology, Institute of Reproductive Biology, University of Texas, Austin, Texas 78712

Anna Marchlewska-Koj (151), Department of Genetics, Institute of Zoology, Jogiellonian University, Krakow, Poland

Michael Meredith (199), Department of Biological Sciences, Florida State University, Tallahassee, Florida 32306

John G. Vandenbergh (95), Department of Zoology, School of Agriculture and Life Sciences, North Carolina State University, Raleigh, North Carolina 27650

* Present address: Duke University Primate Center, Durham, North Carolina 27705

Preface

Specific molecules or blends of compounds are used to convey information both within the body of an organism and between organisms. Within the body, these chemical messengers have become specialized as hormones, neurotransmitters, or other compounds with highly specific actions. Chemical communication among organisms has also resulted in the specialization of certain chemicals or blends of substances having highly specific effects on the recipient, which are termed "pheromones." Pheromones can induce changes in the recipient leading to prompt behavioral responses: these substances are designated as "signalling pheromones." Or, the effects can induce physiological changes that may have a long-term influence on the recipient: these are termed "priming pheromones." Considerable discussion has surrounded the definition of the term pheromone, and some have suggested that it should be abandoned. New fields tend to be subject to semantic controversy; ours has not been an exception. "Pheromone" seems to be a useful term and it is used freely in this volume. Some chapter authors are more comfortable with it than others, and therefore its use varies among chapters.

Research on pheromones is a relatively young field, especially in regard to work on mammals. The discoveries that stimulated the development of this field grew out of basic research on reproductive physiology. Hilda Bruce, working at Cambridge, discovered that pregnancy could be blocked in newly mated female mice by exposure to a strange male or urine from such a male. Wesley Whitten, then at the Australian National University, Canberra, found that estrus was suppressed in a group of female mice and that its appearance was synchronized by male urine. These findings, plus work on insects showing the important role played by pheromones in the control of behavior and developmental physiology, stimulated much of the work reported in this volume.

Progress in the field since its beginnings about 25 years ago has been rapid. Several signalling pheromones in a variety of mammals have been characterized as to the glandular source and the effect on the recipient, and a few have been identified. Although progress has been slow in chemically identifying priming pheromones, several physiological functions related to reproduction and development have been shown to be modified by them; recently, the vomeronasal organ has been identified as the primary receptor organ in a few pheromonal systems. The basic research on pheromones in mammals is beginning to result in some practical applications, particularly with our domestic farm animals.

The purpose of this volume, therefore, is to review current research findings on the role of chemical communication in mammalian reproduction. Investigators, chosen because of their active and pertinent research programs, review the background information in their areas, present up-to-date results of their work and related studies, and attempt to place their work into a historical and theoretical perspective. Through this examination of the current state of the field of pheromones and reproduction, we hope to provide a comprehensive review for the general reader and to identify areas of continuing interest for the specialist.

John G. Vandenbergh

Part I

Signalling Pheromones

1

Chemical Signals and Reproductive Behavior

Robert E. Johnston

Department of Psychology
Cornell University
Ithaca, New York

I. INTRODUCTION

The domain of olfactory sensation, perception, and communication in mammals is a world of gentle suggestions, urgent demands, and seductive entreaties that is largely foreign to human observers. Partly because of this we have just barely begun to understand communication by chemical signals. What we do know concerns a limited set of questions, ones that we

PHEROMONES AND REPRODUCTION IN MAMMALS
Copyright © 1983 by Academic Press, Inc.
All rights of reproduction in any form reserved.
ISBN 0–12–710780–0

as outsiders to this world think are important. By necessity we have had to test most of our ideas in a laboratory setting, which tends to limit the range of discovery to those questions posed by the scientist rather than those suggested by the animals. Nonetheless, real progress has been made in recent years, as the chapters in this book make apparent.

In this chapter I describe some of the ways in which animals actively deploy scent to facilitate sexual interactions, and then I review the functions served by scent signals during these interactions. I have drawn material from both quantitative laboratory studies and selected observational field studies and have attempted to be thorough but not necessarily encyclopedic. Several reviews serve these more general functions (Brown, 1979; Thiessen and Rice, 1976; and see volumes edited by Doty, 1976; Müller-Schwarze and Mozell, 1977; Birch, 1974). This chapter covers all mammals except for primates and domestic farm animals, but of course it cannot make contact with all the relevant literature. There is a heavy bias toward rodents that have been used in laboratory studies.

II. SCENT MARKING AND SCENT DISPLAYS

A. Courtship Scent Marking by Females

It is widely believed that many female mammals advertise their readiness to mate by olfactory signals. The most likely sources of such signals are urine, which contains the metabolic products of many hormones, and secretions of the reproductive organs themselves. The secretions of specialized scent glands may also be influenced by changes in the reproductive states of females (Ebling, 1964).

Some scent-marking behaviors seem to function primarily to signal the female's reproductive state and to attract sexual partners for mating. Several criteria should distinguish sexual advertisement marking from other scent-marking behaviors. First, the frequency of marking should correlate with reproductive state in a way that suggests a sexual function. Second, such marking should be selectively directed at or stimulated by males. Third, the cues from males that stimulate marking should be dependent on reproductive hormones, so that only males in breeding condition should elicit scent marks from females. Fourth, scent marks functioning as sexual advertisements ought to elicit appropriate responses from males such as approach or courtship behaviors.

Table I summarizes reports containing quantitative data on scent marking by females in different reproductive states. Most of the species listed in this table show correlations between marking frequency and reproductive state that suggest a sexual advertisement function. In the two hamster spe-

TABLE I

Scent Marking by Females: Correlations with Reproductive Condition

Species	Diestrous	Proestrous	Estrous	Pregnant	Lactating	Reproductively quiescent	Scent source	Ref.[a]
Mesocricetus auratus (golden hamster)	Moderate	High (3–5 × DE)[b]	Rare	Rare	Low to moderate	Rare	Vaginal secretions	1
Mesocricetus brandti (Turkish hamster)	Moderate	High	Rare	?	?	?	Vaginal secretions	2
Meriones unguiculatus (Mongolian gerbil)	?	?	High?	Low to high	High to moderate	?	Ventral gland	3
Meriones hurrianae (Indian Desert gerbil)	Moderate	High (1.4 × DE)	High (1.4 × DE)	?	?	?	Ventral gland	4
Rattus norvegicus (domestic Norway rat)	Moderate	?	High (2 × DE)	?	?	?	Anogenital and urine	5
Mus musculus (house mouse)	Moderate	High	High	?	?	?	Urine	6
Cavia porcellus (domestic guinea pig)	Moderate	?	High (1.5 × DE)	?	?	?	Anogenital	7
Canis familiaris (domestic dog)	Low to moderate	?	High (2.5 × DE)	?	?	?	Urine	8
Leontopithecus rosalia (golden lion tamarin)	?	?	Low	High	Low at birth and 2 weeks following	?	Sternal gland and circumgenital gland	9

[a] References: 1, Johnston (1977a, 1979, 1983b), Leonard (1972); 2, Frank and Johnston (1981); 3, Wallace *et al.* (1973), Roper and Poliodakis (1977); 4, Kumari and Prakash (1981); 5, Birke (1978); Calhoun (1963); 6, Wolf and Powell (1979); 7, Birke (1981); 8, Dunbar (1978); 9, Kleiman and Mack (1980).

[b] Three to five times greater than marking during diestrus.

cies females mark most frequently the day before estrus, whereas in most of the remaining species females mark most frequently when they are in estrus (house mouse, Norway rat, guinea pig, and dog). There are two exceptions to this pattern. Golden lion marmosets mark most when pregnant, a pattern that is not easy to interpret. In gerbils the high level of marking seen late in pregnancy and early in lactation suggests a function relating to maternal behavior, and one experiment provided further support for such an interpretation: Pups that were scented with a female's sebum were retrieved in preference to washed pups (Wallace *et al.,* 1973). However, there is a postpartum estrus in gerbils, and marking at this time could have a sexual advertisement function as well.

A wealth of qualitative observations indicates that females of many other mammalian species scent mark most around the period of estrus. In some canid species females urine mark more frequently when estrous than when diestrous (e.g., racoon dogs, coyotes, and bat-eared foxes), whereas in other species they do not seem to (e.g., cape hunting dogs, wolves, red foxes, and black-backed jackals) (Kleiman, 1966). African wild dogs mark most frequently shortly before and during heat, and males often engage in simultaneous or nearly simultaneous marking over the marks of estrous females (Van Lawick-Goodall and Van Lawick-Goodall, 1971). Female marten mark with urine and possibly scent glands more frequently during estrus (Markley and Basset, 1942), and Ewer (1973) claims that in all carnivore species that she knows of marking is more frequent during the mating period. Ewer also states that in all felid species females become attractive to males several days before they are receptive, but Schaller (1967, 1972) found no evidence that female lions or tigers marked more at this time.

In most of the species listed in Table I the females were studied only during estrous cycles. Females of most mammalian species spend more time pregnant, lactating, or reproductively quiescent than they do cycling, however, and to understand the significance of changes in scent-marking frequency females should be studied during all of their reproductive states. The only species that has been studied this thoroughly is the golden hamster (see Fig. 1). Vaginal scent marking by golden hamsters rarely if ever occurs during pregnancy or early lactation; as lactation proceeds it becomes more and more frequent, so that by the end of lactation it is as frequent as during the diestrous days of the estrous cycle. Vaginal-marking frequency reaches its peak the day before estrus but then drops to zero on the estrous day (Leonard, 1972; Johnston, 1977a, 1979). We have found that females that are reproductively regressed because they have been placed on short days also rarely if ever vaginal mark. This pattern may be particularly adaptive for a solitary species. The female begins advertising well before she is actually receptive to ensure the presence of a male when she is receptive. An

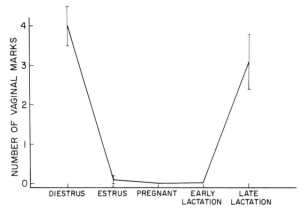

Fig. 1. Mean number of vaginal marks (±SE) by 56 females tested when they were estrous, diestrous, pregnant (day 7–9), early in lactation (day 7–9), or late in lactation (day 21–23) in one of four stimulus conditions. (From Johnston, 1979.)

advance advertising system might also facilitate female "choice" by promoting attraction of several males before the female is actually receptive.

Other rodents that nest solitarily may show similarities in the pattern of changes in marking frequency. Female Indian Desert gerbils mark more frequently during proestrus and estrus than during diestrus (Kumari and Prakash, 1981). Behavioral observations of the solitarily nesting gray tree squirrel indicate that males begin to engage in bouts of "sexual trailing" (i.e., following) 5 days before estrus and locate females apparently by following a scent trail (Thompson, 1977). In more gregarious species advertisement might be concentrated in the time immediately preceding receptivity to avoid unnecessary courtship and aggressive interactions on the days before copulation is possible. For example, Norway rats seem to confine their sexual marking to the period just before copulation (Calhoun, 1963; Birke, 1978). Finally, species with a postpartum estrus should engage in sexual scent marking and become attractive to males near the end of pregnancy, whereas species without postpartum estrus should not begin advertising until the end of lactation or until they begin to cycle again.

One aspect of the hamster marking pattern that is not intuitively obvious is the low level of marking during estrus, especially since the vaginal secretions deposited are known to be highly attractive and sexually arousing (Murphy, 1973; Johnston, 1974, 1975). Several observations help to explain this phenomenon. First, females studied in naturalistic laboratory enclosures are most active in soliciting males and attempting to entice them into their burrows the day before the estrus. Males are confined there until the female becomes receptive; then the pair mates and the female drives the male out (Lisk *et al.*, 1983). The peak in solicitation behavior the day before estrus corresponds with the peak vaginal-marking frequency. Second, estrous females make use of vaginal secretions in another way. They extrude a large quantity of vaginal secretion when males approach. The males sniff, lick, and consume the secretion, thus stimulating copulatory behavior (Johnston, 1975; Murphy, 1973). Third, odors in a female's nest area are more attractive to males when the female is estrous as opposed to diestrous, and this depends on the presence of vaginal secretions (Johnston, 1980). It is not clear whether this is due to a high level of marking on the day before estrus or due merely to leakage of secretions into the nest environment. Wild males probably monitor females' burrows, and they should be aware of a female's approaching estrus. If a female has not obtained a mate before she is estrous, her best strategy may be to stay near her burrow and wait for males to visit her.

The other criteria proposed as characteristic of sexual advertisement scent marking have not been much investigated. Selective orientation toward or stimulation by males has been demonstrated for golden hamsters and dogs. Female hamsters mark least in the presence of other females or their odors, at intermediate levels in clean areas, and most frequently in the presence of males or male odors (Johnston, 1977a). Estrous female dogs urinate more frequently in response to male urine than to female urine (Dunbar, 1978). Hormonal control of the cues from males that elicit sexual marking by females has not been investigated. Responses of males to sexual scent marks of females have likewise received little attention; males responses to sexual odors, some of which are deposited by females when marking, have been studied and are discussed in Section III.

B. Scent Displays during Courtship

Male and female mammals often engage in "olfactory displays" during courtship sequences; that is, they may expose, flaunt, or spray scents at potential partners.

Males of nearly all mammalian species attempt to sniff the genital region of potential sexual partners. This seems to be a means of gathering information about the female's reproductive state rather than a means of determining sex, since in most species only females are inspected in this manner. In many species females that are in estrus or approaching it allow males to investigate their genital region, whereas females that are not in this state avoid or repel such attempts (e.g., for carnivores see Ewer, 1973; for ungulates see Leuthold, 1977). Thus, permission to investigate can be considered a subtle but important courtship display since it indicates an approaching readiness to mate.

More active and conspicuous scent displays also occur. Estrous female golden hamsters extrude a relatively large quantity of vaginal secretions when a male approaches and begins sniffing in the genital region (Murphy, 1973; Johnston, 1975). Male-stimulated urination is common in ungulates, and males of such species sniff and lick the urine or collect it directly in the mouth as the female urinates (Fraser, 1968; Leuthold, 1977; Grau, 1976). Male ungulates often engage in the flehmen response when investigating females, which may facilitate access of the odorants to the vomeronasal organ (Estes, 1972; Ladewig and Hart, 1980; see Chapter 8 by Meredith). Observers usually assume that flehmen allows males to determine a female's reproductive condition, but I am not aware of any proof of this assumption. Male sheep prefer estrous to nonestrous ewes on the basis of unspecified odor cues (Lindsay, 1965), but male goats spend more time sniffing, licking, and engaging in flehmen toward urine from diestrous females than that from estrous females (Hart, 1983).

In a few species of ungulates females may advertise their sexual condition by using and marking in wallows. Female moose, for example, use wallows only during the mating season and compete among themselves for wallows that have been freshly made by bulls (Altmann, 1959), whereas female deer during the rut urinate in scrapes made by bucks (Moore and Marchinton, 1974). Many rodents engage in sand-bathing behaviors (e.g., Eisenberg, 1963), and it has often been suggested that sand-bathing loci may be a focus of chemical marking and communication; I have not found any examples, however, of females engaging in sand bathing differentially during different stages of their reproductive cycle.

Males may also scent mark or scent display during courtship or copulatory sequences. Male European hamsters flank mark the female's nest before attempting to mate with her (Eibl-Eibesfeldt, 1953), and male Norway rats urine mark both before copulation and between bouts of mounting (McIntosh *et al.,* 1979). Both male and female squirrel monkeys of a pair engage in "urine washing" between copulations, at the same time sitting close to one another, purring, and gazing into each other's eyes (Latta *et al.,* 1967). Male and female marmosets also engage in scent marking before and after copulation (Epple, 1970).

A well-known scent display that may have functions in sexual behavior, at least in some species, is the behavior known as enuration (or *harnspritzen*), in which one individual sprays a jet of urine at the other. This behavior has been reported for lagomorphs and South American rodents (see Kleiman, 1971, for a review). In species such as porcupines and pacas a sexual function is clearly indicated since the behavior pattern is different from that used during elimination, the urine is directed at the partner, and the behavior occurs in behavioral sequences that lead to copulation. It is even possible that urine spraying has evolved as a means of stimulating the vomeronasal organ, since the spray would facilitate contact of the chemical signal with the nose and/or mouth, contact that many believe to be necessary for effective vomeronasal stimulation (see Chapter 8).

This brief sample of the relevant literature emphasizes two general points. First, mammals often actively display or present odorants to a partner during courtship, and such presentations may be a crucial step in the sequence of behaviors that culminate in mating. Second, very little is known about the functions of these scent displays or of the odors that the displays make available.

C. Broadcast Scent Marking and Its Potential Sexual Functions

Most scent marking performed by mammals can be categorized as broadcast scent marking, that is, scent marking performed in a wide variety of social contexts or even in apparently asocial contexts such as grooming or walking. Included in this category are all of those scent-marking behaviors that were once regarded as "territorial" marking but are now thought to have no necessary connection with territoriality (Johnson, 1973; Ralls, 1971). Such marking behaviors may be observed at especially high frequencies in agonistic contexts, but they are usually not restricted to these contexts. Broadcast scent marking is functionally analogous to other broadcast communication signals such as song in birds. The functions may differ from species to species, but some of these functions, such as sexual recognition, species recognition, and individual recognition, are important for sexual behavior.

Three characteristics of this type of marking suggest that such behaviors function in reproductive processes. First, the scent glands involved are often sexually dimorphic, the glands in males usually being larger and more active than those in females of the same species. Androgens seem to be the major cause of these sexual differences, especially for glands of the sebaceous type (see Thiessen and Rice, 1976, for review). Second, the marking behaviors are often dependent on sex steroids (Thiessen and Rice, 1976). Third, the frequencies of these marking behaviors are often observed to be highest during the reproductive season (e.g., Ewer, 1973).

Mate Choice and Pair Bond Maintenance

There is some evidence suggesting that broadcast scent marks may be used as many visual and auditory courtship signals are, namely, to promote familiarity and reduce aggressive tendencies of unpaired animals. In studies of two Saharan gerbils, *Meriones libicus* and *Psammomys obesus,* Daly and

Daly (1975a,b) observed that females restricted their movements to relatively small areas around their burrows and the nearby bushes, whereas males moved over a larger home range and visited and scent marked in the home areas of a number of females on a regular basis. Daly (1977) hypothesized that this marking might be a means by which a male became familiar to a female and thus increased his likelihood of mating with her when she was receptive. Using Mongolian gerbils, *Meriones unguiculatus,* Daly showed that males were stimulated to ventral mark more by the odors of females than by the odors of males, indicating that male gerbils direct their marks toward females. Then he showed that a female that had been repeatedly exposed to the scent of the ventral gland of one male was more attracted to and less aggressive toward that male than a male with an unfamiliar odor. These results suggest that familiarity with a male's odors by exposure to his scent marks can influence female behavior and that a male with a familiar scent may be more readily tolerated and accepted as a mate than a male with an unfamiliar scent.

Related experiments with golden hamsters suggest a similar conclusion (Johnston, unpublished observations). Each of nine females were exposed to a male for 5 min (or one intromission) on 5 estrous days and exposed to the male's empty home cage on the intervening days of those estrous cycles. On the female's sixth estrous day she was tested in a neutral arena for her preference of the odors of the familiar male versus those of an unfamiliar male. The odors were presented by anesthetizing the males and placing them behind screened doors at opposite ends of an arena. Estrous females spent more time sniffing at the odors of the familiar male (21.9 ± 5.8 sec) than at the odors of the unfamiliar male (12.2 ± 3.1 sec, $p < .05$; Wilcoxon matched pairs, signed ranks test).

Field observations of pair-bonding mammals also suggest the importance of scent communication in the initial stages of courtship. Male and female pottos (*Perodictus potto*) and galagos (*Galago demidovii*) form bonds, often several months before any overt sexual activity occurs or before the female is sexually mature. Scents may play a role in the series of interactions leading to pairing. Males visit females, scent mark, and may chase them. Only after repeated visits does the female accept the male. At the time of acceptance the pair spends several hours in mutual licking, grooming, scent exchange, and scent marking, yet the sexes are still "solitary" in the sense that they do not have congruent home ranges and do not nest together. Males seem to "control" several females, and maintenance of the bond between the male and his females seems to be dependent on the male's scent marking (Charles-Dominique, 1977). A male and female rufous elephant shrew share a mutually defended territory but are rarely if ever seen in close proximity or to interact directly. They mark their territory, and one would expect that in such a system olfactory information must play an important role in maintenance of the pair (Rathbun, 1979).

III. FUNCTIONS OF SCENT SIGNALS

A. Species Recognition

Communication signals functioning in courtship and mating are likely to be species specific, because selection for specificity to maximize reproductive efficiency and minimize nonfunctional reproductive effort is likely. Females should be particularly sensitive to species differences, because acceptance of a heterospecific male partner has a higher cost than does acceptance of a heterospecific female by a male. Females, for example, could become pseudopregnant or have nonviable or infertile offspring, whereas males that attempted to mate with a heterospecific female would lose much less time and energy.

Table II presents the known cases in which species-specific sexual preferences for odors of closely related species have been investigated. In the majority of studies individual animals were more attracted to the odors of conspecifics of the opposite sex than to the odors of heterospecifics of the opposite sex.

The assumption behind the use of a preference test is that a preference reflects a tendency toward selective pairing or mating in natural circumstances. However, a preference for an odor may be shown for a variety of underlying reasons (Johnston, 1981). Confidence in the meaning of observed preferences can be enhanced if courtship behaviors are selectively oriented toward conspecific odors or if actual mating preferences can also be demonstrated. For example, male bank voles and male and female lemmings and hamsters all preferentially attempt to mate with conspecifics in laboratory situations (see references in Table II). Male Syrian hamsters attempted to mount anesthetized conspecific females much more than anesthetized heterospecific females, a test situation that emphasizes the importance of chemical cues over visual and auditory ones (Murphy, 1980). The elicitation of courtship behaviors by odors is particularly useful as an indicator of sexual interest because in nature scent marks may normally elicit such behaviors. Female hamsters of several species display a kind of solicitation or prelordosis posture in response to confined conspecifics but not to heterospecifics (Murphy, 1977), and golden hamster females engage in vaginal scent marking more frequently in the presence of odors of conspecific males than those of heterospecific males (Johnston and Brenner, 1982). Perhaps the most dramatic example of the species specificity of mat-

TABLE II

Species Specificity of Preferences for Potential Sexual Partners

Test species	Heterospecies	Reproductive state	Attraction: conspecific preferred?	Mating: conspecific preferred?	Odor source	Population sympatric (S) or allopatric (A)	Ref.[a]
		A. Male Preferences					
Clethryonomys, sp. (bank vole)	Subspecies[b]	Estrus	Yes	Yes	Whole body	A	1
Dicrostonyx groenlandicus (lemming)	Lemmus	Estrus and diestrus	Yes	Yes	Whole body	A[c]	2
Lemmus trimucronatus (lemming)	Dicrostonyx	Estrus and diestrus	Yes	Yes	Whole body	A	2
Peromyscus maniculatus bairdi	P. leucopus	Estrus and diestrus	No	No	Urine	S	3
P. leucopus novaboracensis	P. maniculatus	Estrus and diestrus	No	No	Urine	S	3
P. maniculatus rufinus	P. polionotus	Estrus and diestrus	Yes	?	Whole body	A	4
P. polionotus	P. maniculatus	Estrus and diestrus	No	?	Whole body	A	4
P. eremicus	P. californicus	Unknown	Yes	?	Whole body	A and S	5
P. californicus	P. eremicus	Unknown	Yes	?	Whole body	A and S	5
Mesocricetus auratus (golden hamster)	M. brandti	Estrus	Yes	Yes[d]	Vaginal secretion sufficient; other odors also involved	A	6
M. brandti (Turkish hamster)	M. auratus	Estrus	Yes	Yes[d]	Vaginal secretion sufficient; other odors also involved	A	6
Cavia porcellus (guinea pig)	Galea musteloides	Nonreceptive	Yes	?	Whole body	A	7

(continued)

TABLE II *(continued)*

Test species	Heterospecies	Reproductive state	Attraction: conspecific preferred?	Mating: conspecific preferred?	Odor source	Population sympatric (S) or allopatric (A)	Ref.[a]
			B. Female Preferences				
Dicrostonyx groenlandicus (lemming)	*Lemmus*	Estrus and diestrus	Yes	Yes	Whole body	A	2
Lemmus trimucronatus (lemming)	*Dicrostonyx*	Estrus and diestrus	Yes	Yes	Whole body	A	2
Spalax ehrenbergi (mole rat)	Two chromosome forms of super-species complex	Estrus	Yes	?	Urine	A but narrow hybrid zone between populations	8
Peromyscus maniculatus bairdi	*P. leucopus novaboracensis*	Estrus and diestrus	Yes	?	Urine	S	3
Peromyscus leucopus novaboracensis	*P. maniculatus bairdi*	Estrus and diestrus	No	?	Urine	S	3
P. maniculatus rufinus	*P. polionotus*	Estrus	Yes	?	Whole body	A	4
P. polionotus	*P. maniculatus rufinus*	Estrus	No	?	Whole body	A	
Mesocricetus auratus (golden hamster)	*M. brandti*	Estrus	Yes	?	Whole body plus sight and sound	A	9
M. brandti (Turkish hamster)	*M. auratus*	Estrus	Yes	Yes	Whole body plus sight and sound	A	9
M. newtoni (Roumanian hamster)	*M. auratus*	Estrus	Yes	?	Whole body plus sight and sound	A	9

[a] References: 1, Godfrey (1958); 2, Huck and Banks (1980a, b); 3, Doty (1973); 4, Moore (1965); 5, Smith (1965); 6, Murphy (1980); 7, Beauchamp (1973); 8, Nevo et al. (1976); 9, Murphy (1977, 1978).

[b] Four subspecies tested: two different populations of one subspecies; two F_1 hybrids.

[c] Populations studied were allopatric, although other populations are sympatric.

[d] Tested with anesthetized female.

ing preference comes from a study of the white-footed mouse, *Peromyscus maniculatus;* males from one population (subspecies) actually kill a high percentage of females from another population (Perrigo and Bronson, 1983).

A correlation of reproductive state with species preferences may also help with interpretation of the data. Females of two species, *Spalax ehrenbergi* and *Peromyscus maniculatus,* showed preferences for odors of conspecific males only when they were estrous, suggesting a rather highly specific sexual function for attraction responses (Nevo *et al.,* 1976; Doty, 1972, 1973). The lack of a correlation with reproductive state in the other species in which females were tested when estrus and diestrus does not necessarily imply the lack of a sexual function, since courtship and pairing may take place before estrus. Investigations that examine an even wider range of reproductive states would be valuable and would help to make the meaning of species-specific preferences clearer.

If species-specific odor preferences are important in reproductive isolation, one would predict that closely related sympatric species should show clear preferences, whereas closely related but allopatric species might be less prone to demonstrate such preferences. To examine this prediction Smith (1965) tested males of two species of *Peromyscus* for preferences between conspecific and heterospecific females from the males' own geographic area and from other areas. Males of both species preferred conspecific females over heterospecific females regardless of the area from which the females came, but males of one species (*P. eremicus*) showed a significantly weaker preference for the allopatric conspecific females over the allopatric heterospecific females than they did with the sympatric females. Similarly, Moore (1965) showed that *P. maniculatus,* which lives sympatrically with other *Peromyscus* species, showed clear species-specific preferences, whereas a population of *P. polionotus* that is geographically isolated from other *Peromyscus* species did not. The mole rats *Spalax ehrenbergi,* studied by Nevo *et al.* (1976), came from subspecific populations that were allopatric (although the populations came within 3 km of one another with a 300-m-wide hybrid zone between them). These two subspecies demonstrated clear subspecific olfactory and mating preferences. Female Turkish hamsters, *Mesocricetus brandti,* are more discriminating toward conspecific and heterospecific males than their Syrian counterparts, *M. auratus* (Murphy, 1977). Syrian hamsters come from a population that is geographically isolated from other hamsters, whereas Turkish hamsters belong to a widespread "species" that includes populations with different chromosome numbers, populations that might even be classified as different species if a thorough study were done (Todd *et al.,* 1972).

The sources of the odors that influence species-specific preferences are largely unknown. In several studies one source of odor was shown to be sufficient for such preferences, namely, urine for mole rats and several species of mice and vaginal secretions for hamsters (Doty, 1973; Nevo *et al.,* 1976; Murphy, 1980). Only Murphy looked a little farther into the question and showed that the vaginal secretion was not the only odor that provided such information but that other, as yet unspecified odors were also important. Identifying the sources of the relevant odors is important, because if only a few specific scents are involved evolutionary specialization for this purpose is suggested, whereas if all body odors are involved opportunistic use of general biochemical differences between species appears to be more likely.

Development of Species Preferences

Both the perceptual mechanisms underlying preferences and the chemical composition of the signals are a product of gene–environment interactions. Godfrey's studies (1958) on bank voles illustrated the importance of genetic factors when he demonstrated that males prefer females of their own race over F_1 hybrid females. Males of the F_1 generation did not prefer females of either parent stock.

Several cross-fostering studies suggest that social environment does influence, but by no means completely determines, species-specific preferences. Huck and Banks (1980a,b) cross-fostered litters of one species of lemming onto a mother of another species of lemming. When the cross-fostered males became adults, they actually preferred the odors of females of the foster species over those of conspecific females. In sexual behavior tests the effects of cross-fostering were less dramatic: Cross-fostered, in-fostered, and nonfostered males all mated readily with conspecific females. Males of one species (*Dicrostonyx*) also attempted to mate with females of the foster species (*Lemmus*), but *Lemmus* males did not attempt to mate with *Dicrostonyx* females. The cross-fostering procedure had a smaller effect on females than it did on males. Odor preferences of females were affected, but only to the extent of eliminating the normal preference for conspecific males, not to the extent of reversing the preference. Cross fostered, in-fostered, and nonfostered females were equally antagonistic toward heterospecific males and rarely made contact with them or engaged in sexual behavior. Cross fostered females did, however, engage in less contact and less social and sexual behavior with conspecific males than control females did. Female sexual preferences may be more heavily biased by genetic mechanisms than those of males, perhaps because in nature there are less reliable opportunities for female pups to learn about adult males of the species than there are opportunities for male pups to learn about adult females. Alternatively, females may be no more genetically biased than males are but in this experiment were less influenced than males because male pups had massive exposure to an adult female whereas female pups had no experience with an adult male. In nature there would presumably be at least occasional exposures of young pups to adult males or their odors, which might be sufficient for females to learn what conspecific males were like.

B. Sexual Recognition and Elicitation of Courtship Behaviors

Individuals of most mammalian species treat conspecifics differently depending on their sex. In some cases this differential treatment may be restricted to the breeding season, whereas in others it may last throughout the year. Information obtained through several sensory channels is no doubt used for such discriminating, but the olfactory channel is likely to be predominant for many species.

In two early studies it was shown that both mice and gerbils *can* distinguish the odors emanating from males and females when such cues were used as discriminative stimuli in learning tasks (Bowers and Alexander, 1967; Dagg and Windsor, 1971). Of more relevance to social behavior, however, is whether animals *do* respond differentially to such odors. In virtually all species that have been tested odors from males and females cause different behavioral responses in conspecifics, and often the kinds of responses observed suggest a role in reproductive behavior. The most common question that has been asked is whether an animal is more attracted to the odors of one sex or the other. The most prevalent methods employed to answer this question are preference tests (two or more odorants present simultaneously) or attraction tests (only one stimulus present in each test). With male mammals as the test subjects, preferences for the odors of females over the odors of males have been demonstrated in dogs (Dunbar, 1977, 1978), wood rats (August, 1978), hamsters (Landauer et al., 1978), mice (Johnston and Bronson, 1982), rats (Brown, 1977), and guinea pigs (Beauchamp, 1973). In some cases males show stronger preferences when the females are estrous, lending support to the argument that the preference reflects sexual motivation, at least in part. In addition, male preferences for the odors of females over those of males have been shown to be dependent on testicular androgens in hamsters (Landauer and Carter, 1974) and on the presence of the testes in rats (Brown, 1977).

Female mammals have also been tested for their preferences and usually are more attracted to the odors of males than those of other females, as shown, for example, by dogs (Dunbar, 1977, 1978), wood rats (August, 1978), hamsters (Johnston, 1979), and laboratory rats (Brown, 1977). The reproductive state of females can have substantial effects on these preferences. Intact female rats show the strongest attraction to odors of intact males, a lesser attraction to those of castrated males, and yet lower attraction to intact and ovariectomized females, whereas ovariectomized females do not display any preferences (Brown, 1977). Dunbar (1977, 1978) has shown that when female dogs are nonestrus they are more attracted to estrous and nonestrous female urine than to male urine, but when they become estrus they prefer male urine. In hamsters the effect of the female's reproductive state on her attraction to male odors has been investigated in even more detail (Johnston, 1979). Estrous, diestrous, and lactating females are more attracted to the odors of intact males than pregnant females are and all but the pregnant females are more attracted to odors of intact males than odors of castrated males. Estrous females are most highly attracted to male odors, suggesting three levels of attraction to male odors: estrous females > diestrous females and lactating females > pregnant females. This pattern of changes with reproductive state differs from changes in female aggressiveness, vaginal marking, ultrasonic courtship calling, and overtly sexual behaviors in a way that suggests different hormonal mechanisms for each.

Although the factors responsible for the elicitation of courtship behaviors in mammals have not been studied in much detail, a few studies have demonstrated sexual discrimination and selective orientation of courtship behaviors on the basis of odor cues. As discussed in Section II,A the courtship scent marking of female hamsters is stimulated by the odors of males and inhibited by the odors of other females (Johnston, 1977a). Female hamsters also use ultrasonic calls in sexual contexts, apparently to attract males at short range (Floody and Pfaff, 1977a,b; Floody et al., 1977). Female hamsters call more frequently when estrous than when diestrous, and in both states calling is facilitated by the odors of male hamsters but not by the odors of other females. Ablation of the olfactory bulbs drastically reduces the frequency of calling by females (Kairys et al., 1980). Preliminary experiments suggest that females call more in response to the odors of intact males than in response to the odors of castrated males, but attempts to find the source of the androgen-dependent odor have so far been unsuccessful (R. E. Johnston, unpublished observations). Male hamsters also call in sexual contexts, and their calls seem to function as a means of both attracting females and prolonging the duration of lordosis. Calling by males is facilitated by the odors of females but not by those of males (Floody et al., 1977), and the primary scent that stimulates calling is the scent of vaginal secretions of females (Kwan, 1978; Johnston and Kwan, 1983).

In house mice males produce ultrasonic calls in sexual contexts, and at least one of the cues that stimulates male calling is found in the urine of females but not in the urine of males. This cue or cues is under endocrine control, occurring in the urine of estrous females, diestrous females, and ovariectomized females but not in the urine of hypophysectomized females

(Whitney and Nyby, 1979; Nyby *et al.*, 1979). In contrast, the urinary cue that is behaviorally attractive to male mice is dependent on the presence of the ovary (Johnston and Bronson, 1982).

The sources of sex-specific odors have not been thoroughly worked out for any species. Most species have a variety of sexually dimorphic scent glands (Schaffer, 1940; Thiessen and Rice, 1976), and the chemical composition of the secretions of these glands is often strikingly different in males and females (e.g., Stoddart, 1977). Similarly, the chemical composition of excretory products such as urine is quite different in the two sexes. In the instances described above scents that are *sufficient for* sexual discrimination are known, but in no case have both the sufficient and necessary odors been elucidated. In hamsters, for example, males are most attracted to intact females, less attracted to vaginectomized females and castrated males, and least attracted to intact males (Kwan and Johnston, 1980). Since males do not seem to prefer odors of vaginectomized females over those of castrated males, there seem to be just two classes of factors that influence male preferences: vaginal secretions and some androgen-dependent odors. Hamsters have three known sexually dimorphic scent glands that are influenced by androgens (Harderian glands, ear glands, and flank glands). In addition, other apparently nonspecialized sources such as saliva, urine, or sebaceous glands could be involved. The functional significance of multiple, sexually dimorphic scent glands is unknown.

C. Individual Identity, Social Status, Group Membership, and Genetic Relatedness

1. Individual Recognition and Mate Choice

Individual recognition or discrimination may be important for reproductive behavior in a number of contexts, such as mate selection or recognition. As with species or sex discrimination, cues in a variety of modalities may be used to discriminate among individuals, but chemical cues seem likely to be important in most mammals and may be the only cues used by at least some species. Although it is known that a variety of mammalian species can discriminate among individuals on the basis of olfactory cues (see Halpin, 1980, for review), the mechanisms underlying such recognition are not clearly understood. The products of scent glands vary in the ratios of concentrations of components across individuals, and this variation presumably imparts a different quality to the odor of individuals and allows olfactory discrimination (e.g., Stoddart, 1977; Williams, 1956). One species of mongoose is able to discriminate among anal gland scents from different individuals and to discriminate among artificial scents prepared by varying the ratios of six carboxylic acids that occur in the anal gland secretion (Gorman, 1976).

In species in which males and females form long-term associations members of a pair presumably recognize one another, and a few observations suggest that scent is important in such recognition. Galagos and elephant shrews are likely prospects, as described in Section II. Male and female beavers form lifelong pairs; they sleep curled up together and spend a large amount of time in contact with one another, sniffing, grooming, and making soft contact sounds. They respond quite dramatically to strange scent introduced into their living area (Aleksiuk, 1968; Wilsson, 1968; Butler and Butler, 1979). Prairie dogs and ground squirrels of many species greet each other by mutual olfactory investigation of lip-angle scent glands, presumably identifying one another (see Steiner, 1975, for review). Male Columbian ground squirrels respond differentially to the odors of the oral glands of strange and familiar males (Harris and Murie, 1982). Dwarf mongooses clearly distinguish group members from strangers on the basis of scent and are capable of distinguishing anal gland secretions from different individuals (Rasa, 1973).

In species that have a promiscuous or potentially promiscuous mating system, individuals often display preferences for some partners over others, either by selective mating or by differences in the vigor or completeness of mating with different partners. For example, such results have been described for rhesus monkeys (Michael, 1971), dogs (LeBoef, 1967; Beach 1970), and wolves (Rabb et al., 1967; Mech, 1970). Proof for the sensory basis of such preferences is lacking, but in some species scent cues are no doubt important. Dogs and wolves investigate each other first by mutual face sniffing and then by mutual genital-region sniffing (Mech, 1970). Male dogs are capable of distinguishing familiar from strange males on the basis of odor cues (Dunbar and Carmichael, 1981), and dogs and wolves readily distinguish between urine from different individual conspecifics (Brown and Johnston, 1983). In the latter study, dogs and wolves discriminated between two urine samples when they were presented a day apart, demonstrating a memory of at least 24 hr for the smell of an individual.

In a promiscuous mating system, individuals also must be able to discriminate between new and old partners. In a number of species individuals that have mated to satiety with one partner are reinvigorated when placed with a new partner (known as the *Coolidge effect*; see Dewsbury, 1981, for a review). Evidence that this may be an adaptive characteristic comes from comparative studies of rodents, in which the effect appears to occur more frequently in species with a promiscuous mating system than in species that form monogamous pairs.

In two species that show the Coolidge effect, rats and hamsters, odors are sufficient for males to distinguish a new female. Male rats were more attracted to the odors of a novel female than to the odors of the female with which they had just mated to satiety. Since the odors were collected before the mating test, odors from the male or odors produced during copulation were not present, indicating that the males were basing their preferences on discrimination between the two females (Carr *et al.*, 1970a). In the hamster experiments males were tested with anesthetized females following mating to satiety, thus allowing the possibility of attempted copulation with the anesthetized females (Johnston, 1983a; Johnston and Rasmussen, 1983). Males directed more sniffing and mounts at novel unmated females than at familiar females, and similarly preferred novel females that had just mated with another male over familiar females, but showed no preference when presented with two novel females, one of which had mated with another male. Thus, males demonstrated a choice of a novel female, regardless of whether or not she had mated recently. The results could not be explained by the male smelling his own odors on the familiar female, since rubbing the experimental male's odors on one of two novel females did not induce a preference for the unscented female. In addition, males showed preferences for the flank gland odor of novel females over that of familiar females but did not show preferences for odors from the head region (ear glands, Harderian glands) or vaginal secretions, suggesting that the cues for individual recognition may come primarily from the flank gland.

2. Social Status

High rank in a dominance hierarchy and reproductive success are often correlated. If females are exerting some choice, they may base their preference on one of two different mechanisms. Females could choose high-ranking males by being able to recognize all of the males in the group as individuals and know what rank each occupied. Alternatively, males of high and low ranks might produce different cues (behavior, odors, vocalizations, etc.), and females could choose on the basis of the signal emitted. The males' status may be correlated with endocrine differences among males, and these endocrine differences could influence the males' odors or other signals.

Female brown lemmings may in fact choose males on the basis of testosterone-mediated dominance and odor cues (Huck *et al.*, 1981). Estrous female lemmings were more attracted to the odors of males that had been dominant on 9 successive days in encounters with another male than to odors of the defeated males. Dominant males had heavier testes and seminal vesicles than subordinate males, suggesting the possibility that different testosterone levels resulted in different amounts of an androgen-dependent odor. Estrous females also preferred the odors of males that had not yet fought but that eventually became dominant over the odors of males that eventually became subordinate, suggesting that there may have been differences in testosterone levels in males which determined both their attractiveness to females and their success in agonistic encounters. An apparently similar phenomenon was reported for mice, in which females preferred the odors of dominant males over those of subordinate males (at least during the first hour of a 20-hr test). These results are somewhat less convincing, however, since the females preferred a compartment with no odors to both the compartments containing male odors (Mainardi and Pasquali, 1973).

3. Social Group and Genetic Relatedness

Mate choices may be influenced by affiliation or lack of affiliation with a social group. Among European rabbits, for example, young females of another group are attacked by the dominant male of the home group. If a young female is scented with the odors of a strange group and then reintroduced to her own group, she is attacked as if she were a stranger (Mykytowycz, 1968).

Preferences could be based on genetic factors. Yamazaki *et al.* (1976) demonstrated that male mice, given the opportunity to mate with females that are either genetically identical or differ only at the H-2 locus of the major histocompatibility complex, prefer to mate with females that differ at this one locus. Both males and females can distinguish the odors of individuals that differ at this locus (Yamazaki *et al.,* 1979; Yamaguchi *et al.,* 1981). This exceptional ability indicates that discriminations made on the basis of small differences in genetic relatedness are possible. Whether this ability is reflected in actual mate preferences in natural populations is not known, but it is becoming increasingly apparent that genetic relatedness is an important variable influencing social interactions (e.g., Sherman, 1981; Holmes and Sherman, 1982). A positive correlation between degree of relatedness and degree of preference could be one of the mechanisms by which local populations become genetically isolated from one another, despite living in close proximity. Selander (1970) found little evidence of gene flow between two or more populations of mice living in the same barn or in different barns on the same farm. A preliminary report suggests one possible mechanism: Female house mice of two inbred strains were more attracted to the odors of males of their own strain than to odors of males of another strain (Gilder and Slater, 1978). It has been shown that weanling spiny mice, *Acomys cahirinus,* preferred to huddle together with siblings than with nonsiblings of the same age, suggesting discrimination on the basis of kinship (Porter and Wyrick, 1979).

D. Chemical Signalling of Reproductive State

The odors of females of most mammalian species probably vary with their reproductive state; the chemical constituents of scent glands, vaginal secretions, and urine may all vary with the estrous cycle (Ebling, 1964; O'Connell *et al.*, 1981; Novotny, 1982).

Table III summarizes what is known about differential responses of males to the odors of females in different reproductive conditions. Most of these studies showed that males were more attracted to estrous females than to diestrous or nonestrous females. It is surprising that so few species have been investigated, especially considering the belief that nearly all male mammals can detect estrus on the basis of female odors. More work must also be done on the endocrine control of and experiential influences on such responses. The preference for estrous over diestrous urine odors in male rats is dependent on males having both sexual experience and normal androgen levels (Carr *et al.*, 1965, 1970b). Castration and testosterone replacement apparently affect the males' motivation and not their ability to discriminate between the two types of urine (Carr and Caul, 1962).

Other male behaviors should also be differentially influenced by odors of females in different reproductive states, but little information is available. The urination scent-marking frequency of male dogs is increased in the presence of urine from estrous females (Dunbar, 1978), whereas the aggressively motivated scent marking of male hamsters is decreased by estrous odors (Johnston, 1980).

An instructive variation on the general pattern is the golden hamster. Males are equally attracted to the odors of estrous and diestrous females when the females themselves are used as the odor source (Landauer *et al.*, 1977; Johnston, 1980). Male hamsters are not unresponsive to differences in the females' reproductive state, however, because they are much more attracted to odors from both estrous and diestrous females than they are to pregnant or lactating females. This pattern makes sense for a species that lives solitarily and has no postpartum estrus. It is to the advantage of both males and females to get together for mating, and perhaps one way to accomplish this is for the female to be attractive before she is actually receptive (see also Sections II,A and III,B, subsection on female preferences). On the other hand, it is not to the advantage of either sex to be in contact during pregnancy and lactation, when females are very aggressive toward males (Wise, 1974).

Much more subtle differences in attractiveness toward the odors of estrous and diestrous female hamsters can be observed if bedding material from the nest and home cage is used as the odor source. In a simultaneous choice test males prefer odors of bedding from estrous females over those of diestrous females, and they also show less flank marking in the cage of

TABLE III

Responses of Males to Odors of Females in Different Reproductive Conditions

Species	Odor source	Hierarchy of attractiveness of females' reproductive states	Relative stimulation of other male behaviors	Ref.[a]
Rats (*Rattus norvegicus*)	Whole body	Estrus > diestrus		1
	Urine	Estrus > diestrus		2
	Preputial gland	Estrus = proestrus > diestrus		3
Mice (*Mus musculus*)	Vaginal secretions (not urine, preputial glands, or uterus)	Estrus > diestrus	Mount diestrus female scented with vaginal secretions; Estrus > diestrus	4
Gerbils (*Meriones unguiculatus*)	Saliva, ventral gland	Estrus > diestrus		5
Guinea pigs (*Cavia porcellus*)	Vaginal secretion	Can discriminate between estrus and diestrous; preference not tested		6
Hamsters (*Mesocricetus auratus*)	Whole body	Estrus[b] = diestrus > Pregnant = lactating		7,8
	Bedding material, quantity of vaginal secretion[b]	Estrus[b] > diestrus	Aggressive scent marking; diestrus > estrus	7
Dogs (*Canis familiaris*)	Urine and vaginal secretions (not anal glands, saliva, or ear wax)	Estrus > nonestrus	Urination scent marking; estrus > nonestrus	9
Sheep (*Ovis aries*)	Whole body	Estrus > nonestrus		10

[a] References: 1, Carr *et al.* (1965); 2, Pfaff and Pfaffman (1969); 3, Thody and Dijkstra (1978); Gawienowski (1977); 4, Hyashi and Kimura (1974); 5, Block *et al.* (1981); 6, Ruddy (1980); 7, Johnston (1980); 8, Landauer *et al.* (1977); 9, Dunbar (1977, 1978); 10, Lindsay (1965).
[b] See text.

an estrous female (Johnston, 1980). These differences are dependent on the presence of the vagina in the stimulus females. Although the quantity of one attractant in hamster vaginal secretions (dimethyl disulfide) is greatest on the estrous day, the amount of this attractant in the secretions of females is sufficient to attract males throughout the estrous cycle (O'Connell *et al.,* 1981). The level of attractiveness of the secretion does not appear to change over the estrous cycle, during pregnancy and lactation, or even in ovariec-tomized females (Johnston, 1974; Darby *et al.,* 1975). The critical variable in differential responses of males to bedding from females cages may be the quantity of secretion that is deposited by marking or that leaks out of the vagina (Johnston, 1980). These observations indicate that chemical information about estrous and diestrous conditions is available and that this information may influence males in some circumstances, but the importance of this discrimination is small compared to the difference in attractiveness of estrous and diestrous females, on the one hand, and pregnant and lactating females, on the other.

E. Aphrodisiac Functions

Signals that specifically influence the tendency to copulate may be either the same as or different from those that allow sexual discrimination, serve as sexual attractants, or allow discrimination of reproductive state. Although it might seem efficient to use the same substances as both attractants and aphrodisiacs, chemicals with optimal properties for one function may not be optimal for another. Attractants must be highly volatile to be effective over relatively great distances, whereas aphrodisiacs should be larger molecules that are effective only at very short range so that the male or female would be stimulated to copulate only when in contact with a partner. It would certainly not be in one female's interest to release a highly volatile aphrodisiac that might increase the probability of a male mating with another female. Research on the chemical nature of sexual attractants and aphrodisiacs in hamsters is so far consistent with these speculations (see Section IV,A.).

The only male-produced aphrodisiacs so far discovered are those from the salivary secretions of boars (see Chapter 9). Aphrodisiacs produced by females have been described as part of the vaginal secretions of dogs, mice, hamsters, and monkeys (Goodwin *et al.,* 1979; Hyashi and Kimura, 1974; Murphy, 1973; Johnston, 1975; see also Chapter 3). In mice, vaginal secretions taken from estrous females and placed on nonestrous females cause increased mating attempts by sexually experienced males, whereas vaginal secretions taken from nonestrous females have no such effects (Hyashi and Kimura, 1974). In dogs, one component of vaginal secretions has been identified as having sexually arousing effects (Section IV), although the entire vaginal secretion has apparently not been tested (Goodwin *et al.,* 1979). Previous reports that anal gland secretions of dogs had aphrodisiac functions (Donovan, 1969) are apparently incorrect (Dunbar, 1977).

Aphrodisiac functions of odors have been most thoroughly investigated in the golden hamster. Male hamsters require intact olfactory and vomeronasal systems in order to mate (Devor and Murphy, 1973; see also Chapter 8). Presumably, this reflects a necessity for olfactory information, although such lesions also eliminate the rhythmic input from the olfactory system to the brain that occurs regardless of the olfactory environment. This nonspecific input may have general arousal functions that, when eliminated, could cause depression of most behavioral activities. The loss of mating behavior that follows destruction of all olfactory input may be due to both the lack of specific olfactory information and to the lack of nonspecific arousal. Nonetheless, the experiments cited indicate that male hamsters rely on olfactory information for their mating behavior to a greater extent than most other mammals tested; elimination of olfaction in mice may have similar effects (cf. Murphy, 1976).

Vaginal secretions are one source of chemicals that facilitate copulatory behavior of male hamsters. When secretions from females are placed on intact or castrated stimulus males, either awake or anesthetized, experimental males will attempt to copulate with them (Murphy, 1973; Darby *et al.,* 1975; Johnston, 1975). Without the application of vaginal secretions males investigate and then either ignore or attack these same stimulus animals. Males require no sexual experience with females in order to show this facilitation of their copulatory behavior, indicating that the "meaning" of the signal is either acquired while the male is still with the mother in the nest or is genetically determined or both. A sensitive period for developing responsiveness to vaginal secretions and other odors is suggested by a peak in olfactory investigation that occurs between about 10 and 16 days of age (Johnston and Coplin, 1979).

Vaginal secretions are not sufficient to elicit copulatory behavior toward inanimate models of hamsters, thus suggesting the importance of other odor cues (Darby *et al.,* 1975; Johnston, 1977b). Furthermore, vaginal secretions are not necessary for the males' copulatory behavior. Males still attempt to mate with vaginectomized females that lack vaginal secretions, but they do so less quickly and less vigorously than with intact females (Kwan and Johnston, 1980; Johnston and Kwan, 1983; see Fig. 2). I have recently completed a series of experiments attempting to determine what other cues might be involved (Johnston, 1983b). Visual cues are not the only extra cues that are necessary, since males mate equally readily in the light and in the dark with either intact females or vaginectomized females. Neither auditory cues

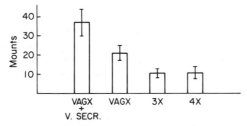

Fig. 2. Mean number of mounts by males ($N = 12$ per stimulus condition) that encountered estrous females during a 10-min trial. Females lacked various sources of scent, as follows: (1) VAGX females were vaginectomized and lacked vaginal secretions; (2) 3X females in addition lacked flank glands and Harderian glands; and (3) 4X females also lacked ear glands. Control females (VAGX and SECR) had been vaginectomized but were scented with vaginal secretions from another female.

nor movements of females are necessary, since males do attempt to copulate with anesthetized intact or vaginectomized females. As might be expected males' mating activities are not as vigorous as with awake females, indicating that an active female does provide cues that are influential. Removal of the Harderian gland, the flank gland, and the ear glands in addition to the vagina does reduce male copulatory performance below that shown toward females that lack just the vagina, but males still attempt to mate with either awake or anesthetized females lacking these scents (Fig. 2).

Thus, although hamsters are perhaps not typical mammals in that they require olfactory input for their sexual behavior, they may be typical in the complexity and redundancy of the cues that influence copulatory performance. Vaginal secretions have a powerful aphrodisiac function on sexually naive males, yet these secretions are neither sufficient nor necessary for copulatory behavior. Other odors and cues in other modalities all contribute to the level of general sexual arousal. Different cues do not seem to have any specific influences on particular components of copulatory behavior. Such complexity of control demonstrates that simple releaser models of communicative behavior are woefully inadequate, even for this relatively simple set of behaviors for which olfactory information appears to be necessary.

IV. CHEMICAL ANALYSIS OF SEXUAL CHEMOSIGNALS

A difficult aspect of research in chemical communication is the chemical identification of the signals. We do not know enough about how the olfactory system works or how chemical signals are constituted, and consequently it is not even clear what the most appropriate research strategy

is. Does one attempt successive fractionations to discover "the" pheromone, or does one attempt to identify all of the constituents and later try
to put them together to discover how they interact to produce the signal?
In this section I discuss the progress that has been made in attempts to
identify compounds important for sexual communication and some of the
difficulties in this endeavor.

A. Chemical Analysis of Scent Sources

Much early work on the chemical content of mammalian scent glands
was done by perfume chemists with such species as civets, musk deer, musk-
rats, and beavers (Lederer, 1950; Kingston, 1965). These species were investigated because their scent glands were thought to contain unique
substances useful in perfumes; many of the musklike compounds, for example, are large macrocyclic molecules that were used as chemical fixatives.
Despite considerable knowledge about the chemistry of these secretions there
has been little research on the functions of the various identified constituents. More recently, with the advent of interest in chemical communication, the chemistry of a variety of other scent glands, secretions, and
excretions has been investigated in detail (see Müller-Schwarze and Mozell,
1977; Müller-Schwarze and Silverstein, 1980).

Suggestive evidence of communicative functions can be obtained by
correlational studies in which the presence of certain compounds is related
to some relevant variable, such as the reproductive state or the sex of the
donor. For example, a compound (2-methylquinoline) has been identified
in the urine of male red foxes which apparently does not occur in the urine
of females, whereas several other compounds occur in greater concentrations in urine from females (Jorgenson *et al.*, 1978). Likewise, a set of seven
compounds whose presence seems to be dependent on estrogen has been
identified in female house mouse urine, whereas another set of compounds
that are dependent on androgens has been identified in male urine (Novotny, 1982). Such substances could be involved in sexual recognition.
Qualitative differences in the composition of scent gland secretions of several other rodent species have been observed that suggest a basis for discrimination and recognition of genera, species, populations, and individuals
(e.g., Stoddart, 1977).

Theoretically, it should be possible to identify the substances that are
important for different messages by a complete analysis of the glandular
secretions from different individuals, sexes, species, and reproductive states.
For example, secretions used for species recognition ought to have components that are unique to a particular species yet are constant among all
individuals of that species; a closely related species should use different

compounds or different ratios of the same compounds. Similarly, a scent gland whose function is to signal "male" should have some components that do not vary greatly from one male to the next but that do vary considerably from the scent gland components of females. A relatively invariant set of concentrations of compounds in males could signal "male" even if the same compounds were found in different ratios in secretions from females. Unfortunately, there are a number of problems with this approach: The enormous number of compounds in each secretion makes their identification extremely time-consuming, and even after identifying a large number of compounds one does not know which ones are important for communication. Furthermore, substances present in only trace amounts may be the most important ones for communication. The mammalian nose is more sensitive than our analytical tools, and for substances of biological significance we do not know how much more sensitive. Scent glands may also have functions not related to communication, such as maintenance of the pelage or thermoregulation (Thiessen and Kittrell, 1980), making the chemical analysis of the communication component more difficult. This type of problem is not encountered in the analysis of communication in other modalities, such as bird song. Finally, "noise" may be introduced into the signal itself by other variables such as diet, which may differ across individuals, sexes, or populations.

A more direct approach to identifying the compounds used as chemical signals is to fractionate the biological material repeatedly and attempt to isolate the active components with bioassays of the fractions. Among programs that have investigated nonprimate mammals, several have met with partial success, notably the work on boar aphrodisiac odors (see Chapter 9), dog aphrodisiacs, and hamster sex attractants and aphrodisiacs.

Gas chromatographic analysis of vaginal secretions of domestic dogs indicated several peaks that were characteristic of estrus but not other reproductive states (Goodwin et al., 1979). One of these peaks was identified as methyl p-hydroxybenzoate; this compound was tested for its behavioral effects by placement on the genital region of nonestrous female dogs. Males attempted to mount the females scented with this compound in 18 of 21 trials, whereas control trials with a number of other compounds did not lead to mounting attempts. This exciting preliminary finding should be investigated more thoroughly, especially since there are many questions to be answered. The aphrodisiac properties of whole vaginal secretions should be established, as should the effectiveness of methyl p-hydroxybenzoate relative to whole vaginal secretions. A methodological difficulty also must be explored. In this study the same group of dogs was used in a long series of experiments, and it is possible that they were inadvertently trained or sensitized to odors or particular types of odors or even that they were keying in on the behavior of the experimenters. A curious aspect of the males' responses to methyl *p*-hydroxybenzoate is that they responded strongly to it when it was placed on the genital region of a female but not when it was presented by itself in an open field (F. Regnier and M. Goodwin, personal communications). It is not known how males would respond if this substance were placed on another part of the female's body or on another male, and thus the degree of effectiveness of this compound in eliciting sexual responses from males is uncertain.

The most thoroughly investigated source of mammalian sex pheromones is the vaginal secretion of hamsters (Singer *et al.*, 1976, 1980; Macrides *et al.*, 1977; O'Connell *et al.*, 1978, 1979, 1981). Vaginal secretions have a variety of effects on the behavior of males, including elicitation of approach, sniffing, licking, copulatory behavior and hormonal responses as well as the reduction of aggressive tendencies and flank-marking frequency (see Johnston, 1977b, for review). The attraction of males to vaginal secretions can be eliminated by castration and reinstated by testosterone therapy but is not dependent on sexual experience (Johnston, 1974; Gregory *et al.*, 1974; Johnston and Coplin, 1979). The only functions so far investigated at the chemical level of analysis are the sexual attractant and aphrodisiac ones.

Singer *et al.* (1976) initially reported that dimethyl disulfide is one component of hamster vaginal secretion that is active in attracting males. This compound elicits approach and prolonged sniffing when it is presented in a bottle underneath a male's cage, when it is placed on the genital region of an anesthetized stimulus male, and when it is placed in a bottle inside a male's home cage (Singer *et al.*, 1976; Macrides *et al.*, 1977). Males are extraordinarily sensitive to dimethyl disulfide, being attracted to it when it is presented in quantities of 500 fg in an under-the-cage assay (O'Connell *et al.*, 1979). Furthermore, the concentration of this compound varies with the estrous cycle, being highest on the estrous day (O'Connell *et al.*, 1981). The function of this variation is not entirely clear, however, since (*a*) even at its lowest levels during the cycle there is roughly 1400 times more than is necessary to attract males in standard laboratory tests (Singer *et al.*, 1980) and (*b*) males do not seem to be differentially attracted to estrous and diestrous females (Landauer *et al.*, 1978; Johnston, 1980). It may be that under field conditions the increased output of this compound does have important consequences for attracting males (O'Connell *et al.*, 1981).

Because dimethyl disulfide is one of the biggest success stories in attempts to characterize mammalian pheromones chemically, it is important to recognize two limitations in our knowledge. First, dimethyl disulfide does not account for all of the attractiveness of hamster vaginal secretions. In every experiment some males fail to respond at all [e.g., in

O'Connell *et al.* (1978) 6 of 13 males failed to respond], and those males that are attracted sniff at the odor for shorter durations than at whole vaginal secretions (O'Connell *et al.,* 1978; Macrides *et al.,* 1977). A variety of volatile acids and alcohols have also been identified in the vaginal secretion, but mixtures of these compounds are not attractive to males, nor do these compounds enhance the response to dimethyl disulfide (O'Connell *et al.,* 1978). Thus, sexual attraction in hamsters is not entirely mediated by a single attractant molecule. Second, the attractiveness of dimethyl disulfide has been tested primarily in a single type of bioassay procedure. This type of test has recently been shown to be a relatively poor one for discriminating between attractiveness due to biological function and that due to other factors such as novelty (Johnston, 1981).

Considerable progress has been made in characterizing the nature of the chemicals in vaginal secretions that act as aphrodisiacs. Dimethyl disulfide attracts males but has no influence on copulatory tendencies, indicating a clear separation of function of some chemical constituents of the vaginal secretion (Macrides *et al.,* 1977). Although the total volatiles do stimulate mounting attempts (Johnston, 1977b), mixture of the acids and alcohols in the proportions found in the secretion is without effect (Singer *et al.,* 1980). Mounting activity is also stimulated by the relatively nonvolatile fraction, and Singer *et al.* (1980) found that these effects are associated with substances having molecular weights between 15,000 and 60,000. At this point it is not known whether the crucial components are large molecular weight molecules, are part of such molecules, or are simply bound to such molecules. As described in Section III,B,4, odors from sources other than the vaginal secretion also facilitate male sexual behavior, but no chemical analysis has yet been undertaken.

B. Speculations on the Nature of Chemical Signals and Olfactory Perception

Although progress has been made in the analysis of chemical signals in mammals, many researchers in this area feel a sense of dissatisfaction because the mammalian work does not have the clarity of results found for insects. Behavioral responses to insect pheromones tend to be less variable, more predictable, and more all-or-none than those in mammals. At the same time it is clear that in many insect species responses are not as automatic as was originally implied by the term "releaser." Responses of insects often depend on the time of day, the experience of the insect, and other variables. Still, situations can usually be arranged so that specific behavioral responses will be elicited. In contrast, mammalian scents do not often elicit behavioral responses other than sniffing. Müller-Schwarze (1977) dealt with this problem by classifying many mammalian scents as "informer" pheromones, that is, social odors that provide information but that do not cause a directly functional response. A related way of thinking about mammalian social odors is that they may change the bias of a response hierarchy or provide the context within which other signals are effective. This kind of subtlety and complexity makes the discovery of communicatory functions and the development of reliable bioassays exceedingly difficult.

Some of the problems of analysis may be due to fundamental differences in the nature of the signals, the nature of the olfactory apparatus, and the degree to which the signals and the sensory systems have been specialized during the course of evolution. There are two logical extremes for olfactory signals and the associated sensory mechanisms of response. One is the original insect "releaser" model, in which a single chemical constitutes the signal and a specific receptor detects the molecule. At the other extreme is what I will call the "odor-quality" model. In this model the signal consists of a complex mixture of substances that is experienced by the organism as an odor quality or *gestalt,* which depends on all of the constituents for its essence. At least some of the quality of each odor must be dependent on nonspecialized receptors, although the model does not rule out specific receptors for some components of a scent signal. Thus, there might be a small number of components that determine the basic character of the odor but other components that gave it richness, depth, and complexity. A direct analogy is that of flavor chemistry. The substances that impart flavor to dry red wine are numerous. Some relatively small number of these (say, 10–15), when mixed together in exactly the right proportions, might allow the flavor to be correctly identified as "red wine," but it would still be disappointing to a sophisticated wine drinker, because the mixture would lack all the subtle nuances and characteristics that, for example, would identify it as cabernet sauvignon or a particular chateau and vintage of cabernet sauvignon. Similarly, a chemist might put together the main components of a mammalian scent, which would elicit a low level of appropriate responses. This synthetic scent might never yield a full-fledged response, however, because it would lack the subtle nuances that make a scent realistic to an animal.

Both these extremes, as well as many cases that fall in between, may exist in mammals. Some types of functions, such as a specific behavioral response or a hormone release, may be more biased toward the specific-signal end of the continuum, whereas other functions, such as species or individual recognition, may necessarily tend to occur toward the odor-quality end. However, in cases in which there may be a chemical that is used for a particular function, such as sexual arousal, it may function only in the context of the pervasive odor quality that belongs to a member of a particular species. Using a musical analogy, the note that is the aphrodisiac may be effective only if it occurs within the framework of the hamster symphony in the key of "female."

This odor-quality model is not at all the same as the one that seems to be emerging from the insect work. Among insects that have more than one component in their signals, these components seem to work at precise ratios and to have specific functions. This is just a slightly more complex version of the one-pheromone–one-receptor model; the specificity and the relatively automatic elicitation of behavioral responses are still there, but now several precise response mechanisms must be integrated rather than a simple yes-or-no response. In the mammalian case I am suggesting a very different model, one that is additive but nonlinear; many components contribute to the overall odor quality, but no individual component is either necessary or sufficient. If this odor-quality model is correct in some cases, it may not be practical to do much more than identify compounds that yield partial activity in a bioassay and discover some additive relationships. On the other hand, if some mammalian systems approach the specific-signal type of model, it ought to be possible to characterize the chemical signal thoroughly.

REFERENCES

Aleksiuk, M. (1968). *J. Mammal.* **49**, 759–762.
Altmann, M. (1959). *J. Mammal.* **40**, 420–424.
August, P. V. (1978). *Am. Midl. Nat.* **99**, 206–218.
Beach, F. A. (1970). *Behaviour* **36**, 131–148.
Beauchamp, G. K. (1973). *Physiol. Behav.* **10**, 589–594.
Birch, M. C., ed. (1974). "Pheromones." North-Holland Publ., Amsterdam.
Birke, L. I. A. (1978). *Anim. Behav.* **26**, 1165–1166.
Birke, L. I. A. (1981). *Z. Tierpsychol.* **55**, 79–89.
Block, M. L., Volpe, L. C., and Hayes, M. J. (1981). *Science* **211**, 1062–1064.
Bowers, J. M., and Alexander, B. K. (1967). *Science* **158**, 1208–1210.
Brown, D., and Johnston, R. E. (1983). *In* "Chemical Signals in Vertebrates III" (D. Müller-Schwarze and R. M. Silverstein, eds.), pp. 343–346. Plenum, New York.
Brown, R. E. (1977). *J. Comp. Physiol. Psychol.* **91**, 1190–1206.
Brown, R. E. (1979). *Adv. Study Behav.* **10**, 103–162.
Butler, R. G., and Butler, L. A. (1979). *Behav. Neural Biol.* **26**, 442–454.
Calhoun, J. B. (1963). *DHEW Pub. (HSA) (V.S.) Pub.* HSA No. 1008.
Carr, W. J., and Caul, W. F. (1962). *Anim. Behav.* **10**, 20–27.
Carr, W. J., Loeb, L. S., and Dissinger, M. L. (1965). *J. Comp. Physiol. Psychol.* **59**, 370–377.
Carr, W. J., Krames, L., and Costanzo, D. J. (1970a). *J. Comp. Physiol. Psychol.* **71**, 216–222.
Carr, W. J., Wylie, N. R., and Loeb, L. S. (1970b). *J. Comp. Physiol. Psychol.* **72**, 51–59.
Charles-Dominique, P. (1977). "Ecology and Behaviour of Nocturnal Primates." Columbia Univ. Press, New York.

Dagg, A. I., and Windsor, D. E. (1971). *Can. J. Zool.* **49**, 283–285.

Daly, M. (1977). *J. Comp. Physiol. Psychol.* **91**, 1082–1094.

Daly, M., and Daly, S. (1975a). *Mammalia* **39**, 289–311.

Daly, M., and Daly, S. (1975b). *Z. Tierpsychol.* **37**, 298–321.

Darby, E. M., Devor, M., and Chorover, S. L. (1975). *J. Comp. Physiol. Psychol.* **88**, 496–502.

Devor, M., and Murphy, M. R. (1973). *Behav. Biol.* **9**, 31–42.

Dewsbury, D. A. (1981). *Psychol. Bull.* **89**, 464–482.

Donovan, C. A. (1969). *J. Am. Vet. Med. Assoc.* **155**, 1995–1996.

Doty, R. L. (1972). *J. Comp. Physiol. Psychol.* **81**, 191–197.

Doty, R. L. (1973). *J. Comp. Physiol. Psychol.* **84**, 296–303.

Doty, R. L., ed. (1976). "Mammalian Olfaction, Reproductive Processes, and Behavior." Academic Press, New York.

Dunbar, I. F. (1977). *Behav. Biol.* **20**, 471–481.

Dunbar, I. F. (1978). *Biol. Behav.* **3**, 273–286.

Dunbar, I., and Carmichael, M. (1981). *Behav. Neural Biol.* **31**, 465–470.

Ebling, F. J. (1964). *J. Endocrinol.* **10**, 147–154.

Eibl-Eibestfeldt, I. (1953). *Z. Tierpsychol.* **10**, 204–254.

Eisenberg, J. F. (1963). *Behaviour* **22**, 16–23.

Epple, G. (1970). *Folia Primatol.* **13**, 48–62.

Estes, R. D. (1972). *Mammalia* **36**, 315–341.

Ewer, R. F. (1973). "The Carnivores." Cornell Univ. Press, Ithaca, New York.

Floody, O. R., and Pfaff, D. W. (1977a). *J. Comp. Physiol. Psychol.* **91**, 794–806.

Floody, O. R., and Pfaff, D. W. (1977b). *J. Comp. Physiol. Psychol.* **91**, 820–829.

Floody, O. R., Pfaff, D. W., and Lewis, C. D. (1977). *J. Comp. Physiol. Psychol.* **91**, 807–819.

Frank, D. H., and Johnston, R. E. (1981). *Behav. Neural Biol.* **33**, 514–518.

Fraser, A. F. (1968). "Reproductive Behaviour in Ungulates." Academic Press, New York.

Gawienowski, A. M. (1977). *In* "Chemical Signals in Vertebrates" (D. Müller-Schwarze and M. M. Mozell, eds.), pp. 45–60. Plenum, New York.

Gilder, P. M., and Slater, P. J. B. (1978). *Nature (London)* **274**, 364–365.

Godfrey, J. (1958). *Proc. R. Phys. Soc. Edinburgh* **27**, 47–55.

Goodwin, M., Gooding, K. M., and Regnier, F. (1979). *Science* **203**, 599–561.

Gorman, M. L. (1976). *Anim. Behav.* **24**, 141–145.

Grau, G. A. (1976). *In* "Mammalian Olfaction, Reproductive Processes, and Behavior" (R. L. Doty, ed), pp. 219–242. Academic Press, New York.

Gregory, E., Engel, K., and Pfaff, D. (1975). *J. Comp. Physiol. Psychol.* **89**, 442–446.

Halpin, Z. T. (1980). *Biol. Behav.* **5**, 233–248.

Harris, M. A., and Murie, J. O. (1982). *Anim. Behav.* **30**, 140–148.

Hart, B. L. (1983). *In* "Chemical Signals in Vertebrates III" (D. Müller-Schwarze and R. M. Silverstein, eds.), pp. 87–104. Plenum, New York.

Holmes, W. G., and Shermm, P. W. (1982). Am. Zool. **22**, 491–517.

Huck, W. U., and Banks, E. M. (1980a). *Anim. Behav.* **28**, 1046–1052.

Huck, U. W., and Banks, E. M. (1980b). *Anim. Behav.* **28**, 1053–1062.

Huck, U. W., Banks, E. M., and Wang, S. C. (1981). *Behav. Neural Biol.* **33**, 364–371.

Hyashi, S., and Kimura, T. (1974). *Physiol. Behav.* **13**, 563–567.

Johnson, R. P. (1973). *Anim. Behav.* **21**, 521–535.

Johnston, R. E. (1974). *Behav. Biol.* **12**, 111–117.

Johnston, R. E. (1975). *Anim. Learn. Behav.* **3**, 161–166.

Johnston, R. E. (1977a). *Anim. Behav.* **25**, 317–327.

Johnston, R. E. (1977b). *In* "Chemical Signals in Vertebrates" (D. Müller-Schwarze and M. M. Mozell, eds.), pp. 225–249. Plenum, New York.

Johnston, R. E. (1979). *Horm. Behav.* **13**, 21–39.
Johnston, R. E. (1980). *J. Comp. Physiol. Psychol.* **94**, 894–904.
Johnston, R. E. (1981). *J. Comp. Physiol. Psychol.* **93**, 951–960.
Johnston, R. E. (1983a). *In* "Chemical Signals in Vertebrates III" (D. Müller-Schwarze and R. M. Silverstein, eds), pp. 245–258. New York.
Johnston, R. E. (1983b). In preparation.
Johnston, R. E., and Brenner, D. (1982). *Behav. Neural Biol.* **35**, 46–55.
Johnston, R. E., and Bronson, F. H. (1982). *Biol. Reprod.* **27**, 1174–1180.
Johnston, R. E., and Coplin, B. (1979). *Behav. Neural Biol.* **25**, 473–489.
Johnston, R. E., and Kwan, M. (1983). Submitted for publication.
Johnston, R. E., and Rasmussen, K. (1983). In preparation.
Jorgenson, J. W., Novotny, M., Carmack, M., Copland, G. B., Wilson, S. R., Katona, S., and Whitten, W. K. (1978). *Science* **199**, 796–798.
Kairys, D. J., Magalhaes, H., and Floody, O. R. (1980). *Physiol. Behav.* **25**, 143–146.
Kingston, B. H. (1965). *Proc. Int. Congr. Endocrinol. 2nd, 1964,* Part 1, pp. 209–214.
Kleiman, D. G. (1966). *Symp. Zool. Soc. London* **18**, 167–177.
Kleiman, D. G. (1971). *Z. Tierpsychol.* **29**, 259–278.
Kleiman, D. G., and Mack, D. S. (1980). *Folia Primatol.* **33**, 1–14.
Kumari, S., and Prakash, I. (1981). *Anim. Behav.* **29**, 1269–71.
Kwan, M. (1978). *Diss. Abstr. Int.* **39**, 433b (University Microfilms No. 78–09, 810).
Kwan, M., and Johnston, R. E. (1980). *J. Comp. Physiol. Psychol.* **94**, 905–913.
Ladewig, J., and Hart, B. L. (1980). *Physiol. Behav.* **24**, 1067–1071.
Landauer, M. R., and Carter, C. S. (1974) *Pap., Meet. Am. Psychol. Assoc.*
Landauer, M. R., Banks, E. M., and Carter, C. S. (1977). *Horm. Behav.* **9**, 193–202.
Landauer, M. R., Banks, E. M., and Carter, C. S. (1978). *Anim. Behav.* **26**, 611–621.
Latta, J., Hopf, S., and Ploog, D. (1967). *Primates* **8**, 229–246.
LeBoef, B. J. (1967). *Behaviour* **29**, 268–295.
Lederer, E. (1950). *Prog. Chem. Org. Nat. Prod.* **6**, 87–153.
Leonard, C. M. (1972). *J. Comp. Physiol. Psychol.* **80**, 208–215.
Leuthold, W. (1977). "African Ungulates." Springer-Verlag, Berlin.
Lindsay, D. R. (1965). *Anim. Behav.* **13**, 75–78.
McIntosh, T. K., Davis, P. G., and Barfield, R. J. (1979). *Behav. Neural Biol.* **26**, 161–168.
Macrides, F., Johnson, P. A., and Schneider, S. P. (1977). *Behav. Biol.* **20**, 377–386.
Mainardi, M., and Pasquali, A. (1973). *Acta Nat.* **9**, 3–12.
Markley, M. H., and Bassett, C. F. (1942). *Am. Midl. Nat.* **28**, 604–616.
Mech, L. D. (1970). "The Wolf." Am. Mus. Nat. Hist. Press, Garden City, New York.
Michael, R. P. (1971). *In* "Frontiers in Neuroendocrinology" (L. Martini and W. F. Ganong, eds), pp. 359–398. Oxford Univ. Press, London and New York.
Moore, R. E., (1965). *Am. Midl. Nat.* **73**, 85–100.
Moore, W. G., and Marchinton, R. L. (1974). *In* "Behaviour of Ungulates and its Relation to Management," New Ser. No. 24, pp. 447–456. IUCN Publications, Morges, Switzerland.
Müller-Schwarze, D. (1977). *In* "Chemical Signals in Vertebrates" (D. Müller-Schwarze and M. M. Mozell, eds.), pp. 413–431. Plenum, New York.
Müller-Schwarze, D., and Mozell, M. M., eds. (1977). "Chemical Signals in Vertebrates." Plenum, New York.
Müller-Schwarze, D., and Silverstein, R. M., eds. (1980). "Chemical Signals in Vertebrates and Aquatic Invertebrates." Plenum, New York.
Murphy, M. R. (1973). *Behav. Biol.* **9**, 367–375.
Murphy, M. R. (1976). *In* "Mammalian Olfaction, Reproductive Processes, and Behavior" (R. L. Doty, ed.), pp. 95–117. Academic Press, New York.

Murphy, M. R. (1977). *J. Comp. Physiol. Psychol.* **91**, 1337–1346.

Murphy, M. R. (1978). *Anim. Behav.* **26**, 312.

Murphy, M. R. (1980). *Behav. Neural Biol.* **30**, 323–340.

Mykytowycz, R. (1968). *Sci. Am.* **218**, 116–126.

Nevo, E., Bodmer, M., and Heth, G. (1976). *Experientia* **32**, 1511–1512.

Novotny, M. (1982). Paper presented at Chemical Signals in Vertebrates III, Sarasota, 1982.

Nyby, J., Wysocki, C. J., Whitney, G., Dizinno, G., and Schneider, J. (1979). *J. Comp. Physiol. Psychol.* **93**, 957–975.

O'Connell, R. J., Singer, A. G., Macrides, F., Pfaffmann, C., and Agosta, W. C. (1978). *Behav. Biol.* **24**, 244–255.

O'Connell, R. J., Singer, A. G., Pfaffmann, C., and Agosta, W. C. (1979). *J. Chem. Ecol.* **5**, 575–585.

O'Connell, R. J., Singer, A. G., Stern, F. L., Jesmajian, S., and Agosta, W. C. (1981). *Behav. Neural Biol.* **31**, 457–464.

Perrigo, G., and Bronson, F. (1983). *In* "Chemical Signals in Vertebrates III" (D. Müller-Schwarze and R. M. Silverstein, eds.), pp. 195–210. Plenum, New York.

Pfaff, D., and Pfaffmann, C. (1969). *Olfaction Taste, Proc. Int. Symp., 3rd, 1968,* pp. 258–267.

Porter, R. H., and Wyrick, M. (1979). *Anim. Behav.* **27**, 761–766.

Rabb, G. B., Woolpy, J. H., and Ginsburg, B. E. (1967). *Am. Zool.* **7**, 305–312.

Ralls, K. (1971). *Science* **171**, 443–449.

Rasa, O. A. E. (1973). *Z. Tierpsychol.* **32**, 293–318.

Rathbun, G. (1979). *Adv. Ethol.* **20**, 1–84.

Roper, T. J., and Polioudakis, E. (1977). *Behaviour* **61**, 207–237.

Ruddy, L. L. (1980). *J. Comp. Physiol. Psychol.* **94**, 767–774.

Schaffer, J. (1940). "Die Hautdrusenorgane der saugetiere." Urban & Schwarzenberg, Berlin.

Schaller, G. B. (1967). "The Deer and the Tiger." Univ. of Chicago Press, Chicago, Illinois.

Schaller, G. B. (1972). "The Serengeti Lion." Univ. of Chicago Press, Chicago, Illinois.

Selander, R. K. (1970). *Am. Zool.* **10**, 53–66.

Sherman, P. W. (1981). *Behav. Ecol. Sociobiol.* **8**, 251–259.

Singer, A. G., Agosta, W. C., O'Connell, R. J., Pfaffmann, C., Bowen, D. V., and Field, F. H. (1976). *Science* **191**, 948–950.

Singer, A. G., Macrides, F., and Agosta, W. C. (1980). *In* "Chemical Signals in Vertebrates and Aquatic Invertebrates" (D. Müller-Schwarze and R. M. Silverstein, eds.), pp. 365–375. Plenum, New York.

Smith, M. H. (1965). *Evolution* **19**, 430–435.

Steiner, A. L. (1975). *Nat. Can.* **102**, 737–751.

Stoddart, D. M. (1977). *In* "Chemical Signals in Vertebrates" (D. Müller-Schwarze and M. M. Mozell, eds.), pp. 333–356. Plenum, New York.

Thiessen, D. D., and Kittrell, M. W. (1980). *Physiol. Behav.* **24**, 417–424.

Thiessen, D. D., and Rice, M. (1976). *Psych. Bull.* **83**, 505–539.

Thody, A. J., and Dijkstra, H. (1978). *J. Endocrinol.* **77**, 397–403.

Thompson, D. C. (1977). *Can. J. Zool.* **55**, 1176–1184.

Todd, N. B., Nixon, C. W., Mulvaney, D. A., and Connelly, M. E. (1972). *J. Hered.* **63**, 73–77.

Van Lawick-Goodall, H., and Van Lawick-Goodall, J. (1971). "Innocent Killers." Houghton-Mifflin, Boston, Massachusetts.

Wallace, P., Owen, K., and Theissen, D. D. (1973). *Physiol. Behav.* **10**, 463–466.

Whitney, G., and Nyby, J. (1979). *Am. Zool.* **19**, 457–463.

Williams, R. J. (1956). "Biochemical Individuality." Univ. of Texas Press, Austin.

Wilsson, L. (1968). "My Beaver Colony." Doubleday, New York.

Wise, D. A. (1974). *Horm. Behav.* **5,** 235–250.

Wolf, P. R., and Powell, A. J. (1979). *Behav. Neural Biol.* **27,** 379–383.

Yamaguchi, M., Yamazaki, K., Beauchamp, G. K., Bard, J., Thomas Z., and Boyse, E. A. (1981). *Proc. Natl. Acad. Sci. U.S.A.* **78,** 5817–5820.

Yamazaki, K., Boyse, E. A., Mike, V., Thaler, H. T., Mathieson, B. J., Abbott, J., Boyse, J., Zayas, Z. A., and Thomas, L. (1976). *J. Exp. Med.* **144.** 1324–1335.

Yamazaki, K., Yamaguichi, M., Baronoski, L., Bard, J., Boyse, E.A., and Thomas, L. (1979). *J. Exp. Med.* **150,** 755–760.

2

Chemical Communication in Mother–Young Interactions

Michael Leon

Department of Psychobiology
University of California
Irvine, California

I. INTRODUCTION

Not only must mammalian mothers reliably identify, defend, and nurse their offspring throughout the dependent phase of the young, but they must do so as their progeny change rapidly in their physical, physiological, and behavioral characteristics. At the same time the offspring must deal effectively with the new social and environmental situations that they face if they are to survive their dependent phase.

What has emerged from the many careful studies of mother–young in-

PHEROMONES AND REPRODUCTION IN MAMMALS
Copyright © 1983 by Academic Press, Inc.
All rights of reproduction in any form reserved.
ISBN 0-12-710780-0

teractions that have been reported in this century is a partial understanding of the methods for communicating the present status of the interacting mother and offspring, as well as methods for inducing responses that will meet the future needs of those changing individuals. Indeed, there appear to be intricate programs of closely meshed signals between parent and progeny that induce both the rapid and the prolonged responses essential for coping with the complexities of motherhood and infancy.

The importance of signal modality in mediating mother–young interactions varies both with the specialized characteristics of each species and with the type of interaction for which the signal is required. In this chapter I discuss the role of a single modality, olfaction, in the mediation of nurtural interactions of mammals. It is my hope that the reader will be struck by the variety of situations in which olfactory signals take preeminence in ensuring the success of the maternal episode.

II. OLFACTORY MEDIATION OF MATERNAL BEHAVIORS

A. Initiation of Maternal Responsiveness to the Young

Mammalian mothers and their offspring use a number of olfactory-based mechanisms that allow the complex, changing needs of developing offspring to be met. Indeed, pup odors may allow mothers of some species to begin caring for the strange, new individuals to whom they have given birth.

When virgin female Norway rats (*Rattus norvegicus*) initially encounter rat pups, they begin to alternate tentative approaches, at which time they sniff the pups, with an active avoidance of the pups (Fleming and Luebke, 1981; Fleming and Rosenblatt, 1974a,b; Terkel and Rosenblatt, 1971). Two lines of evidence indicate that strange pups emit an odor that females find aversive.

First, and most directly, anosmia was produced in virgin females by destruction of the olfactory bulb or by lateral olfactory tract damage. Those females that did not cannibalize fostered pups began caring for them fairly rapidly after their initial introduction. Destruction of the olfactory mucosa by means of zinc sulfate application induced rapid maternal responsiveness without inducing cannibalism, presumably because this procedure avoided the production of the elevated reactivity seen in bulbectomized rats (Cain, 1974; Fleischer *et al.*, 1981; Fleming and Rosenblatt, 1974a,b; Mayer and Rosenblatt, 1975, 1977, 1979).

Destruction of the vomeronasal organ of virgin females similarly facilitated their acceptance of the young, and the combined destruction of the vomeronasal organ and the olfactory bulbs further reduced the latency of such females to care for the foster young (Fleming *et al.*, 1979). Moreover, either destruction of the amygdala, which is the projection site of both primary and accessary olfactory systems (Scalia and Winans, 1975), or destruction of the stria terminalis, which is the major efferent projection of the amygdala to the medial preoptic area (Heimer and Nauta, 1969), similarly accelerated the onset of maternal behavior in virgin female rats (Fleming et al., 1981). These data are particularly interesting because the intact medial preoptic area has been shown to be critical for the onset of maternal behavior (Numan, 1974; Numan et al., 1977).

The second, indirect line of evidence arises from the observation that continued forced cohabitation of foster pups with intact virgin females will eventually induce the adults to care for the young (Cosnier and Couturier, 1966; Rosenblatt, 1967; Wiesner and Sheard, 1933). These data are consistent with the idea that forced proximity familiarizes the females with the odor of the pups, perhaps decreasing its aversive quality, and thereby allows the adults to approach and care for the young. Virgin females had an even shorter latency to behave maternally when the proximity was further increased by housing the pups with the adults in small cages (Terkel and Rosenblatt, 1971).

Rat mothers, of course, normally do not have the opportunity to gain gradual olfactory familiarity with the pups before maternal care is initiated; they uniformly begin to care for the pups as they emerge from the birth canal (Rosenblatt and Lehrman, 1963; Wiesner and Sheard, 1933). It has been suggested, however, that the dams may become familiar with the odor of their own young during pregnancy by experiencing the odors of the secretions emanating from the birth canal (Birch, 1956). To date, there has been no adequate test of that proposal.

Rather than finding the odor of the pups aversive, puerperal females may need the olfactory stimulation provided by the pups to initiate maternal care; that is, pup odor may be a releaser for maternal behavior. The available data indicate that, although such olfactory stimulation may contribute to the uniformly immediate maternal responsiveness of parturient female rats, it is probably not critical for its onset.

Benuck and Rowe (1975) and Schwartz and Rowe (1976) found that olfactory bulbectomy interfered with the normal onset of maternal behavior in parturient females, but these results were likely due to the nonolfactory consequences of bulb removal. Dams that experienced bulb removal as neonates or experienced bilateral bulb destruction in two stages—both procedures that typically minimize side effects of neutral destruction—exhibited normal maternal behavior following delivery of their young (Fleming and Rosenblatt, 1974b; Pollack and Sachs, 1975). Similarly, Benuck and Rowe (1975) found normal onset of maternal behavior after prepartum destruction of the olfactory mucosa by means of zinc sulfate application. Again, this procedure produces anosmia with minimal central nervous system injury, thereby minimizing behavioral side effects (Alberts, 1974; Cain, 1974). Olfactory bulbectomy performed either 1 or 2 days before parturition also did not prevent the onset of maternal care (Herrenkohl and Rosenberg, 1972; Schlein *et al.,* 1972). Pup odors may still be aversive to parturient females, but other factors may prime the females to act maternally, such that neither an aversion to pup olfactory cues nor a lack of pup olfactory releasing stimuli would delay the initiation of maternal behavior.

The internal state created by the hormones associated with the termination of pregnancy does prime Norway rat females to begin behaving maternally at birth (for detailed reviews, see Moltz and Leon, 1972; Slotnick, 1975; Rosenblatt *et al.,* 1979). It may be that this hormonal state decreases the threshold for maternal responses or that the hormones induce the females to be less reactive to any aversive aspect of contact with the strange pups or that hormones may alter the actual perception of pup olfactory cues. All of these factors may contribute to the normal rapid onset of maternal responsiveness, and all may interact with olfactory experience obtained during previous pregnancies or lactations (Cohen and Bridges, 1981).

In contrast to Norway rats, mouse (*Mus musculus*) mothers subjected to olfactory bulbectomy did not become maternal toward their young at birth, and often cannibalized their litters. Moreover, bulbectomized virgin mice did not come to accept cohabiting foster pups (Gandelman *et al.,* 1971a,b, 1972; Zarrow *et al.,* 1971). Even if anosmia was produced by application of zinc sulfate either in late gestation or before conception, the females neglected or ate their offspring at term (Seegal and Denenberg, 1974; Vandenbergh, 1973). The effects of bulbectomy on maternal behavior were, however, more severe than those of zinc sulfate administration (Vandenbergh, 1973). In addition, multiparous mice cared for their pups when made peripherally anosmic, in contrast to their behavior following bulbectomy (Seegal and Denenberg, 1974). Although the partial congruence of centrally and peripherally induced anosmias suggests a common mediation of their consequences by olfactory cues, the differences in performance are sufficient to withhold judgment on that point. It would seem, however, that olfactory cues may serve as a critical part of the pup releasing stimulus complex for maternal behavior, at least in primiparae.

Nonlactating golden hamsters (*Mesocricetus auratus*) typically react immediately to the appearance of foster pups, either by caring for them or by cannibalizing the young (Marques and Valenstein, 1976; Rowell, 1961). Olfactory bulbectomy reduced the occurrence of both maternal and cannibalistic behaviors, whereas anosmia induced by zinc sulfate treatment (which probably spared the vomeronasal organ; see Winans and Powers, 1977) had little effect on the occurrence of either behavior pattern

(Marques, 1979). Cutting the vomeronasal nerve, however, induced most killers to care for foster pups, and those females that continued to cannibalize pups postoperatively were induced to become maternal after zinc sulfate administration. The reduction in pup killing was not due to an overall deficit in attack behaviors following these procedures, for the animals continued to attack and kill insects (Marques, 1979).

Pup olfactory cues seem to have different roles in different species regarding the onset of parental care. Rats and hamsters appear to find pup odors aversive, and suppression of their perception of pup odors disinhibits their caretaking behaviors. Rats appear to use both the main and accessory olfactory systems to register the aversive pup odor, whereas the accessory system seems to play the major processing role in hamsters. Mice, on the other hand, appear to respond to the pup odor as a releaser of maternal care, with the main olfactory system possibly principally involved.

B. Maternal Recognition of Offspring

Although some mammalian mothers may care for offspring of other dams, many care only for their own, and mothers involved in such exclusive relationships must have some means by which they can distinguish their own young. Solitary species may accomplish this task by default; mothers who have young that remain in isolated nests may simply restrict their care to those within their nest. Group-living mothers that normally restrict maternal care to their own offspring must employ specific cues to identify them, and in some cases these cues have been shown to be olfactory.

Norway rat dams are found only with their own young in the wild (Telle, 1966) and kill alien pups when they are presented to them in the laboratory (King, 1939). If the dam is barred from the nest, however, and the alien young are allowed to mingle with the resident pups in the nest, the dams care for the pups (King, 1939). Although rat dams may simply accept the occupants of their relatively isolated maternal nest (Calhoun, 1962) as their own, they may be responding to olfactory cues specific to the mother–young unit. Data suggestive of the latter possibility come from work on laboratory strains of Norway rats, which are somewhat more tolerant of alien young than their wild counterparts. These dams simply prefer to retrieve their own young before aliens, a preference that is eliminated by destruction of the olfactory bulbs (Beach and Jaynes, 1956). If alien pups are allowed to spend considerable time in the nest, the preference for own young is also eliminated (Misanin *et al.*, 1977). These data suggest that the discrimination by mother rats is based on differential olfactory cues emitted by or placed on the young. Rat mothers emit odors that change with their diet (Leon, 1975), and the pups may be marked by these maternal odors (Leon, 1974).

There is yet another aspect of rat offspring recognition. Mother rats lick the anogenital region of their male offspring more than that of the female pups (Moore and Morelli, 1979), a difference that can be reversed by the application of male pup urine onto the female pups or by the application of a masking odor onto the males or by the occlusion of the perineal area with collodion (Moore, 1981). These data indicate not only that rat dams can discriminate between own and alien young, but that they can distinguish the sex of their own pups. Given that at least one rodent species (*Neotoma floridana*) differentially rears females in times of diet restriction (McClure, 1980), the sexual discrimination made by Norway rat mothers may have some important functional value under certain environmental circumstances.

Wild guinea pigs (*Cavia aperea*) nurse only their own precocial offspring (Rood, 1972), whereas laboratory strains (*Cavia porcellus*) care for alien young (Rood, 1972). In a choice situation, however, the domesticated guinea pigs preferred their own litter to an unfamiliar litter of similar age (Porter *et al.,* 1973) and nursed their own young more frequently than the strange young (Fullerton *et al.,* 1974). These dams even preferred an artificial odor that had been experienced in the presence of pups (Porter *et al.,* 1973). Differences in pup odors may arise from differences in individual maternal odors, which themselves may be based on diet variations that have been shown to produce differences in odors emitted by adult guinea pigs (Beauchamp, 1976).

Another rodent species that may identify its own young through olfactory cues is the spiny mouse (*Acomys cahirinus*), the only murid rodent that bears precocial young. When these mothers are on the same diet, they retrieve alien young as quickly as their own, but if the maternal diet differs the dams gather up their own faster than they retrieve strange young (Doane and Porter, 1978). Since spiny mouse mothers produce diet-specific odors (Doane and Porter, 1978; Porter and Doane, 1977) and it is not unlikely that dams normally eat at least somewhat different diets, it may be that the young acquire a distinctive odor from their mother.

Gerbils increase scent marking with their ventral gland when lactating (Wallace *et al.,* 1973; Yahr, 1976), and the odors from these secretions have been shown to have signaling capabilities in adults (Thiessen *et al.,* 1970; Yahr, 1977). Gerbil dams mark the pups with the sebum from the gland, marking cleaned pups more vigorously than pups that already have sebum on them (Wallace *et al.,* 1973). Moreover, the mothers retrieve marked pups before unscented pups (Wallace *et al.,* 1973), suggesting that the odors deposited on the pups may serve to identify the pups of a particular mother. Gerbil ventral gland odor also varies with the adult's diet (Skeen and Thiessen, 1977), and it is possible that individuals mark their litters with their own odor and use that cue as a means of litter recognition.

Rabbits (*Oryctolagus cuniculus*) mark their own young (Mykytowycz, 1968), and although they are only somewhat aggressive toward strange young from the same colony they attack alien offspring who are not colony members (Mykytowycz and Dudzinski, 1972). Moreover, the mothers attack their own young if they have been marked with the odor of females from another colony (Mykytowycz, 1968).

Sheep (*Ovis aries*) accept both their own and alien young for a brief period after parturition, subsequently rejecting alien lambs (Bouissou, 1968; Poindron and LeNeindre, 1980; Smith *et al.*, 1966). Destruction of the olfactory mucosa or olfactory bulbs prevented the development of maternal rejection responses toward the alien young (Baldwin and Shillito, 1974; Bouissou, 1968; Poindron, 1974, 1976). Sheep mothers also use olfactory cues, along with visual and auditory cues, for continued recognition of the young (Alexander, 1977; Lindsay and Fletcher, 1968; Morgan *et al.*, 1975; Poindron and LeNeindre, 1980). Wild Corsican sheep (*Ovis ammon*) lose the capacity to recognize their own offspring if the anus of the young is covered (Pfeffer, 1967), suggesting an olfactory mechanism for identification of own young in these animals.

Goats (*Capra hircus*) also recognize their own offspring and reject aliens (Collias, 1956; Hersher *et al.*, 1958; Klopfer *et al.*, 1964). Olfactory cues appear to be involved in mediating this phenomenon, for mothers with impaired chemoreception continued to accept aliens (Klopfer and Gamble, 1966). The chemical cues involved in the recognition of own young seem to be deposited on the kids during maternal licking of the kids and during ingestion of milk by the kids (Gubernick *et al.*, 1979; Gubernick, 1980, 1981).

Pigs (*Sus domesticus*) can identify their own offspring shortly after their birth (Signoret *et al.*, 1975). Rejection of alien offspring appears to be due to differential olfactory cues, since sows subjected to olfactory bulb damage cared for an alien piglet, whereas intact mothers rejected it (Meese and Baldwin, 1975).

Human beings can discriminate between their own offspring and unfamiliar children by means of olfactory cues and are even able to discriminate between one of their own children and their other child using olfactory cues (Porter and Moore, 1981). Human odors vary with diet (Wallace, 1977), a factor that may allow familial identification, given a common family diet. Identical twins are more difficult to discriminate between by their odor than unrelated adults or siblings that are not twins (Kalmus, 1955; Wallace, 1977), and the olfactory discriminability of the identical twins can be magnified if they have very different diets (Wallace, 1977). The ability of parents to discriminate among siblings, given that the siblings have had similar diets, may therefore be based on inherent differences between the odors produced by individual siblings.

There are other species in which olfactory recognition of young has received suggestive but, in some cases, very limited support. For example, parents of several species are known to mark their young (Autrum and von Holst, 1968; Martin, 1968; Rasa, 1973; Schultze-Westrum, 1969) or to discriminate between their young and alien young (Fogden, 1971; Grau, 1976; Klopfer, 1970; LeBoeuf *et al.,* 1972; Michener and Sheppard, 1972) or to have chemical differences in the secretions of glands that are specific to different litters (Stoddart *et al.,* 1975) or to attack alien young (Gandelman and Davis, 1973; Goodall, 1977) or to have offspring that appear to mark themselves (Brockie, 1976), but the extent to which olfactory stimuli actually influence recognition of own young has not yet been established in these situations.

C. Nest Defense

Mammalian mothers typically defend their young from both predators and conspecifics, and there is some evidence that olfaction is involved in the control of the behavior in at least one species. House mouse (*Mus musculus*) mothers vigorously defend their nest site against conspecific intrusion by either males or females (Crowcroft and Rowe, 1963; Gandelman, 1972; Svare and Gandelman, 1973).

These mice do not attack conspecifics indiscriminately, for lactating females tolerate other mothers and even engage in communal care of their offspring (Crowcroft and Rowe, 1963; Gandelman *et al.,* 1970; Saylor and Salmon, 1971). Not only are such community members accepted, but community males may also enjoy safe conduct in the nest area. Svare and Gandelman (1973) reported that lactating female mice did not attack males that had been housed within their cage behind a wire partition, although they continued to attack unfamiliar males. Familiarity tempered the defensive responses of mouse mothers to both familiar and unfamiliar colony males (Green, 1978), and olfactory cues may be involved in the differential attack by mothers against familiar and unfamiliar intruders (Lynds, 1976). Strange male mice were cleaned and then were anointed with water, the urine of the resident female, or the urine of a colony female before they were introduced into the cage. The resident females were far more likely to defend their nest against males painted with the unfamiliar urine than against males painted with the urine of the resident female or against cleaned males with water applied to their coats.

Although males marked with different odors may act differently when placed into the resident dam's cage, and thus elicit differential attack, it may be that the female allows other mice to pass unattacked if they emit a familiar odor. The familiar odor may arise from the familiar mouse, or the familiar odor may be the odor of the resident, placed on the familiar mouse, thereby conferring immediate olfactory familiarity on the other mouse.

D. Maintenance of Maternal Behaviors

1. Retrieving

Although hormonal stimulation is critical for the normal onset of maternal behavior in Norway rats, hormones do not seem to play such a role after the dams have initiated maternal care (Rosenblatt *et al.,* 1979). Rather, the changes occurring in the mother rats seem to be induced by the cues emanating from the developing pups themselves (Reisbeck *et al.,* 1975; Rosenblatt, 1969).

Olfactory cues have been implicated in controlling maternal retrieval of stray Norway rat pups back to the nest. Stray pups were shown to emit ultrasonic calls under certain circumstances, and dams oriented toward, but did not approach, recordings of those calls (Allin and Banks, 1972). The mothers were able to locate the pups in a maze if they were both to hear the ultrasonic calls and to smell the odors of the pups (Smotherman *et al.,* 1974, 1978). The authors suggested that the odor aroused the dams to search and the ultrasonic calls guided the mothers to the precise location of their strays. Indeed, bilaterally bulbectomized rat dams did quite poorly when given retrieval tests relative to the performance of dams sustaining unilateral damage or sham-operated dams (Benuck and Rowe, 1975; Schwartz and Rowe, 1976). These differences persisted through day 16 postpartum, when retrieving normally declines (Brewster and Leon, 1980; Rosenblatt, 1965, 1969). Dams made anosmic by application of zinc sulfate on day 20 of gestation similarly had poor retrieval performance after parturition (Benuck and Rowe, 1975), reinforcing the idea that efficient retrieval requires the presence of pup olfactory cues. Herrenkohl and Rosenberg (1972) also reported that bulbectomized dams spent less time than controls retrieving pups during the first 3 days postpartum. No deficit in any aspect of mother–young interactions in bulbectomized multiparous females was found, even when detailed parametric tests of maternal care were taken over a prolonged period (Schwartz and Rowe, 1976). The importance of olfactory cues may therefore decline with maternal experience.

2. Endocrine Release

Whereas rat mothers remain maternal in the absence of direct endocrine facilitation, the initiation of lactation and the continued provision of milk to the young clearly require the action of a variety of hormones (Tucker, 1974). Suckling stimulation provided by the pups normally stimulates the release of maternal prolactin (Sar and Meites, 1969; Simpson *et al.,* 1973)

252724

and corticosterone (Simpson *et al.,* 1973; Voogt *et al.,* 1969), both of which are essential for lactation. There is also evidence that both may be released by the odor of the pups in the absence of suckling stimulation.

Zarrow *et al.* (1972) found that lactating rats had a sustained elevation of circulating levels of adrenal corticosteroids when exposed to a pup behind a mesh screen. Plasma corticosteroid levels remained elevated following blinding and deafening but were markedly reduced following bilateral olfactory bulb destruction. Similarly, mothers separated from their day 14 young by a mesh floor experienced a release of hypophyseal prolactin (Grosvenor, 1965; Grosvenor *et al.,* 1970). Deafening or blinding of the dams, either alone or in combination, did not alter the pup-induced release of prolactin, but anosmia produced by bulb ablation substantially prevented the release of the hormone in response to the pups (Mena and Grosvenor, 1971). Moreover, intact dams exposed to selectively presented visual and/or auditory pup cues did not experience a release of prolactin, but olfactory cue presentation alone was sufficient to induce a significant release of that hormone (Mena and Grosvenor, 1971).

3. Survival and Weight Gain of Pups

Benuck and Rowe (1975) found that bulbectomized dams had a high proportion of pups that died early in the perinatal period, but the mediating factors have not yet been identified. It may be, however, that the pups suffered from insufficient maternal attention. Specifically, pup urine has been found to be attractive to adult rats, and bulbectomized dams tend to lick the perineal region of their pups less than control dams (Charten *et al.,* 1971). Pederson *et al.* (1982) noted that 40% of Cesarean-delivered pups died within 1 hr of delivery if they had not received mechanical stimulation that mimicked maternal licking during that period. It is therefore possible that bulbectomized mothers did not administer sufficient stimulation to their pups to ensure their survival. It should be noted that females made anosmic by means of zinc sulfate did not have any more deaths than control dams (Benuck and Rowe, 1975), calling into question the specificity of the phenomenon to olfactory cues. Benuck and Rowe (1975) and Schwartz and Rowe (1976) also found that the young of bulbectomized dams grew at a significantly slower rate than the young of control dams. The depressed pup growth might have been due to a depression of circulating hormone levels in dams that could not smell their pups, a situation that might have adversely affected milk production. Bulbectomized dams also spent less time in contact with their pups (Benuck and Rowe, 1975; see also Mena and Grosvenor, 1971), a situation that might have limited the amount of milk and/or warmth that the mothers delivered to their nursing, ectothermic young. Rosenblatt *et al.* (1979) suggested that anosmia may have chronically raised the temperature of mother rats, as it does in young male rats (Söderberg and Larsson, 1976) and, because the amount of time that Norway rats spend in contact with their young is limited by the elevated heat load of mother rats (Leon *et al.,* 1978; Woodside and Leon, 1980; Woodside *et al.,* 1980), such a chronic rise in body temperature would be expected to limit maternal contact time. The limited opportunity for heat and milk transfer might have adversely affected pup growth.

III. OLFACTORY MEDIATION OF FILIAL BEHAVIORS

A. Development of Olfactory Systems

1. Anatomy

By day 17 of embryonic life of the mouse (*Mus musculus*) the olfactory neurons, which are the receptors that transduce incoming chemical information, have the same cytological features as those of adults (Cuschieri and Bannister, 1975a,b). By the time of birth electroolfactographic recordings of olfactory neurons in the Norway rat revealed activity patterns similar to those of adults (Gesteland and Sigwart, 1977).

The prenatal anatomical development of the Norway rat vomeronasal organ and its projection site, the accessory olfactory bulb, seems to precede that of the main olfactory bulb (Smith, 1935; Kratzing, 1971). The division of the mitral cells in the mouse accessory olfactory bulb is completed by embryonic day 13 and precedes that of the mitral cells in the main olfactory bulb by about 2 days (Hinds, 1968a,b, 1972a,b; Hinds and Ruffett, 1973). Synapse formation in the mouse olfactory bulb starts at about day 14 of gestation, and exponential growth continues for several weeks postpartum (Hinds and Hinds, 1976). An examination of the ultrastructure of the mitral cells of the rat main bulb showed that the cells were still cytologically immature at birth, with a rapid growth and development occurring during the first week postpartum (Singh and Nathaniel, 1977). Mitral cell dendritic bundles are also elaborated during the postnatal period (Scheibel and Scheibel, 1975), and the glomeruli, which are the synaptic structures formed by the incoming olfactory neurons and the mitral cells, increase in number by an order of magnitude over the first 2 months of life (Meisami and Shafa, 1978). Although the volume of the mitral cell layer expands postnatally, the actual number of mitral cells apparently declines, indicating that the growth of the individual cells is responsible for the expansion of the layer (Rosselli-Austin and Altman, 1979). It should be noted, however, that Meisami and Shafa (1978) reported that the number of mitral cells remains constant from birth through the first 2 months postpartum at about 70,000 per bulb.

Although the number of synaptic connections increases postnatally, at least some of all of the different kinds of normal olfactory bulb connections appear to be formed by the time of birth, suggesting that the afferent circuit within the bulb may be demonstrably functional by that time (Hinds and Hinds, 1976). The afferents from the bulb in Norway rats also appear to be present but not in their mature number by the time of birth, and a number of the synaptic connections in the olfactory cortex are functional at that time (Westrum, 1975). The maturation of the olfactory cortex therefore predates the maturation of other cortical systems (Caley and Maxwell, 1968; Peters and Feldman, 1973). The innervation from the bulb to the rat olfactory cortex occurs just before the time of birth and is preceded by the innervation from the accessory olfactory bulb (Schwob and Price, 1978). The innervation continues to expand in the postnatal period (Schwob and Price, 1978).

The granule cells are interneurons that mediate much of the inhibition in the olfactory system (Shepherd, 1972). Whereas granule cell division and migration seem to be complete by the time of birth in the accessory olfactory bulb (Hinds, 1968a; Smith, 1935), most of the granule cells in the main olfactory bulb are acquired postnatally (Altman and Das, 1966; Hinds, 1968a; Rosselli-Austin and Altman, 1979). The growth of these cells is rapid until about day 12 postpartum, with a slower addition of cells occurring thereafter into adulthood (Altman and Das, 1966; Kaplan and Hinds, 1977).

2. Physiology

Math and Davrainville (1980) found spontaneous activity in the mitral cell layer of rats within a few hours of birth; the frequency of firing increased until day 7, with little change thereafter. The number of spontaneously active units for each electrode penetration was found by Shafa *et al.* (1981) to be low at day 4, increasing after day 7, and peaking at day 17, with most of the activity located in the caudal third of the bulb. Iwahara *et al.* (1973), Salas *et al.* (1969), and Shafa *et al.* (1981), however, did not find much activity in the bulb during the first 4 or 5 days postpartum. If these differences were not due to technical features of the recording methods but were real differences in the rate of olfactory development, they might have been due to differential housing (Math and Desor, 1974), nutrition (Cousin and Davrainville, 1980), or endocrine state of the young (Brunjes and Alberts, 1980; Johanson, 1980; Johanson *et al.,* 1980).

The pattern of evoked responses to both high-frequency and low-frequency electrical stimulation of the contralateral bulb during the first 35 days postpartum was consistent with the notion that the excitatory capabilities of the mitral cells are present at birth and that the modulation of those responses by inhibitory input from granule cells begins after the first week (Math and Davrainville, 1980). This conclusion is supported by EEG patterns in developing rats (Salas *et al., 1969*), with observation of adult patterns beginning with the twelfth day postpartum, when the granule cell population plateaus in the bulb (Altman and Das, 1966). Salas *et al.* (1969) found the full adult pattern to arise at about day 24, whereas Schönfelder and Schwartze (1971) found the adult pattern to emerge several weeks later.

Uptake of radiolabeled 2-deoxyglucose, a measure of neural metabolic activity and presumably proportional to neural firing rates (see Kennedy *et al.*, 1975), has been used to study the neural function in the rat olfactory bulb (Jourdan *et al.*, 1980; Sharp *et al.*, 1975; Stewart *et al.*, 1979). Astic and Saucier (1982b) found that olfactory stimulation produced increased uptake in specific glomeruli as early as the first day of life, although many fewer glomeruli were affected in the neonate than in older animals, and the labeling was not as dense as it was in older rats. In addition, as the pups grew older, the uptake patterns became more clearly defined, and it was possible to differentiate spatially distinct glomerular uptake patterns for nest odor and for an artificial odor. The locus of uptake for the rats as young as 9 days old was similar to that of adult uptake patterns when adults and young were exposed to the same odor (Jourdan *et al.*, 1980). The primary projections of the 1-day-old olfactory bulb are labeled and presumably functional, and the connections become more extensive by day 9 (Astic and Saucier, 1982a).

The picture that emerges from these data is that the rat and mouse olfactory systems are almost certainly functional *in utero,* with the vomeronasal organ maturing before the main olfactory bulb. The young rodents should therefore be able to use this sense from birth and to make more and more sophisticated use of their olfactory capabilities.

There are, in fact, behavioral indications that the system is functional early in life. Alberts and May (1980a,b) followed the development of odor-induced polypnea, which is a stereotyped burst of sniffing, throughout the early life of young rats. They found that both amyl acetate and adult rat urine elicited responses that were roughly proportional to the concentration of the odors and that the sensitivity of the animals to the odors increased as they grew older. Other indications of the use of olfactory cues are discussed in the following sections.

B. Suckling

Perhaps the critical facet of maternal care in mammals is the provision of milk for the offspring, and a reliable mechanism is needed to ensure that nipple location and attachment are made by the young animals. The young of altricial species are particularly interesting because they must attach and reattach to the nipples with their limited sensorimotor capabilities. The young must repeatedly manage to engage the nipples over the course of both their own developmental changes and the systematic changes in maternal behaviors that occur during the lactational period.

The first indication that olfactory cues are critically involved in facilitating nursing interactions came from experiments in which the olfactory bulbs of young rats were damaged. This procedure led to retarded growth (Hill and Almi, 1981; King, 1964; Rouger et al., 1967; Singh and Tobach, 1975; Singh et al., 1976), although not always the death, of the young pups (Pollack and Sachs, 1975; Shafa et al., 1980; Teicher et al., 1978). Destruction of the olfactory mucosa by infusion of zinc sulfate solution similarly disrupted the normal pattern of pup weight gain and mortality (Alberts, 1976; Shafa et al., 1980; Singh et al., 1976; Tobach, 1977). Although these data are consistent with the notion that the increased weight loss and mortality were specifically the result of anosmia rather than a nonspecific trauma, the use of these invasive procedures did not rule out alternative explanations of the retardation of pup growth (see Alberts, 1974; Cain, 1974).

The key demonstration that olfactory cues stimulate nipple attachment in young rats came from studies in which the nipple attachment to an anesthetized dam was virtually eliminated when the entire ventrum (Hofer et al., 1976) or only the nipples (Teicher and Blass, 1976) were cleaned with organic solvents. Washing disrupted nipple attachment by pups from their first opportunity (Teicher and Blass, 1977) through 30 days postpartum (Blass et al., 1977; Bruno et al., 1980). Not only did the pups fail to locate the nipples when placed on the anesthetized ventrum of the dams, but they did not even attach when their head was held close to the washed nipples. Application of a small quantity of the organic solvent to the nipples without engaging in the cleaning procedure to remove resident organic compounds did not deter the young from attaching to the nipples, indicating that the elimination of nipple attachment was not due to any aversive taste of residual solvents (Teicher and Blass, 1976).

Teicher and Blass (1976) were then able to reinstate nipple attachment to previously cleaned nipples in 4- to 5-day-old rat pups by painting the nipples either with an extract taken from the fluid previously used to clean the nipples or with saliva taken from the pups that were deprived of suckling for 24 hr. Other fluids, such as maternal urine, cow milk, saline, amyl acetate, vanilla extract, saliva from virgin female rats (Teicher and Blass, 1976), or milk from rat mothers (Singh and Hofer, 1976), were clearly ineffective in restoring nipple attachment to cleaned nipples, data indicative of a specific chemical cue present both on the nipple of mother rats and in the saliva of the pups.

That rat milk itself did not induce nipple attachment suggests that the effectiveness of the pup saliva was not due to its association with an attractant contained in mother's milk, a conclusion reinforced by the prolonged period between milk intake and pup saliva collection. Indeed, recent work has implicated a particular component of pup saliva, dimethyl disulfide, as the probable specific attractant that comes to localize the nipple for the pups (Pederson and Blass, 1979, 1982). Interestingly, this substance is an attractant present in the vaginal secretions of both adult rats and hamsters during estrus (Gawienowski *et al.,* 1976; Gawienowski and Stacewicz-Sapuntzakis, 1978; see also Chapter 1).

Teicher *et al.* (1980) even presented evidence suggesting that a special neural mechanism may be involved in the response to the odors associated with suckling. Using the 2-deoxyglucose autoradiographic method for the measurement of ongoing neural activity, Teicher *et al.* (1980) identified a specific site within the olfactory bulb of young rats that has increased activity associated with suckling. The elevated activity was observed in an enlarged glomerulus located at the junction of the main and accessory olfactory bulbs. These data are particularly intriguing because they parallel the findings of specialized macroglomeruli in insects for the processing of species-typic chemical cues (Boeckh and Boeckh, 1979; Hildebrand *et al.,* 1979).

If the attractant were only placed on the nipple by contact with the saliva of the pups, it would be difficult to imagine the means by which the pups could locate the nipples for the first time. Clearly, there must be another mechanism that slows initial identification of the nipple and that also involves chemical cues. In this instance, however, the cues come not from the saliva of the pups, but from the amniotic fluid and the saliva of the mother. Specifically, pups did not attach to nipples for their first suckling bout when the nipples were washed with organic solvents but did attach when the washed nipples were painted with an extract from the wash, mother's saliva, or amniotic fluid (Teicher and Blass, 1977). Several other substances were ineffective in restoring the attachment behavior of the pups.

One possibility is that the pup saliva, maternal saliva, and amniotic fluid all contain dimethyl disulfide and that the pups respond to a single cue throughout lactation. Indeed, a single cue would be consistent with the fact that puerperal females lick both the amniotic fluid and their own nipples during the birth of the young, before the young begin to suckle (Roth and Rosenblatt, 1967), and a common chemical could be deposited on the nipple during that time.

Dimethyl disulfide does not, however, appear to be a normal constituent of rat amniotic fluid (see Pederson *et al.,* 1982). Nonetheless, Pederson and Blass (1981, 1982; Pederson *et al.,* 1982) have presented evidence consistent with the idea that the initial location of the nipple is specified for the young through perinatal experience with chemical cues that are contained in amniotic fluid. Such experience may be gained while the young are bathed in amniotic fluid within the uterus and/or from the amniotic fluid that saturates the nest during the birth process (Rosenblatt and Lehrman, 1963). Specifically, Pederson and Blass (1982) placed citral into the amniotic fluid near the head of the fetus during the last 2 days postpartum and then exposed the newborn pups to the citral odor while stimulating them with a soft brush to mimic the maternal licking that precedes the first nipple attachment. When the pups received both prenatal and postnatal exposure to the odor, they subsequently attached for the first time to nipples scented with citral but would not attach to the naturally scented nipples of mother rats. Just prenatal or just postnatal chemical experience was not effective in establishing the prepotency of the artificial cue. These data are notable in that they constitute the first demonstration in a mammal that behavioral organization can be directed by prenatal events.

There are several possible routes by which chemical cues could influence the development of nipple attachment behavior. If the cues are in the fluid surrounding the fetus, they may well stimulate the vomeronasal organ, a structure responsive to fluid-borne chemical cues (see Chapter 8). Alternatively, the odors may stimulate the olfactory bulb directly, by bathing the olfactory mucosa *in utero,* or may even be taken up in the blood and transported to the bulb, thereby stimulating the main olfactory system (Maruniak *et al.,* 1980).

Pederson *et al.* (1982) also found that exposure of citral to 2–3 day old pups could induce the pups to attach to a washed nipple treated with citral only if the citral was experienced when the pups were aroused. Pups are normally aroused as the mother licks them (Rosenblatt and Lehrman, 1963) and comes into contact with them (Hofer, 1975; Hofer and Shair, 1978), and the pups were experimentally aroused either with a soft brush or by amphetamine injection to mimic the situation in which they normally experience nipple odors. The pups were induced by the citral to attach to the nipple only if they had been exposed to the odor while aroused; odor alone or arousal alone was insufficient to induce the pups to attach to a citral-scented nipple. Pups exposed to another odor (benzaldehyde) while being stimulated manually or pharmacologically attached to nipples scented with that odor but did not attach to citral-scented nipples, indicating a further specificity of the olfactory-based attachment.

Taken as a whole, these data suggest the possibility that neither the amniotic chemical cues nor the dimethyl disulfide present in pup saliva are inherent releasers of nipple attachment behavior by young rats. These data support the idea that both cues in turn must acquire their significance for the pups through exposure to the odor under specific neural states. Although these experiences are certain to be gained under normal circumstances, their capacity to release nipple attachment behavior appears to require perinatal experience.

C. Recognition of Siblings

In addition to maternal recognition of young, the young may come to recognize each other by their individual or litter odors. Spiny mice, for example, initially seek contact both with littermates and with strangers but subsequently preferentially huddle and share food with their siblings, even when from different generations (Porter et al., 1978, 1980; Porter and Wyrick, 1979). Recognition here seems to be based on olfactory cues, for when young mice were made anosmic they no longer preferred to huddle with their littermates (Porter et al., 1978). The young do not, however, prefer littermates that have been reared apart from them (Porter et al., 1980, 1981), suggesting that the ability to identify siblings is acquired postnatally, rather than being an inherent capacity of the pups (Porter et al., 1981).

Norway rats also approach the odor of siblings, although they have not been observed to prefer them to strange pups that have been reared by mothers having the same diet as their own mother (Leon, 1974). The pups, however, appear to be marked by the odor of the mother, for when the odor of the mother was suppressed, or when the pups were washed, pups no longer approached the odor of littermates (Leon, 1974, also unpublished observations). Pups with experimentally induced peripheral anosmia also did not prefer to huddle with pups (Alberts, 1978a), and rat pups chose to huddle with other rat pups in preference to gerbil pups (Alberts and Brunjes, 1978). Mother rats produce a diet-specific attractant (Leon, 1975), and it may be that pups would prefer to approach the odor of littermates if their dams are on different diets. Experience with different artificial odors induced an olfactory bias in the congregating behavior of young rats (Brunjes and Alberts, 1979), as well as in the approach behavior to the odors alone (Leon et al., 1977). The point here is that olfactory-based sibling preferences have not yet been ruled out in this species.

Block et al. (1981) found that gerbils (Meriones unguiculatus) identify and prefer the chemical cues present in the saliva of their siblings. Given that these animals normally investigate and lick the snout area of conspecifics, such cues may form the basis for preferential treatment of kin throughout their lives.

Human beings also appear to be able to discriminate the odor of siblings (Porter and Moore, 1981). This ability may be based on postnatal experience with a diet-specific family odor, for, as noted before, human odors vary with diet (Wallace, 1977) and family members may well have similar diets. Again, there may also be inherent components in a family odor, given the similarity of the odors that exist in human identical twins on identical diets (Wallace, 1977).

In different species there may be a greater or lesser role played by experience in the establishment of the ability of siblings to identify each other. Autenrieth and Fichter (1975) reported that two unrelated pronghorn antelope (*Antilocarpa americana*) subsequently behaved as siblings after being brought together as fawns. Sherman (1980) noted that the young of Belding's ground squirrels (*Spermophilus beldingi*) appear to obtain a knowledge of closely related squirrels from postnatal experience. The young occasionally enter a strange mother's nest after their first day above ground. When these individuals subsequently reemerge with their new, unrelated siblings, they treat the unrelated individuals as kin and the genetically related individuals as aliens.

Although olfaction has yet to be implicated in these cases, chemical cues have been identified as the means by which a primitively social sweat bee (*Lasioglossum zephyrum*) identifies kin (Kukuk *et al.,* 1977). Greenberg (1979) went on to find not only that these bees identified kin that they had never met, allowing them entrance to the nest, but that there was a positive linear relationship between the coefficient of relationship of the bees tested and the probability of allowing entering bees to pass.

D. Attraction to the Nest

Newborn kittens (*Felis domesticus*) initially rarely vocalize and tend to become inactive when in the nest area, subsequently orienting toward and approaching the nest area. These animals seem to use both olfactory and thermal cues to locate the nest (Freeman and Rosenblatt, 1978; Rosenblatt *et al.,* 1969; Rosenblatt, 1971).

During the first week of life, young Norway rats are capable of pivoting and orienting toward stimuli but do not move easily through their environment until near the end of the second week postpartum (Altman and Sudarshan, 1975; Altman *et al.,* 1971). By 2 to 4 days postpartum, however, young rats reliably orient toward the odor of their home bedding or nest material (Altman and Sudarshan, 1975; Bolles and Woods, 1964; Cornwell-Jones and Sobrian, 1977; Sczerzenie and Hsiao, 1977).

Although most of the pups oriented toward the nest odor most of the time during the test period on day 8, the pups did not reach the home cage until after the first week of life (Altman and Sudarshan, 1975). Gregory and Pfaff (1971) reported that 9- to 12-day-old rats began to move away from littermates and toward home bedding in preference to either clean bedding or bedding soiled by a nonlactating female rat. They also found that 13- to 19-day-old pups did not prefer home bedding to the bedding of a strange dam and litter. Carr *et al.* (1979), however, found a home preference on day 12, no preference on day 16, and a preference for alien bedding on day 20.

Syrian hamster pups begin to approach home bedding by 4 to 8 days postpartum, and the pups become less attracted to the odor after day 10, their choice becoming random by day 19 (Devor and Schneider, 1974; Gregory and Bishop, 1975). Hamster pups are probably kept within the confines of their nest by their need for warmth (Alberts, 1976; Leonard, 1974), which is provided by the other pups and the mother within the insulated nest. As their own thermoregulatory systems mature, they are less and less attracted to the warmth, and they begin to approach the home odor (Alberts, 1976; Devor and Schneider, 1974; Leonard, 1974). When the pups' olfactory bulbs are removed, the pups continue to seek out warmth at the time when such behavior normally declines (Leonard, 1978). Devor and Schneider (1974) suggested that the pups' attraction to home odor cues may "tether" the young to the nest site, thus facilitating the continuation of maternal care by keeping the mobile pups close to home.

Spiny mice are precocial murid rodents that are capable of coordinated movement through their environment from the day of birth. One might therefore imagine that the need for some kind of olfactory "tether" would be immediate. Indeed, within 26 to 36 hr after birth, these mice prefer the bedding taken from their home cage to clean bedding or bedding taken from either a nonlactating female or an adult male (Porter and Ruttle, 1975; Porter and Doane, 1976). The home nest bedding was not preferred to that of another lactating female when both females were on the same diet (Porter and Ruttle, 1975), but bedding soiled by a dam on the same diet as the mother was preferred, even if the dam was a member of another species (*Mus musculus*) (Doane and Porter, 1978; Porter *et al.,* 1977; Porter and Doane, 1977).

Gerbil pups began to prefer home bedding in preference to clean bedding at 15 days of age, and they also preferred maternal bedding to that of nonlactating females or adult males (Gerling and Yahr, 1982). Coincidently, it is at about 2 weeks postpartum that there is an increase in the proportion of gerbil pups returning to the nest site after being scattered (Waring and Perper, 1979). No preference was shown for the odor of their own mother compared with that of a strange mother, and pups were not attracted to the odor of their father, even if he participated in their care. Pups reared with both parents, however, preferred the odor of their own parents, suggesting an avoidance of unfamiliar male odors. The preference continued through days 30–38 and, although there were no clear indications that the attraction waned in weanlings, by the time the gerbils reached adulthood they no longer preferred the maternal bedding to clean bedding (Gerling and Yahr, 1982). These data suggest a long-lasting olfactory bond between mother gerbils and their young, and, as it happens, gerbil pups overwinter with their parents before they emerge from the burrow (Bannikov, 1954).

E. Attraction to Maternal Odors

1. Emission of Maternal Odors

Mother gerbils increase their ventral scent-marking behavior during gestation and lactation (Yahr, 1976; Wallace et al., 1973), and the gland itself is enlarged during that time (Wallace et al., 1973). Gerbil pups reared by intact dams prefer the nest odors of intact dams to those of dams whose ventral scent glands have been removed, and pups raised by dams without their ventral glands do not prefer the odor of their home cage to that of nonlactating females (Gerling and Yahr, 1982). These data indicate both that the ventral gland is the site of the emission of the attractant and that the attraction to the odor by the pups appears to be under experiential control.

Norway rat mothers have also been found to be the source of an odor that attracts their young. Shapiro and Salas (1970) found that rat pups would briefly inhibit their movement in response to the odor of their mother during the first week postpartum. Bolles and Woods (1964) observed that a rat pup crawled toward its mother in the home cage as early as day 4 postpartum, and others reported that pups would approach their mother in the home cage by days 10 to 12 (Donaldson, 1924; Small, 1899).

Pups reliably approached the odor of their dam from a distance in preference to nonlactating rats on day 10 (Nyakas and Endröczi, 1970) and day 16 postpartum (Leon and Moltz, 1971). Anesthesia of the olfactory mucosa blocked the pups' preference for the mother (Nyakas and Endröczi, 1970).

Leon and Moltz (1972) went on to find that there was a clear increase in the proportion of the young that approached their own mother beginning at 12 to 14 days postpartum. This attraction remained high through day 27, and by day 41 there was no preference evidenced by the pups for the odor of the dam. The time period during which the pups are normally attracted to the mother corresponds quite well to the period during which the pups can venture from the nest while continuing to have periodic nursing bouts with their dam (Rosenblatt and Lehrman, 1963).

To trace the development of the attraction of pups to maternal odor separately from the development of odor emission by dams, two procedures were employed. In the first, pups of different ages were allowed to approach either standard colony mothers that were 16 days postpartum, or nonlactating females. The pups began to approach the standardized attractive odor source at about days 12 to 14 postpartum and continued to approach the odor until about 27 days. In the second procedure, day 16 pups were used as standard odor detectors and allowed to choose between dams of different lactational stages and nonlactating females. These pups did not evidence a significant attraction with an approach response until day 14, with the attraction waning by day 27 postpartum (Leon and Moltz, 1972). These data suggest that there is a close synchrony between the time during which the mother produces the attractant and the time during which the young actually approach the odor. Mothers may also emit the attractant in low quantities during the first 2 weeks postpartum, a situation sufficient to induce the pups to orient toward the mother and the nest material during that time.

2. Synthesis of Maternal Odors

The principal source of the odor was found to be the anal excreta emitted by the attractive dams, particularly that portion of the material designated as cecotrophe (Harder, 1949; Leon, 1974). Harder (1949) described the morphology and function of the ceca of a wide range of rodents and lagomorphs, including both the wild Norway rat (*Wanderratte,* called *Epimys norvegicus,* using the classification of Simpson, 1945) and the albino strain of that species (*Weisse Ratte*). The cecotrophe is thought to be differentiated from the feces in the cecum, a large structure of the gastrointestinal tract located at the junction of the small and large intestines. Material taken directly from the cecum of lactating female rats that were attractive to pups, lactating females that were not as yet attractive to pups, nonlactating females, and males was highly attractive to the young, whereas material taken from the gastrointestinal tract above the level of that structure was not attractive to the pups (Leon, 1974, 1978). These data indicate both that the site of synthesis of the odor is the cecum and that the attractant is synthesized in adult Norway rats regardless of their sex or reproductive state.

The mechanism of synthesis appears to involve the action of cecal bacteria. Antibiotic suppression of gut bacterial population or restriction of the dams to a sucrose-based diet suppressed the attractiveness of the dams (Leon, 1974, 1975). Moreover, the cecal material of both nonlactating and lactating females subjected to bacterial suppression was not attractive to the test pups. These data suggest both that the experimental procedures interfered directly with odor synthesis rather than with odor emission alone and that lactating and nonlactating rats have a common mechanism for odor synthesis. It would therefore seem that one important difference between lactating dams and other rats in terms of attractiveness to pups lies in a differential emission of the odor-bearing cecotrophe to the external environment.

3. Mechanism of Odor Emission

a. Role of Food Intake. The partially digested food entering the cecum is acted on by resident microorganisms to break down cellulose, to increase the efficiency of diet utilization, and to synthesize vitamins (Hoetzel and Barnes, 1966; Mikelson, 1956). Normally, rats ingest virtually all of the cecotrophe that they defecate (Leon, 1974; Lutton and Chevallier, 1973), but lactating females defecate more than they reingest, thereby normally emitting more of the attractive material to the external environment than do nonlactating rats (Leon, 1974). When the defecated cecotrophe of non-lactating rats is collected, as can occasionally be done, this material is quite attractive to the pups, indicating that the attractive odors are normally not inactivated in the gut (Leon, 1974, 1978). The odor is therefore not synthesized in the cecum and inactivated in nonlactating rats. Since both lactating and nonlactating rats normally synthesize and emit the attractive odor, the difference between attractive mother rats and their relatively unattractive nonlactating counterparts would appear to be due to the much greater probability that dams will emit significant amounts of cecotrophe to the environment.

The increased defecation of uningested cecotrophe appears to be due, in part, to the greatly increased food intake of lactating females (Brody and Nisbet, 1938; Cotes and Cross, 1954; Fleming, 1976; Ota and Yokoyama, 1967a,b; Slonaker, 1925). Decreasing the amount of food available to mother rats decreases the amount of cecotrophe that they defecate while allowing them to continue to lactate. Diet restriction decreased the attractiveness of the rat dams to the point that the mobile young no longer preferred to approach their odor in preference to that of nonlactating females (Leon, 1975). That the effects of the diet restriction were mediated by a suppression of emission rather than a suppression of odor synthesis was demonstrated by the continued attractiveness of the material taken directly from the ceca of diet-restricted dams (Leon, 1975). This is not to say that the increased food intake by dams produces the emission of cecotrophe; cecotrophe is emitted even when the rats, lactating or not, are not eating very much. Nevertheless, the increased food intake of lactating females greatly increases the likelihood that the cecotrophe, and hence the attractive odor, will be reliably emitted to the external environment in quantities sufficient to attract the pups from a distance.

Mother rats are able to process the greatly elevated amount of food that they consume because the food is transported through the gastrointestinal tract at an elevated rate (Adams *et al.,* 1976). The facilitation of diet processing during lactation is probably mediated by at least two factors. The first involves changes in both the macrostructure and the microstructure of the tract itself, induced directly or indirectly by the increased food intake of the dams (Boyne *et al.,* 1953; Campbell and Fell, 1964; Cripps and Williams, 1975; Elias and Dowling, 1976; Fell *et al.,* 1963; Poo *et al.,* 1939; Souders and Morgan, 1957). Increased food intake also stimulates the secretion of bile into the gastrointestinal tract of rats (Merle *et al.,* 1978). The bile serves as a natural laxative, with an increase in bile acid secretion associated with a linear increase in the amount defecated (Bergmann, 1952; Bloomfield, 1963; Forth *et al.,* 1966; Meyer and McEwen, 1948). Kilpatrick *et al.* (1980) found that an elevation in the concentration of gastrointestinal tract cholic acid (which seems to be the active laxative substance in the bile of lactating rats) induced nonlactating females to become attractive to rat pups, presumably by increasing the amount of cecotrophe that was defecated but not reingested by them.

Lee and Moltz (1980) found that the emission of maternal odor was also influenced by the acidity of the maternal gut, which was in turn affected by the acidity of the pup feces ingested by the dams. Dams attracted pups only when gut acidity was low, but it is unclear whether gut acidity affects odor synthesis, emission, or both processes. Kilpatrick and Moltz (1981) also found that lesions of the ventromedial area of the hypothalamus of nonlactating rats did not render nonlactating females attractive to pups, despite their increased food intake, presumably because the lesions induced the rats to increase the acidity of the gastrointestinal tract (Weingarten and Powley, 1980).

b. Pup Stimulation. Pups also appear to affect maternal odor emission by stimulating food intake by their mothers. Mother rats kept with day 1 pups did not increase their food intake or cecotrophe defecation and did not attract pups at 16 days postpartum (M. Leon, unpublished observations; Moltz and Leon, 1973). Mother rats kept with somewhat older pups continued to lactate (Bruce, 1961; Nicoll and Meites, 1959), to eat large quantities of food (Ota and Yokoyama, 1967a), and to attract pups (Holinka and Carlson, 1976; Moltz *et al.,* 1974). Mothers kept with still older pups, which were presumably weaned, decreased their food intake (Ota and Yokoyama, 1967b) and were not attractive to the pups (Holinka and Carlson, 1976).

c. Endocrine Mediation of Pup Stimuli. The ability of pups to stimulate odor emission via stimulation of maternal food intake seems to be mediated by the pups' ability to induce the release of maternal prolactin. Circulating prolactin levels are elevated during lactation and prolactin release has been found to be stimulated by the pups (Amenomori *et al.*, 1970; Grosvenor *et al.*, 1970; Mena and Grosvenor, 1972; Moltz *et al.*, 1969; Terkel *et al.*, 1972). Suppression of prolactin by means of ergot derivatives or by antiserum to prolactin suppressed maternal food intake (Leon, 1978; Shani *et al.*, 1975; Tindal, 1956; Tomagane *et al.*, 1976). Whereas prolactin suppression inhibited cecotrophe defecation and odor emission (Leon, 1974; Leon and Moltz, 1973), odor synthesis remained unaffected (Leon, 1974). Prolactin replacement therapy partially restored elevated food intake, cecotrophe defecation, and attractiveness of the mothers (Leon, 1974, 1978; Leon and Moltz, 1973). Elevation of circulating prolactin levels in nonlactating female rats by means of injection stimulated an increase in food intake, cecotrophe defecation, and attractiveness of the females to test pups (Leon, 1974). Elevation of maternal prolactin levels by means of continued association with pups of advancing age similarly induced nonlactating females to become attractive to rat pups (Koranyi *et al.*, 1977; Leidahl and Moltz, 1977; Marinari and Moltz, 1978).

d. Role of Experience. Since synthesis of the cecal odor is dependent on cecal bacteria and since enteric bacterial populations and their metabolic products differ with different diets (Draser *et al.*, 1973; Lampen and Peterjohn, 1951; Porter and Rettger, 1940; Rettger and Horton, 1914), it seemed possible that the cecal odor would change with a change in diet. Indeed, it did. Leon (1975) found that pups raised with mothers on diet A would approach the anal excreta of nonlactating diet A colony dams in preference to the odor of the anal excreta of nonlactating diet A females or lactating dams on diet B. Moreover, diet A pups did not preferentially approach diet B mothers even when opposed to diet B nonlactating females. Pups reared with diet B mothers preferred the diet B maternal odor to that of diet B nonlactating females or diet A mothers. Similarly, diet B pups did not even prefer diet A dam odor to that of diet A nonlactating females.

The first point to be made regarding these data is that changes in diet induce changes in cecal odor. The second point is that the pups must acquire their attraction to the odor that they will approach postnatally, since there is no single "maternal" odor invariably present in the maternal anal excreta that they come to approach. In fact, pups reared with mothers on the sucrose-based diet, which suppressed cecal odor, did not approach the odor of the anal excreta produced by dams on diet A (Leon, 1974, 1975). If these pups were reared with such mothers, but in a room in which diet A mothers reared their own pups and produced a distinctive odor, the pups reared with the sucrose-diet dams preferentially approached the diet A cecal odor (Leon, 1975).

Familiarity with maternal odors would then be gained by the pups during the first 2 weeks postpartum, when mothers are emitting cecotrophe in small amounts. Even brief exposure to maternal odors during that period would appear to be sufficient to induce the pups subsequently to approach maternal odors. When pups are kept with mothers on control diets for the first week, or even the first 3 or 4 days postpartum, they subsequently prefer maternal odors even if maternal cecal odors are then suppressed (Schumacher and Moltz, 1982) or if the pups are then reared in isolation from their dams (Galef and Kaner, 1980). In addition, familiarity with maternal odors other than those emanating from maternal anal excreta also may come to attract the young, particularly in the absence of the salient cecal odor. Rat pups are attracted to such alternative cues (Galef and Heiber, 1976), and the authors suggested that the bacterially altered urinary odors emitted by adult rats that have been found to be highly attractive to adult rats (von Reiff, 1956) may also be the source of this alternative pup attractant. Such cues continue to attract weanling pups after the attraction to the cecal odor has waned (Galef and Heiber, 1976).

The observed attraction of pups to odors may be the final result of inherent olfactory biases, mere familiarity, and associations between odors and the mother; that is, different maternal odors, cecally or otherwise derived, may hold differential attraction for pups in the absence of experience, but familiarity with or without maternal associations may alter inherent biases. Leon et al. (1977) found that rat pups reared by dams whose cecal odor was suppressed and exposed in isolation to the odors of dams on diet A preferentially approached the odor, but pups preexposed only to the fresh air did not preferentially approach the maternal odor. Pups similarly exposed to an arbitrarily selected odor also became attracted to that odor. These data suggest that simple exposure of the pups to the maternal odors, even in the absence of the mothers, was sufficient to induce attraction to those odors. The data also indicate that the attraction of pups to odors is limited neither to a single maternal odor nor to naturally produced maternal odors.

Maternal associations with natural or arbitrarily selected olfactory cues experienced by pups appear, however, to play a role in reinforcing the attraction of pups to odors (Galef, 1981; Galef and Kaner, 1980). There is also some evidence that natural odors evoke a stronger attraction than do arbitrarily selected odors (Schumacher and Moltz, 1982), although Alberts and May (1980b), Brunjes and Alberts (1979), and Alberts (1981) found little evidence for such a bias.

Alberts (1981) found that the specific loss of the nutritional experiences associated with maternal contact did not affect the development of attraction to an odor experienced concurrently with maternal care. However, odor experienced in the presence of warmth was clearly preferred to odor experienced in contact with a cooler substrate. Given the critical importance of thermal considerations both for the development of rat pups (Alberts, 1978b; Levine, 1969; Taylor, 1960) and for the limitation of maternal contact time (Leon *et al.,* 1978; Woodside *et al.,* 1980, 1981; Woodside and Leon, 1980), it may well be that odor–temperature associations play an important role in the development of odor preferences.

e. Neural Basis for Development of Olfactory Preferences. The neural basis for the development of olfactory preferences are still obscure. Doving and Pinching (1973) and Pinching and Doving (1974) found that odor-specific, spatially distinct patterns induced morphological alterations in the olfactory bulbs of young rats continuously exposed to any of a number of arbitrarily selected odors. These data suggested that exposure to specific maternal or artificial odors could "imprint" onto the nervous system a special responsiveness to odors experienced early in life. Indeed, Laing and Panhuber (1980) found that such exposure of young rats to odors induced an increased sensitivity to those cues as measures by behavioral means (but see Dalland and Doving, 1981). Exposure of pups to different maternal odors, however, did not induce different patterns of morphological changes in specific areas of the mitral cell layer (Leon, 1980). Given that in pups with severe restriction of olfactory experience the morphological changes were present throughout the layer (Laing and Panhuber, 1978), it would seem that continuous exposure to a single artificial odor constituted a form of olfactory deprivation, and the odor complex generated by either of the two cecal odors was sufficient to allow the normal development of the mitral cells.

Using what may have been a more sensitive assay for differential neural response than morphological changes, Astic and Saucier (1982b) found specific areas of activity in the glomerular layer of the olfactory bulbs of young rats when exposed to nest odors in a test situation. The areas of increased neural activity were distinct from those induced by an artificial odor.

Suppression of the development of the normal population of granule cells in the olfactory bulbs of young rats did not alter the acquisition of approach behavior to maternal nest odors (Yanai and Rosselli-Austin, 1978). It may be, however, that the maturation of the granule cells restricts the period during which the developing system remains plastic in response to environmental odors.

The neural alterations that may occur in the development of olfactory preferences may conform, with some alterations, to the models proposed by Freeman (1981) and Grossberg (1976) dealing with the formation of olfactory representations in the central nervous system. The neural circuits in the olfactory system may develop a template to which incoming odors can be neurally matched, allowing a special responsiveness to meaningful odors. A familiar odor experienced in the presence or absence of the dams may well have a special neural template formed over the course of the first 2 weeks postpartum, allowing both a special neural coding and a special behavioral response to that odor. Young animals may be particularly sensitive to olfactory template formation. Olfactory neural templates may also be more easily or durably formed for naturally occurring odors than for artificial odors. Grossberg (1976) suggested that norepinephrine is involved in the process by mediating the gating of neural impulses, and, indeed, depletion of brain norepinephrine in young rats reduced pup preferences for conspecific but not for familiar artificial odors (Cornwell-Jones, 1981; Marasco *et al.,* 1979; Sobrian and Cornwell-Jones, 1977).

4. Function of Maternal Odors

The most obvious function of maternal attractants is that of an olfactory "tether" to facilitate the union of mother and young over the course of lactation. Given the common need for continuing contact between mother and young, one should be able to identify analogous mechanisms in a wide range of organisms. In fact, attraction of the young to maternal and/or maternal nest olfactory cues has been found in cichlid fish (*Cichlastoma citrinellum,* Barnett, 1977, 1981), crayfish (*Orconectes sanborni, Cambarus virilis, Procambarus clarkii,* Little, 1975, 1976), hamsters (*Mesocricetus auratus,* Devor and Schneider, 1974), spiny mice (*Acomys cahirinus,* Porter and Doane, 1976; Porter and Ruttle, 1975; Doane and Porter, 1978), rabbits (*Oryctolagus cuniculus,* Mykytowycz and Ward, 1971), white-footed mice (*Peromyscus leucopus,* Geyer, 1981), house mice (*Mus musculus,* Breen and Leshner, 1977; Geyer, 1981), pine voles (*Microtus pinetorum,* Geyer, 1979), gerbils (*Meriones unguiculatus,* Gerling and Yahr, 1982; Wallace *et al.,* 1973), cats (*Felis domesticus,* Freeman and Rosenblatt, 1978), squirrel monkeys (*Saimiri sciureus,* Kaplan and Russell, 1974; Kaplan *et al.,* 1977), marmosets (*Callithrix jacchus, Saguinus fuscicollis,* Cebul *et al.,* 1978), and human beings (MacFarlane, 1975; Russell, 1976).

There are also some data from Norway rats suggesting this tether function. Rat pups increase their sniffing and exploratory behavior at the same time that they begin to approach the maternal odor from afar (Bolles and Woods, 1964; Welker, 1964). Furthermore, when pups of this age are placed away from the odor of the mother and the nest, there is a striking increase in pup locomotor activity (Bronstein and Dworkin, 1974; Campbell and Raskin, 1978; Campbell *et al.,* 1969; Randall and Campbell, 1976). Similarly, when the pups are made anosmic at that age, they also have a greatly elevated activity level even in the presence of the mother and littermates (Alberts, 1976; Hofer, 1975, 1976). The elevated activity is independent of thermal and nutritive disruption (Hofer, 1973a,b; Randall and Campbell, 1976) and can be reversed, at least in the young that are separated from their mothers, by the introduction of maternal odor into the testing area (Hofer, 1975, 1976; Randall and Campbell, 1976; Schapiro and Salas, 1970). Nest-related odors have also been found to facilitate milk intake (Johanson and Hall, 1981) and learning (Infurna et al., 1979; Smith and Spear, 1978, 1980) by the pups. The deceleration of pup heart rate after maternal separation is also reversed by the introduction of maternal odor into this isolated test area (Compton et al., 1977). Rat pups increase their ultrasonic distress vocalizations when separated from their dam, and these calls also can be suppressed by the introduction of maternal nest odor (Conely and Bell, 1978; Hofer and Shair, 1978; Oswalt and Meier, 1975). Taken as a whole, then, these data suggest that the maternal odor may keep mobile young in or near the nest by decreasing their activity and arousal levels.

Rat pups appear to be marked by the odor of their mother (Leon, 1974), and Alberts (1978a; Alberts and Brunjes, 1978; Brunjes and Alberts, 1979) has found that mobile pups use olfactory cues to regain contact with littermates. Given the importance of huddling by the pups for maintaining thermal homeostasis (Alberts, 1978b), the function of olfactory cues may be to facilitate both energy conservation and reunions of the entire litter with the dam.

Rat pups are also drawn to the area in which adult conspecifics are eating (Galef and Clark, 1972), and olfactory cues constitute an important portion of the attractive stimulus complex of adults at the feeding site (Galef, 1981; Galef and Heiber, 1976). Pups also prefer to explore in areas previously marked by conspecifics (Galef and Heiber, 1976).

Exposure of pups to a diet-related odor induced the young to prefer the diet associated with that odor over a diet associated with another odor (Bronstein and Crockett, 1980; Leon et al., 1977). Moreover, exposure of rat weanlings to a variety of odors enhanced their subsequent tolerance for variability in their diet (Hennessy et al., 1977). Olfactory cues may therefore guide the young to safe areas and safe food in their new environment.

Leon and Behse (1977) found that rat pups ceased responding to the cecal odor of their own mother when the weanlings had developed their own cecal odor. Moreover, suppression of weanling cecal odor induced the pups to continue to approach the odor of attractive dams. Since weanlings prefer the same diet as their dams (Galef and Clark, 1972) and the young routinely ingest the anal excreta of their dams (Galef, 1979; Leon, 1974), which probably inoculates them with the same enteric flora of their dams, the young appear to produce the same cecal odor as their dams. Weanlings seem to shift their attraction to their own cecal odor when they cease their maternal approach behavior. It may be that pups can process the solid food available to them in their environment only when they have the full complement of cecal bacteria, and the development of the cecal odor signals the end of the weaning process. The development of an individual odor by the pups may also allow them to move easily through areas that their own odor has marked "safe" (Ewer, 1968; Mykytowycz, 1973).

Harder (1949) found that young rabbits allowed to ingest anal excreta were protected from an outbreak of coccidiosis, whereas those deprived of anal excreta succumbed to the disease. Harder concluded that "to deprive the animals of caecotrophe is to reduce their powers of resistance." On the basis of Bertok's (1977) finding that the presence of a bile acid protects the gut against the toxins produced by *Escherichia coli,* Moltz and Kilpatrick (1978) suggested that the ingestion of maternal anal excreta, containing such bile acids, protects the weanlings from disease. Maternal odors may therefore attract the pups to the maternal excreta, the ingestion of which may serve some protective function for the young.

Sexual imprinting involves the acquisition of specific species-typic cues during development that are subsequently used for species identification during mating (see Immelmann, 1972). Early olfactory experience with artificial odors has been shown to alter the social/olfactory preferences of house mice (Goldenblatt, 1978; Mainardi *et al.,* 1965), rats (Marr and Gardner, 1965; Marr and Lilliston, 1969), guinea pigs (Carter, 1972; Carter and Marr, 1970), hamsters (Cornwell-Jones, 1975), and spiny mice (Porter and Etscorn, 1974, 1975).

The possibility that natural olfactory cues normally play a role in the development of species-typic social preferences was reinforced by a group of cross-fostering studies. Here, pups of one species are raised by mothers of another species, and the subsequent olfactory/social preferences are then observed. Olfactory/social preference shifts have been found in offspring cross-fostered between house mice and spiny mice (Porter *et al.,* 1977), southern grasshopper mice (*Onychomys torridus*) and white-footed mice (*Peromyscus leucopus*) (McCarty and Southwick, 1977), house mice and Norway rats (Lagerspetz and Heino, 1970), pygmy mice (*Baiomys taylori*) and house mice (Quadagno and Banks, 1970), and collared lemmings (*Dicrostonyx groenlandicus*) and brown lemmings (*Lemmus trimucronatus*) (Huck and Banks, 1980). Black-tailed deer (*Odocoileus hemiones*) fawns reared by a surrogate mother and exposed to the odor of a pronghorn antelope (*Antilocarpa americana*) similarly shifted olfactory/social preferences (Müller-Schwarze and Müller-Schwarze, 1971) to the species with which they had had early olfactory experience. These data suggest that olfactory cues may be very important in the formation of social interactions with species members and may serve as effective reproductive isolating mechanisms.

IV. SUMMARY AND CONCLUSIONS

The success of the mother–young interaction is critical for mammalian reproduction, and it should be clear that olfactory cues are extensively utilized in virtually every aspect of parental care to ensure the normal growth and development of the offspring. Mothers are influenced by the olfactory cues emanating from offspring in the induction of maternal responsiveness and the maintenance of maternal physiology. Moreover, odors identify their own young for preferential treatment. Unwelcome intruders are also identified by individual olfactory cues.

At the same time that the mother relies on different cues to influence her maternal behaviors, the offspring have a rapid development of their olfactory systems and use a set of olfactory cues to locate and attach to their mother's nipple and subsequently to locate both the nest area and the mother herself. The gradual process of weaning and experience with the surrounding environment also may entail the use of maternal olfactory cues that guide the offspring through unfamiliar experiences.

The characteristics of olfactory cues seem to fit the requirements for effective communication between mother and young. For example, such cues have sufficient diversity to identify individuals, even in the context of a burrow system. The cues can also be long lasting, chronically marking the mother, the nest, the offspring, the surrounding environment, and possibly adult conspecifics. Given that many species have only periodic contact with their offspring, the continuing influence of olfactory cues on both the mother and young allows a continuity of maternal influence, even in her physical absence.

The lack of singular, species-typic olfactory cues in most of the situations that have been discussed may be due to the apparent recruitment of nonspecialized body secretion odors to facilitate the complex interactions between mother and young. Indeed, it would seem that mammalian mothers have adapted the nonspecialized mechanisms that are effective in regulating their nonlactating physiology and social interactions to the task of regulating interactions with their offspring.

Associated with the changing nature of many maternal secretions is the dramatic plasticity in the nervous system of young mammals that allows attraction to maternal odors to be gained with limited experience. Even in the one situation in which a single chemical cue appears to serve as a releaser for a specific behavior, the system develops in such a way as to have that cue invariably present during a period in which the young will develop an attraction to olfactory cues that happen to be in their environment.

The difficulties associated with stimulus identification and control as well as the difficulty of human researchers in comprehending the olfactory world of most mammals have hampered progress in the research on the olfactory control of reproductive behavior. The obvious central role that olfactory cues play in the regulation of these processes should ensure sufficient interest to provoke major advances in our understanding of the problem in the coming years.

ACKNOWLEDGMENTS

This work was supported, in part, by a grant from the National Science Foundation (BNS-8023107) and a Research Scientist Development Award (MH 00371) from ADAMHA, National Institute of Mental Health. I thank Lynda Adrig and Kelli Montgomery for their help in the preparation of this manuscript.

REFERENCES

Adams, S.A., Ajam, I.K., Matthews, B.F., and Sullivan, P.B. (1976). *J. Physiol.* (*London*) **257**, 57P-58P.
Alberts, J.R. (1974). *Physiol. Behav.* **12**, 657-670.
Alberts, J.R. (1976). *In* "Mammalian Olfaction, Reproductive Processes, and Behavior" (R.L. Doty, ed.), pp. 67-94. Academic Press, New York.
Alberts, J.R. (1978a). *J. Comp. Physiol. Psychol.* **92**, 220-230.
Alberts, J.R. (1978b). *J. Comp. Physiol. Psychol.* **92**, 231-245.
Alberts, J.R. (1981). *In* "Development of Perception: Psychobiological Perspectives" (R.N. Aslin, J.R. Alberts, and M.R. Peterson, eds.), Vol. 1, pp. 322-357. Academic Press, New York.
Alberts, J.R., and Brunjes, P.C. (1978). *J. Comp. Physiol. Psychol.* **92**, 897-906.
Alberts, J.R., and May, B. (1980a). *Physiol. Behav.* **24**, 957-963.
Alberts, J.R., and May, B. (1980b). *Physiol. Behav.* **24**, 965-970.
Alexander, G. (1977). *Appl. Anim. Ethol.* **3**, 65-81.
Allin, J.T., and Banks, E.M. (1972). *Anim. Behav.* **20**, 175-185.
Altman, J., and Das, G.D. (1966). *J. Comp. Neurol.* **126**, 337-390.
Altman, J., and Sudarshan, K. (1975). *Anim. Behav.* **23**, 896-920.
Altman, J., Sudarshan, K., Das, G.D., McCormick, N., and Barnes, D. (1971). *Dev. Psychobiol.* **4**, 97-114.
Amenomori, Y., Chen, Y., and Meites, J. (1970). *Endocrinology* **86**, 506-510.
Astic, L., and Saucier, D. (1982a). *Dev. Brain Res.* **2**, 141-156.
Astic, L., and Saucier, D. (1982b). *Dev. Brain Res.* **2**, 243-256.
Autenrieth, R.E., and Fichter, E. (1975). *Wildl. Monogr.* **42**, 1-111.
Autrum, H., and von Holst, D. (1968). *Z. Vergl. Physiol.* **58**, 347-355.
Baldwin, B.A., and Shillito, E.E. (1974). *Anim. Behav.* **22**, 220-223.
Bannikov, A.G. (1954). *In* "Mammals of the Mongolian Peoples Republic," pp. 410-415. USSR Acad. Sci., Moscow.

Barnett, C. (1977). *J. Chem. Ecol.* **3**, 436–468.
Barnett, C. (1981). *Z. Tierpsychol.* **55**, 173–182.
Beach, F.A., and Jaynes, J. (1956). *J. Mammal.* **37**, 177–180.
Beauchamp, G.K. (1976). *Nature (London)*, **263**, 587–588.
Benuck, I., and Rowe, F.A. (1975). *Physiol. Behav.* **14**, 439–447.
Bergmann, M. (1952). *Wien. Klin. Wochenschr.* **64**, 704–707.
Bertok, L, (1977). *Perspect. Biol. Med.* **21**, 70–76.
Birch, H.G. (1956). *Am. J. Orthopsychiatry* **26**, 279–284.
Blass, E.M., Teicher, M.H., Cramer, C.P., Bruno, J.P., and Hall, W.G. (1977). *J. Comp. Physiol. Psychol.* **94**, 115–127.
Block, M.L., Volpe, L.C., and Hayes, M.J. (1981). *Science* **211**, 1062–1064.
Bloomfield, D.K. (1963). *Proc. Natl. Acad. Sci. U.S.A.* **50**, 117–124.
Boeckh, J., and Boeckh, V. (1979). *J. Comp. Physiol.* **132**, 235–242.
Bolles, R.C., and Woods, J. (1964). *Anim. Behav.* **12**, 427–441.
Bouissou, M.F. (1968). *Rev. Comp. Anim.* **3**, 77–83.
Boyne, A.W., Chalmers, M.I., and Cuthbertson, D.P. (1953). *Hoppe-Seyler's Z. Physiol. Chem.* **295**, 424–435.
Breen, M.F., and Leshner, A.I. (1977). *Physiol. Behav.* **18**, 527–529.
Brewster, J.A., and Leon, M. (1980). *J. Comp. Physiol. Psychol.* **94**, 69–79.
Brockie, R. (1976). *Anim. Behav.* **24**, 68–71.
Brody, S., and Nisbet, R. (1938). *Res. Bull.—Mo., Agric./Exp. St.* **285**, 5–30.
Bronstein, P.M., and Crockett, D.P. (1980). *In* "Chemical Signals in Vertebrates and Aquatic Invertebrates" (D. Müller-Schwarze and R.M. Silverstein, eds.), pp. 157–172. Plenum, New York.
Bronstein, P.M., and Dworkin, T. (1974). *Bull. Psychon. Soc.* **4**, 124–126.
Bruce, H.M. (1961). *J. Reprod. Fertil.* **2**, 17–34.
Brunjes, P.C., and Alberts, J.R. (1979). *J. Comp. Physiol. Psychol.* **93**, 548–555.
Brunjes, P.C., and Alberts, J.R. (1980). *Horm. Behav.* **14**, 76–85.
Bruno, J.P., Teicher, M.H., and Blass, E.M. (1980). *J. Comp. Physiol. Psychol.* **94**, 15–127.
Cain, D.P. (1974). *Psychol. Bull.* **81**, 654–671.
Caley, D.W., and Maxwell, D.S. (1968). *J. Comp. Neurol.* **133**, 17–44.
Calhoun, J.B. (1962). "The Ecology and Sociology of the Norway Rat." U.S. Public Health Serv., Bethesda, Maryland.
Campbell, B.A., and Raskin, L.A. (1978). *J. Comp. Physiol. Psychol.* **92**, 176–184.
Campbell, B.A., Lytle, L.D., and Fibiger, H.C. (1969). *Science* **166**, 637–638.
Campbell, R.M., and Fell, B.F. (1964). *J. Physiol. (London)* **171**, 90–97.
Carr, W.J., Marasco, E., and Landauer, M.R. (1979). *Physiol. Behav.* **23**, 1149–1151.
Carter, C.S. (1972). *Anim. Behav.* **20**, 54–60.
Carter, C.S., and Marr, J.N. (1970). *Anim. Behav.* **18**, 238–244.
Cebul, M.S., Alveario, M.C., and Epple, G. (1978). *In* "The Biology and Conservation of the Callitrichidae" (D. Keiman, ed.), pp. 141–146. Smithsonian Press, Washington, D.C.
Charten, D., Adrien, J., and Cosnier, J. (1971). *Rev. Comp. Anim.* **5**, 89–94.
Cohen, J., and Bridges, R.S. (1981). *J. Comp. Physiol. Psychol.* **95**, 450–459.
Collias, N.E. (1956). *Ecology* **37**, 228–239.
Compton, R.P., and Koch, M.D., and Arnold, W.J. (1977). *Physiol. Behav.* **18**, 769–773.
Conely, L., and Bell, R.W. (1978). *Dev. Psychobiol.* **11**, 193–197.
Cornwell-Jones, C.A. (1975). *Behav. Biol.* **14**, 175–188.
Cornwell-Jones, C.A. (1981). *Brain Res.* **213**, 379–385.
Cornwell-Jones, C.A., and Sobrian, S.K. (1977). *Physiol. Behav.* **19**, 685–688.
Cosnier, J., and Couturier, C. (1966). *C.R. Seances Soc. Biol. Ses Fil.* **160**, 789–791.
Cotes, M.P., and Cross, B.A. (1954). *J. Endocrinol.* **10**, 363–367.

Cousin, X., and Davrainville, J.L. (1980). *Brain Res.* **193**, 598–603.

Cripps, A.W., and Williams, V.J. (1975). *Br. J. Nutr.* **23**, 17–32.

Crowcroft, P., and Rowe, F.P. (1963). *Proc. Zool. Soc. London* **140**, 517–531.

Cuschieri, A., and Bannister, L.H. (1975a). *J. Anat.* **119**, 277–286.

Cuschieri, A., and Bannister, L.H. (1975b). *J. Anat.* **119**, 471–498.

Dalland, T., and Doving, K.B. (1981). *Behav. Neural Biol.* **32**, 79–88.

Devor, M., and Schneider, G.E. (1974). *Behav. Biol.* **10**, 211–221.

Doane, H.M., and Porter, R.H. (1978). *Dev. Psychobiol.* **11**, 271–277.

Donaldson, H.H. (1924). "The Rat: Data and Reference Tables," 2nd ed. Wistar Inst., Philadelphia, Pennsylvania.

Doving, K.B., and Pinching, A.J. (1973). *Brain Res.* **52**, 115–129.

Draser, B.S., Crowther, J.S., Goddard, P., Hawksworth, G., Hill, M.J., Peach, S., and Williams, R.E.O. (1973). *Proc. Nutr. Soc.* **32**, 49–52.

Elias, E., and Dowling, R.H. (1976). *Clin. Sci. Mol. Med.* **51**, 427–433.

Ewer, R.F. (1968). "The Ethology of Mammals," Plenum, New York.

Fell, B.F., Smith, K.A., and Campbell, R.M. (1963). *J. Pathol. Bacteriol.* **85**, 179–188.

Fleischer, S., Kordower, J.H., Kaplan, B., Dicker, R., Smerling, R., and Ilgner, J. (1981). *Physiol. Behav.* **26**, 957–959. Fleming, A. S. (1976).

Fleming, A.S. (1976). *Physiol. Behav.* **17**, 841–848.

Fleming, A.S., and Leubke, C. (1981). *Physiol. Behav.* **27**, 863–868.

Fleming, A.S., and Rosenblatt, J.S. (1974a). *J. Comp. Physiol. Psychol.* **86**, 221–232.

Fleming, A.S., and Rosenblatt, J.S. (1974b). *J. Comp. Physiol. Psychol.* **86**, 233–246.

Fleming, A.S., Vaccarino, F., Tombosso, L., and Chee, P. (1979). *Science* **203**, 372–374.

Fleming, A.S., Vaccarino, F., and Leubke, C. (1981). *Physiol. Behav.* **25**, 731–743.

Fogden, S.C.L. (1971). *J. Zool.* **164**, 61–92.

Forth, W.W., Rummel, W., and Glasner, H. (1966). *Naunyn Schmiedeberg's Arch. Pharmakol. Exp. Pathol.* **254**, 364–380.

Freeman, N.C.G., and Rosenblatt, J.S. (1978). *Dev. Psychobiol.* **11**, 437–457.

Freeman, W.J. (1981). *Perspect. Biol. Med.* **24**, 561–592.

Fullerton, C., Berryman, J.C., and Porter, R.H. (1974). *(Cavia porcellus) Behaviour* **48**, 145–156.

Galef, B.G. (1979). *J. Comp. Physiol. Psychol.* **93**, 295–305.

Galef, B.G. (1981). *J. Comp. Physiol. Psychol.* **95**, 614–622.

Galef, B.G., and Clark, M.M. (1972). *J. Comp. Physiol. Psychol.* **78**, 220–225.

Galef, B.G., and Heiber, L. (1976). *J. Comp. Physiol. Psychol.* **90**, 727–739.

Galef, B.G., and Kaner, H.C. (1980). *J. Comp. Physiol. Psychol.* **94**, 588–595.

Gandelman, R. (1972). *Horm. Behav.* **3**, 23–28.

Gandelman, R., and Davis, P.G. (1973). *Dev. Psychobiol.* **6**, 251–257.

Gandelman, R., Paschke, R.E., Zarrow, M.X., and Denenberg, V.H. (1970). *Dev. Psychobiol.* **3**, 245–250.

Gandelman, R., Zarrow, M.X., and Denenberg, V.H. (1971a). *Physiol. Behav.* **7**, 583–586.

Gandelman, R., Zarrow, M.X., Denenberg, V.H., and Myers, M. (1971b). *Science* **171**, 210–211.

Gandelman, R., Zarrow, M.X., and Denenberg, V.H. (1972). *J. Reprod. Fertil.* **28**, 453–456.

Gawienowski, A.M., and Stacewicz-Sapuntzakis, M. (1978) *Behav. Biol.* **23**, 267–270.

Gawienowski, A.M., Orsulak, P.J., and Stacewicz-Sapuntzakis, M. (1976). *Psychoneuroendocrinology* **1**, 411–418.

Gerling, S., and Yahr, P. (1982). *Physiol. Behav.* **28**, 667–673.

Gesteland, R.C., and Sigwart, C.D. (1977). *Brain Res.* **133**, 144–149.

Geyer, L.A. (1979). *Am. Zool.* **19**, 420–431.

Geyer, L.A. (1981). *Am. Zool.* **21**, 117–128.

Goldenblatt, A. (1978). *Behav. Biol.* **22**, 269–273.

Goodall, J. (1977). *Folia Primatol.* **28**, 259–282.

Grau, G.A. (1976). *In* "Mammalian Olfaction, Reproductive Processes, and Behavior" (R.L. Doty, ed.), pp. 219–242. Academic Press, New York.

Green, J.A. (1978). *J. Comp. Physiol. Psychol.* **92**, 1179–1187.

Greenberg, L. (1979). *Science* **206**, 1095–1097.

Gregory, E.H., and Bishop, A. (1975). *Physiol. Behav.* **15**, 373–376.

Gregory, E.H., and Pfaff, D.W. (1971). *Physiol. Behav.* **6**, 573–576.

Grossberg, S. (1976). *Biol. Cybernet.* **23**, 187–202.

Grosvenor, C.E. (1965). *Endocrinology* **76**, 340–342.

Grosvenor, C.E., Maiweg, H., and Mena, F. (1970). *Horm. Behav.* **1**, 111–120.

Gubernick, D.J. (1980). *Anim. Behav.* **28**, 124–129.

Gubernick, D.J. (1981). *In* "Parental Care in Mammals" (D.J. Gubernick and P.H. Klopfer, eds.), pp. 243–306. Plenum, New York.

Gubernick, D.J., Jones, K.C., and Klopfer, P.H. (1979). *Anim. Behav.* **27**, 314–315.

Harder, W. (1949). *Ver. Dtch. Zool. Ges.* **2**, 95–109.

Heimer, L., and Nauta, W.J. (1969). *Brain Res.* **13**, 279–284.

Hennessy, M.B., Smotherman, W.P., and Levine, S. (1977). *Physiol. Behav.* **19**, 481–483.

Herrenkohl, L.R., and Rosenberg, P.A. (1972). *Physiol. Behav.* **8**, 595–598.

Hersher, L., Moore, A.U., and Richmond, J.B. (1958). *Science* **128**, 1342–1343.

Hildebrand, J.G., Matsumoto, S.G., Camazine, S.M., Tolbert, L.P., Blank, S., Ferguson, H., and Ecker, V. (1979). *In* "Insect Neurobiology and Pesticide Action (Neurotox, 1979)," pp. 375–382. Soc. Chem. Ind., London.

Hill, D.L., and Almi, C.R. (1981). *Physiol. Behav.* **27**, 811–817.

Hinds, J.W. (1968a). *J. Comp. Neurol.* **134**, 287–304.

Hinds, J.W. (1968b). *J. Comp. Neurol.* **134**, 305–322.

Hinds, J.W. (1972a). *J. Comp. Neurol.* **146**, 233–252.

Hinds, J.W. (1972b). *J. Comp. Neurol.* **146**, 253–276.

Hinds, J.W., and Hinds, P.L. (1976). *J. Comp. Neurol.* **169**, 15–40.

Hinds, J.W., and Ruffett, T.L. (1973). *J. Comp. Neurol.* **151**, 281–306.

Hoetzel, D., and Barnes, R.H. (1966). *Vitam. Horm. (N.Y.)* **24**, 115–171.

Hofer, M.A. (1973a). *Behav. Biol.* **9**, 629–633.

Hofer, M.A. (1973b). *Psychosom. Med.* **35**, 350–359.

Hofer, M.A. (1975). *Psychosom. Med.* **37**, 245–264.

Hofer, M.A. (1976). *J. Comp. Physiol. Psychol.* **90**, 829–838.

Hofer, M.A., and Shair, H., (1978). *Dev. Psychobiol.* **11**, 495–504.

Hofer, M.A., Shair, H., and Singh, P. (1976). *Physiol. Behav.* **17**, 131–136.

Holinka, C.F., and Carlson, A.D. (1976). *Behav. Biol.* **16**, 489–505.

Huck, V.W., and Banks, E.M. (1980). *Anim. Behav.* **28**, 1046–1052.

Immelmann, K. (1972). *Adv. Study Behav.* **4**, 147–175.

Infurna, R.N., Steinert, P.A., and Spear, N.E. (1979). *J. Comp. Physiol. Psychol.* **93**, 1097–1108.

Iwahara, S., Oishi, H., Sano, K., Yang, K.M., and Takahashi, T. (1973). *Jpn. J. Physiol.* **23**, 361–370.

Johanson, I.B. (1980). *Dev. Psychobiol.* **13**, 343–351.

Johanson, I.B., and Hall, W.G. (1981). *J. Comp. Physiol. Psychol.* **95**, 837–847.

Johanson, I.B., Turkewitz, G., and Hamburgh, M. (1980). *Dev. Psychobiol.* **13**, 331–342.

Jourdan, F., Duveau, A., Astic, L., and Holley, A. (1980). *Brain Res.* **188**, 139–154.

Kalmus, H. (1955). *Br. J. Anim. Behav.* **3**, 25–31.

Kaplan, J.N., and Russell, M. (1974). *Dev. Psychobiol.* **7**, 15–19.

Kaplan, J.N., Cubicciotti, D., and Redican, W.K. (1977). *Dev. Psychobiol.* **10**, 447–453.

Kaplan, M.S., and Hinds, J.W. (1977). *Science* **197**, 1092-1094.

Kennedy, C., DesRosiers, M.H., Jehle, J.W., Reivich, M., Sharp, F., and Sokoloff, R. (1975). *Science* **187**, 850-853.

Kilpatrick, S.J., and Moltz, H. (1981). *Physiol. Behav.* **26**, 1129-1131.

Kilpatrick, S.J., Bolt, M., and Moltz, H. (1980). *Physiol. Behav.* **25**, 31-34.

King, H.D. (1939). *Am. Anat. Mem.* **17**, 1-72.

Kling, A. (1964). *Am. J. Physiol.* **206**, 1395-1400.

Klopfer, P.H. (1970). *Folia Primatol.* **13**, 137-143.

Klopfer, P.H., and Gamble, L. (1966). *Z. Tierpsychol.* **23**, 588-592.

Klopfer, P.H., Adams, D.K., and Klopfer, M.S. (1964). *Proc. Natl. Acad. Sci. U.S.A.* **52**, 911-914.

Koranyi, L., Phelps, C.P., and Sawyer, C.H. (1977). *Physiol. Behav.* **18**, 287-292.

Kratzing, J. (1971). *Aust. J. Biol. Sci.* **24**, 787-796.

Kukuk, P.F., Breed, M.D., Sobti, A., and Bell, W.J. (1977). *Behav. Ecol. Sociobiol.* **2**, 319-327.

Lagerspetz, K., and Heino, T. (1970). *Psychol. Rep.* **27**, 255-262.

Laing, D.G., and Panhuber, H. (1978). *J. Comp. Physiol.* **124**, 259-265.

Laing, D.G., and Panhuber, H. (1980). *Physiol. Behav.* **25**, 555-558.

Lampen, J.A., and Peterjohn, H.R. (1951). *J. Bacteriol.* **62**, 281-292.

LeBoeuf, B.J., Whiting, R.J., and Gantt, R.F. (1972). *Behaviour* **43**. 121-156.

Lee, T.M., and Moltz, H. (1980). *Physiol. Behav.* **24**, 983-989.

Leidahl, L., and Moltz, H. (1977). *Physiol. Behav.* **18**, 399-402.

Leon, M. (1974). *Physiol. Behav.* **13**, 441-453.

Leon, M. (1975). *Physiol. Behav.* **14**, 311-319.

Leon, M. (1978). *Adv. Study Behav.* **8**, 117-153.

Leon, M. (1980). *In* "Chemical Signals in Vertebrates and Aquatic Invertebrates" (D. Müller-Schwarze and R.M. Silverstein, eds.), pp. 193-209. Plenum, New York.

Leon, M., and Behse, J. (1977). *Physiol. Behav.* **14**, 311-319.

Leon, M., and Moltz, H. (1971). *Physiol. Behav.* **7**, 265-267.

Leon, M., and Moltz, H. (1972). *Physiol. Behav.* **8**, 683-686.

Leon, M., and Moltz, H. (1973). *Physiol. Behav.* **10**, 65-67.

Leon, M., Galef, B.G., and Behse, J. (1977). *Physiol. Behav.* **18**, 387-391.

Leon, M., Croskerry, P.G., and Smith, G.K. (1978). *Physiol. Behav.* **21**, 793-811.

Leonard, C.M. (1974). *J. Comp. Physiol. Psychol.* **86**, 458-469.

Leonard, C.M. (1978). *J. Comp. Physiol. Psychol.* **92**, 1084-1094.

Levine, S. (1969). *Physiol. Behav.* **4**, 143-145.

Lindsay, D.R., and Fletcher, I.C. (1968). *Anim. Behav.* **16**, 415-417.

Little, E.E. (1975). *Nature (London)* **255**, 400-401.

Little, E.E. (1976). *J. Comp. Physiol.* **112**, 133-142.

Lutton, C., and Chevallier, F. (1973). *J. Physiol. (London)* **66**, 219-228.

Lynds, P.G. (1976). *Physiol. Behav.* **17**, 157-159.

McCarty, R., and Southwick, C.H. (1977). *Behav. Biol.* **19**, 255-260.

McClure, P.A. (1980). *Science* **211**, 1058-1060.

MacFarlane, A. (1975). *In* "The Human Neonate in Parent-Infant Interaction," pp. 103-117. Ciba Found., Amsterdam.

Mainardi, D., Marsan, M., and Pasquali, A. (1965) *Atti Soc. Ital. Sci. Nat. Mus. Civ. Stor. Nat. Milano* **104**, 325-338.

Marasco, E.M., Cornwell-Jones, C.A., and Sobrian, S.K. (1979). *Pharmacol., Biochem. Behav.* **10**, 319-323.

Marinari, K.T., and Moltz, H. (1978). *Physiol. Behav.* **21**, 525-528.

Marques, D.M. (1979). *Behav. Neural Biol.* **26**, 311-329.

Marques, D.M., and Valenstein, E.S. (1976). *J. Comp. Physiol. Psychol.* **90**, 653–657.
Marr, J.N., and Gardner, L.E. (1965). *J. Genet. Psychol.* **107**, 167–174.
Marr, J.N., and Lilliston, L.G. (1969). *Behaviour* **33**, 277–282.
Martin, R.D. (1968). *Z. Tierpsychol.* **25**, 409–495.
Maruniak, J.A., Silver, W.L., and Moulton, D.G. (1980). *Soc. Neurosci. Abstr.* **6**, 242.
Math, F., and Davrainville, J.L. (1980). *Brain Res.* **190**, 243–247.
Math, F., and Desor, D. (1974). *C.R. Hebd. Seances Acad. Sci.* **279**, 931–934.
Mayer, A.D., and Rosenblatt, J.S. (1975). *J. Comp. Physiol. Psychol.* **89**, 701–710.
Mayer, A.D., and Rosenblatt, J.S. (1977). *Physiol. Behav.* **18**, 101–109.
Mayer, A.D., and Rosenblatt, J.S. (1979). *J. Comp. Physiol. Psychol.* **93**, 879–898.
Meese, G.B., and Baldwin, B.A. (1975). *Appl. Anim. Ethol.* **1**, 379–386.
Meisami, E., and Shafa, F. (1978). *Proc. Int. Symp. Olfaction Taste, 6th, 1978,* p. 198.
Mena, F., and Grosvenor, C.E. (1971). *Horm. Behav.* **2**, 107–116.
Mena, F., and Grosvenor, C.E. (1972). *J. Endocrinol.* **52**, 11–22.
Merle, L., Dangoumau, J., and Balabaud, C. (1978). *Experientia* **34**, 764–765.
Meyer, A.E., and McEwen, J.P. (1948). *Am J. Physiol.* **153**, 386–392.
Michener, G.R., and Sheppard, D.H. (1972). *Can. J. Zool.* **50**, 1343–1349.
Mikelson, O. (1956). *Vitam. Horm. (N.Y.)* **14**, 1–95
Misanin, J.R., Zawacki, D.M., and Krieger, W.G. (1977). *Bull. Psychon. Soc.* **10**, 313–316.
Moltz, H., and Kilpatrick, S.J. (1978). *Neurosci. Biobehav. Rev.* **2**, 277–280.
Moltz, H., and Leon, M. (1972). In "Modern Perspectives in Psycho-Obstetrics" (J.G. Howell, ed.), pp. 3–30. Brunner/Mazel, New York.
Moltz, H., and Leon, M. (1973). *Physiol. Behav.* **10**, 69–71.
Moltz, H., Levin, R., and Leon, M. (1969). *Science* **163**, 1083–1084.
Moltz, H., Leidahl, L., and Rowland, D. (1974). *Physiol. Behav.* **12**, 409–412.
Moore, C.L. (1981). *Anim. Behav.* **29**, 383–386.
Moore, C.L., and Morelli, G.A. (1979). *J. Comp. Physiol. Psychol.* **93**, 677–684.
Morgan, P.D., Boundy, C.A.P., Arnold, G.W., and Lindsay, D.R. (1975). *Appl. Anim. Ethol.* **1**, 139–150.
Müller-Schwarze, D., and Müller-Schwarze, C. (1971). *Nature (London)* **229**, 55–56.
Mykytowycz, R. (1968). *Sci. Am.* **218**, 116–126.
Mykytowycz, R. (1973). *J. Reprod. Fertil., Suppl.* **19**, 433–446.
Mykytowycz, R., and Dudzinski, M.L. (1972). *Behaviour* **43**, 97–120.
Mykytowycz, R., and Ward, M.M. (1971). *Forma Funct.* **4**, 137–148.
Nicoll, C.S., and Meites, J. (1959). *Proc. Soc. Exp. Biol. Med.* **101**, 81–82.
Numan, M. (1974). *J. Comp. Physiol. Psychol.* **87**, 746–759.
Numan, M., Rosenblatt, J.S., and Komisaruk, B.R. (1977). *J. Comp. Physiol. Psychol.* **91**, 146–164.
Nyakas, C., and Endröczi, E. (1970). *Acta Physiol. Acad. Sci. Hung.* **38**, 59–65.
Oswalt, G.L., and Meier, G.W. (1975). *Dev. Psychobiol.* **8**, 129–135.
Ota, K., and Yokoyama, A. (1967a). *J. Endocrinol.* **38**, 251–261.
Ota, K., and Yokoyama, A. (1967b). *J. Endocrinol.* **38**, 263–268.
Pederson, P.E., and Blass, E.M. (1979). *Int. Soc. Dev. Psychobiol. Abstr.* p. 22.
Pederson, P.E., and Blass, E.M. (1981). In "The Development of Perception: Psychobiological Perspectives" (R.N. Aslin, J.R. Alberts, and M.R. Peterson, eds.), Vol. 1, pp. 359–381. Academic Press, New York.
Pederson, P.E., and Blass, E.M. (1982). *Dev. Psychobiol.* **15**, 349–356.
Pederson, P.E., Williams, C.L., and Blass, E.M. (1982). *J. Exp. Psychol.* **8**, 329–341.
Peters, A., and Feldman, M. (1973). *Z. Anat. Entwicklungsgesch.* **141**, 3–37.
Pfeffer, P. (1967). *Mammalia* **31**, Suppl., 1–262.
Pinching, A.J., and Doving, K.B. (1974). *Brain Res.* **82**, 195–204.

Poindron, P. (1974). *Ann. Biol. Anim., Biochim., Biophys.* **14**, 411–415.
Poindron, P. (1976). *C.R. Hebd. Seances Acad. Sci.* **282**, 489–491.
Poindron, P., and LeNeindre, P. (1980). *Adv. Study Behav.* **11**, 75–119.
Pollack, E.I., and Sachs, B.D. (1975). *Physiol. Behav.* **14**, 337–343.
Poo, L.J., Lew, W., and Addis, T. (1939). *J. Biol. Chem.* **128**, 69–77.
Porter, J.R., and Rettger, L.F. (1940). *J. Infect. Dis.* **66**, 104–110.
Porter, R.H., and Doane, H.M. (1976). *Physiol. Behav.* **16**, 75–78.
Porter, R.H., and Doane, H.M. (1977). *Physiol. Behav.* **19**, 129–131.
Porter, R.H., and Etscorn, F. (1974). *Nature (London)* **250**, 732–733.
Porter, R.H., and Etscorn, F. (1975). *Behav. Biol.* **15**, 515–517.
Porter, R.H., and Moore, J.D. (1981). *Physiol. Behav.* **27**, 493–495.
Porter, R.H., and Ruttle, K. (1975). *Z. Tierpsychol.* **38**, 154–162.
Porter, R.H., and Wyrick, M. (1979). *Anim. Behav.* **27**, 761–766.
Porter, R.H., Fullerton, C., and Berryman, J.C. (1973). *Z. Tierpsychol.* **32**, 489–495.
Porter, R.H., Deni, R., and Doane, H.M. (1977). *Behav. Biol.* **20**, 244–251.
Porter, R.H., Wyrick, M., and Pankey, J. (1978). *Behav. Ecol. Sociobiol.* **3**, 61–68.
Porter, R.H., Moore, J.D., and White, D.M. (1980). *Behav. Ecol. Sociobiol.* **8**, 207–212.
Porter, R.H., Tepper, V.J., and White, D.M. (1981). *Dev. Psychobiol.* **14**, 375–382.
Quadagno, D.M., and Banks, E.M. (1970). *Anim. Behav.* **18**, 379–390.
Randall, P.K., and Campbell, B.A. (1976). *J. Comp. Physiol. Psychol.* **90**, 453–459.
Rasa, O.A.E. (1973). *Z. Tierpsychol.* **32**, 293–318.
Reisbeck, S., Rosenblatt, J.S., and Mayer, A.D. (1975). *J. Comp. Physiol. Psychol.* **89**, 722–732.
Rettger, L.F., and Horton, G.P. (1914). *Zentralbl. Bakteriol., Parasitenkd., Infektionskr. Hyg., Abt. 1: Orig.* **73**, 362–372.
Rood, J.P. (1972). *Anim. Behav. Monogr.* **5**, 1–83.
Rosenblatt, J.S. (1965). *In* "Determinants of Infant Behavior Vol III" (B.M. Foss, ed.), Vol. III, pp. 3–45. Methuen, London.
Rosenblatt, J.S. (1967). *Science* **156**, 1512–1514.
Rosenblatt, J.S. (1969). *Am. J. Orthopsychiatry* **39**, 36–56.
Rosenblatt, J.S. (1971). *In* "The Biopsychology of Development" (E. Tobach, L.R. Aronson, and E. Shaw, eds.), pp. 345–410. Academic Press, New York.
Rosenblatt, J.S., and Lehrman, D.S. (1963). *In* "Maternal Behavior in Mammals" (H.L. Rheingold, ed.), pp. 8–57. Wiley, New York.
Rosenblatt, J.S., Turkewitz, G., and Schneirla, T.C. (1969). *Trans. N.Y. Acad. Sci.* [2] **31**, 231–250.
Rosenblatt, J.S., Siegel, H.I., and Mayer, A.D. (1979). *Adv. Study Behav.* **10**, 225–311.
Rosselli-Austin, L., and Altman, J. (1979). *J. Dev. Physiol.* **1**, 295–319.
Roth, L.L., and Rosenblatt, J.S. (1967). *J. Comp. Physiol. Psychol.* **63**, 397–400.
Rouger, Y., Tobach, E., and Schneirla, T.C. (1967). *Am. Zool.* **7**, 792–793.
Rowell, T.E. (1961). *Anim. Behav.* **9**, 11–15.
Russell, M. (1976). *Nature (London)* **260**, 520–522.
Salas, M., Guzman-Flores, C., and Schapiro, S. (1969). *Physiol. Behav.* **4**, 699–703.
Sar, M., and Meites, J. (1969). *Neuroendocrinology* **4**, 25–31.
Saylor, A., and Salmon, M. (1971). *Behaviour* **40**, 61–85.
Scalia, F., and Winans, S.S. (1975). *J. Comp. Neurol.* **161**, 31–56.
Schapiro, S., and Salas, M. (1970). *Physiol. Behav.* **5**, 815–817.
Scheibel, M.E., and Scheibel, A.B. (1975). *Brain Res.* **95**, 407–421.
Schlein, P.A., Zarrow, M.X., Cohen, H.A., Denenberg, V.H., and Johnson, N.P. (1972). *J. Reprod. Fertil.* **30**, 39–42.
Schönfelder, J., and Schwartze, P. (1971). *Acta Biol. Med. Ger.* **27**, 103–110.

Schumacher, S.K., and Moltz, H. (1982). *Physiol. Behav.* **28,** 67-71.

Schultze-Westrum, T.G. (1969). *Olfaction Taste, Proc. Int. Symp., 3rd, 1968,* pp. 268-277.

Schwartz, E., and Rowe, F.A. (1976). *Physiol. Behav.* **17,** 879-883.

Schwob, J.E., and Price, J.L. (1978). *Brain Res.* **151,** 369-374.

Sczerzenie, V., and Hsiao, S. (1977). *Dev. Psychobiol.* **10,** 315-321.

Seegal, R.F., and Denenberg, V.H. (1974). *Physiol. Behav.* **13,** 339-341.

Shafa, F., Meisami, E., and Mousaui, R. (1980). *Exp. Neurol.* **67,** 215-233.

Shafa, F., Shineh, S.N., and Bidanjiri, A. (1981). *Brain Res.* **223,** 409-412.

Shani, J., Goldhaber, G., and Sulman, F.G. (1975). *J. Reprod. Fertil.* **43,** 571-573.

Shapiro, S., and Salas, M. (1970). *Physiol. Behav.* **5,** 815-817.

Sharp, F.R., Kauer, J.S., and Shepherd, G.M. (1975). *Brain Res.* **98,** 596-600.

Shepherd, G.M. (1972). *Physiol. Res.* **52,** 864-917.

Sherman, P. (1980). *In* "Sociobiology: Beyond Nature/Nature?" (G. Barlow and J. Silverberg, eds.), pp. 505-544. Westview Press, Boulder, Colorado.

Signoret, J.P., Baldwin, B.A., Frase, D., and Hafez, E.S.E. (1975). *In* "The Behavior of Domestic Animals" (E.S.E. Hafez, ed.), 3rd ed., pp. 295-329. Williams & Wilkins, Baltimore, Maryland.

Simpson, A.A., Simpson, M.H.W., Sinha, Y.N., and Schmidt, G.H. (1973). *J. Endocrinol.* **58,** 675-676.

Simpson, G.G. (1945). *Bull. Am. Mus. Nat. Hist.* **85,** 1-350.

Singh, D.N.P., and Nathaniel, E.J.H. (1977). *Anat. Rec.* **189,** 413-432.

Singh, P.J., and Hofer, M.A. (1976). *Soc. Neurosci. Abstr.* **2,** 163.

Singh, P.J., and Tobach, E. (1975). *Dev. Psychobiol.* **8,** 151-164.

Singh, P.J., Tucker, A.M., and Hofer, M.A. (1976). *Physiol. Behav.* **17,** 373-382.

Skeen, J.T., and Thiessen, D.D. (1977). *Physiol. Behav.* **19,** 11-14.

Slonaker, J.R. (1925). *Am. J. Physiol.* **71,** 362-394.

Slotnick, B.M. (1975). *In* "Hormonal Correlates of Behavior" (B.E. Eleuthériou and R.L. Sprott, eds.), Vol. II, pp. 585-656. Plenum, New York.

Small, W.S. (1899). *Am. J. Psychol.* **11,** 80-100.

Smith, C.G. (1935). *J. Comp. Neurol.* **61,** 477-508.

Smith, F.V., Toller, V., and Boyes, T. (1966). *Anim. Behav.* **14,** 120-125.

Smith, G.J., and Spear, N.E. (1978). *Science* **202,** 327-329.

Smith, G.J., and Spear, N.E. (1980). *Behav. Neural Biol.* **28,** 491-495.

Smotherman, W.P., Bell, R.W., Starzec, J., Elias, J.W., and Zachman, T.A. (1974). *Behav. Biol.* **12,** 55-66.

Smotherman, W.P., Bell, R.W., Hershberger, W.A., and Coover, G.D. (1978). *Anim. Behav.* **26,** 265-273.

Sobrian, S.K., and Cornwell-Jones, C. (1977). *Behav. Biol.* **21,** 329-340.

Söderberg, V., and Larsson, K. (1976). *Physiol. Behav.* **17,** 993-995.

Souders, H.J., and Morgan, A.F. (1957). *Am. J. Physiol.* **191,** 1-7.

Stewart, W.B., Kauer, J.S., and Shepherd, G.M. (1979). *Brain Res.* **185,** 715-734.

Stoddart, D.M., Alpin, R.T., and Wood, M.J. (1975). *J. Zool.* **177,** 529-540.

Svare, B., and Gandelman, R. (1973). *Horm. Behav.* **4,** 323-334.

Taylor, P.M. (1960). *J. Physiol. (London)* **154,** 153-168.

Teicher, M.H., and Blass, E.M. (1976). *Science* **193,** 422-425.

Teicher, M.H., and Blass, E.M. (1977). *Science* **198,** 635-636.

Teicher, M.H., Flaum, L.E., Williams, M., Eckert, S.J., and Lumia, A.R. (1978). *Physiol. Behav.* **21,** 553-561.

Teicher, M.H., Stewart, W.B., Kauer, J.S., and Shepherd, G.M. (1980). *Brain Res.* **194,** 530-535.

Telle, H.J. (1966). *Z. Angew. Zool.* **53,** 129-196.

Terkel, J., and Rosenblatt, J.S. (1971). *Horm. Behav.* **2**, 161-171.

Terkel, J., Blake, C.A., and Sawyer, C.H. (1972). *Endocrinology* **91**, 49-53.

Thiessen, D.D., Blum, S.L., and Lindzey, G. (1970). *Anim. Behav.* **18**, 26-30.

Tindal, J.S. (1956). *J. Endocrinol.* **14**, 268-274.

Tobach, E. (1977). *Ann. N.Y. Acad. Sci.* **290**, 226-269.

Tomogane, H. Ota, K., Unno, H., and Yokoyama, A. (1976). *Endocrinol. Jpn.* **23**, 129-136.

Tucker, H.A. (1974). *In* "Lactation" (B.L. Larson and V.R. Smith, eds.), Vol. 1, pp. 277-326. Academic Press, New York.

Vandenbergh, J.G. (1973). *Physiol. Behav.* **10**, 257-261.

von Reiff, M. (1956). *Acta Trop.* **13**, 289-318.

Voogt, J.L., Sar, M., and Meites, J. (1969). *Am. J. Physiol.* **216**, 655-658.

Wallace, P. (1977). *Physiol. Behav.* **19**, 577-579.

Wallace, P., Owen, K., and Thiessen, D.D. (1973). *Physiol. Behav.* **10**, 463-466.

Waring, A., and Perper, T. (1979). *Anim. Behav.* **28**, 1091-1097.

Weingarten, H.P., and Powley, T.L. (1980). *Am. J. Physiol.* **232**, G221-G228.

Welker, W.R. (1964). *Behaviour* **22**, 223-244.

Westrum, L.E. (1975). *J. Neurocytol.* **4**, 713-732.

Wiesner, B.P., and Sheard, N.M. (1933). "Maternal Behaviour in the Rat." Oliver & Boyd, Edinburgh.

Winans, S.S., and Powers, J.B. (1977). *Brain Res.* **126**, 325-344.

Woodside, B., and Leon, M. (1980). *J. Comp. Physiol. Psychol.* **94**, 41-60.

Woodside, B., Pelchat, R., and Leon, M. (1980). *J. Comp. Physiol. Psychol.* **94**, 61-68.

Woodside, B., Leon, M., Attard, M., Feder, H.H., Siegel, H.I., and Fischette, C. (1981). *J. Comp. Physiol. Psychol.* **95**, 771-780.

Yahr, P. (1976). *Physiol. Behav.* **16**, 395-399.

Yahr, P. (1977). *Anim. Behav.* **25**, 292-297.

Yanai, J., and Rosselli-Austin, L. (1978). *Behav. Biol.* **24**, 539-544.

Zarrow, M.X., Gandelman, R., and Denenberg, V.H. (1971). *Horm. Behav.* **2**, 227-238.

Zarrow, M.X., Schlein, P.A., Denenberg, V.H., and Cohen, H.A. (1972). *Endocrinology* **91**, 191-196.

3

Chemical Communication in Primate Reproduction

Eric B. Keverne

Department of Anatomy
Cambridge University
Cambridge, England

I. INTRODUCTION

Although it is generally accepted that most mammals use all their senses to assess their social environment, some clearly rely on olfactory information more than others, especially in the context of reproduction. Thus, not only do mice identify the sex of an individual by its odor, but their physiological reproductive state is determined largely by chemical cues (see Chapter 4 by Vandenbergh). Mice clearly fit into the category of macrosmatic mammals. Primates, on the other hand, including man, have all of their senses well developed and with the evolutionary enlargement of the neocortex have the capacity to assimilate and integrate information rapidly from a number of sensory channels simultaneously. More pertinently, primates possess the ability to attend to whichever sensory channel is most

PHEROMONES AND REPRODUCTION IN MAMMALS
Copyright © 1983 by Academic Press, Inc.
All rights of reproduction in any form reserved.
ISBN 0-12-710780-0

relevant at the time, and behavior does not come under the obligatory domination of any one sense. In other words, we use our senses intelligently to derive maximal information from the environment. So far as olfaction is concerned, neuroanatomists have traditionally classified primates as microsmatic. What they mean by this term is that a relatively small area of the brain is given over to the olfactory sense, and the peripheral receptors are fewer in number than in a macrosmatic species such as the mouse or rabbit. Indeed, a cursory look at the brain provides convincing anatomical contrasts between what can be seen as representing the olfactory sense, for example, in the mouse and the monkey. In the former the olfactory bulb occupies a large part of the cranial cavity, whereas the olfactory bulbs of a monkey are barely visible, being totally subordinated by the neocortex. Similarly, macrosmatic species have a larger number of receptor cells in the olfactory mucosa than are found in a monkey (contrast the rabbit's 100 million receptors with the monkey's 10 million). Now, if receipt and interpretation of the olfactory message relied on these anatomical features, primates could certainly be considered microsmatic. However, two important findings have invalidated this method of classification. The first came when recordings from single olfactory receptors became possible and it was discovered that such receptors are not narrowly tuned to particular odors but can respond to a number of different odors. This favored the consideration of a pattern of receptor firing as the means of coding odor cues (Gesteland *et al.,* 1965). The second finding came when it was discovered that the neural projections of the olfactory system have access to the neocortex via the thalamus (Powell *et al.,* 1965). The fact that olfactory information is coded as a pattern which requires a higher order of recognition means that animals with a greater neural backup have the potential for a more sophisticated pattern recognition. Since the olfactory bulb seems to be acting mainly as a filter, and decoding of the olfactory message is a more central event, animals with a greater neocortical support system have the greatest ability to make use of this system. Primates do not therefore have a poorly developed sense of olfactory perception, and the ways in which this is employed may well be the most evolved of all species.

II. DO CHEMICAL CUES INFLUENCE PRIMATE REPRODUCTIVE PHYSIOLOGY?

Most of the research that has demonstrated an influence of chemical cues on reproductive physiology has been conducted on rodents, especially the house mouse. In the female such primer pheromones bring their influence to bear on reproductive processes by way of the accessory olfactory system (see Chapter 8). This consists of the vomeronasal organ with its neural projection relaying in the accessory olfactory bulb before entering directly into the limbic brain by way of the amygdala. Although present in prosimian primates, only vestiges of the accessory olfactory system are present in monkeys and apes. It is therefore improbable that primer pheromones exist which influence female reproduction in the higher primates. Indeed, the evolutionary trend has been to emancipate reproduction from the physical environment such that ovulation can occur at any time of year and any time of the day or night. Reproduction is not, however, totally independent of the social environment since the stress of social subordination may reduce the reproductive capacity of some female primates (Bowman *et al.,* 1978). Chemical cues do not appear to be involved in this process, but infertility results from the continuous threat of aggression maintaining high levels of the stress hormone prolactin. It is interesting that many of the pheromonal effects in mice influence reproductive events also by changing the secretion of prolactin (Keverne, 1982), as do the effects of light on seasonal breeding in sheep (Revault and Ortavant, 1977) and tactile cues in rodents (Smith and Neill, 1976). Thus, although the environment influences reproduction in a number of species by neuroendocrine mechanisms that have much in common, in primates we again see an emancipation from the domination of these mechanisms by any one sense. However, after the establishment of social subordination, one could envisage how selective sensory information, even olfactory information, might be sufficient to reinforce the "status quo" and maintain neuroendocrine profiles that characterize subordinate monkeys.

The vomeronasal organ (Schilling, 1970) and accessory olfactory bulb (Stephan, 1965) are present in prosimian primates. Whether chemical cues are important in the reproduction of certain prosimians is a matter of some speculation, but both laboratory (Evans and Goy, 1968) and field studies (Harrington, 1974) of seasonal breeding and estrus synchronization in lemurs have suggested that this might be a useful area to investigate. The Lemuridae and Indriidae are diurnal prosimians and have developed the most elaborate range of scent marking, which involves both visual and olfactory displays. Exactly what information these scent marks convey is little understood, although it has been suggested that they may aid in sexual identification (Clark, 1974; Harrington, 1974). It is further possible that the reproductive status of female lemurs may be communicated from genital marking, since the frequency of this behavior peaks during the period of estrus (Evans and Goy, 1968; Schilling, 1970).

The solitary life of the nocturnal loris is characterized by scent marking with urine, which is performed most frequently on the boundaries of the territory (Charles-Dominique, 1977). This suggests that these nocturnal prosimians utilize urine for attracting the opposite sex and deterring the members of the same sex, a suggestion strongly supported by laboratory studies (Schilling, 1980).

Among New World primates it has been reported that female squirrel monkeys increase urine washing in the breeding season (Latta *et al.,* 1967) and that the frequency of olfactory inspections of females by males increases markedly in the months leading up to and during the seasonal mating peak (Hennessy *et al.,* 1979). Behavioral observations of the spider monkey (*Ateles geoffroyi*) led Klein (1971) to conclude that information concerning sexual receptivity is transmitted via chemical stimuli and that the primary function of the female's hypertrophied clitoris is urine marking. Similar correlative observations have been made for the howler monkey (Altmann, 1959) the Titi monkey (Moynihan, 1966), and marmosets (Epple, 1967, 1976). The reproduction of marmosets is of particular interest, for, in spite of being mated by the alpha male, subordinate females do not become pregnant in the presence of their mother, the alpha female (Epple, 1967; Abbott and Hearn, 1978). Subordinate females suffer from complete ovarian failure due to gonadotropin insufficiency (Abbott *et al.,* 1981). Removal of the subordinates from the group reinstates ovarian cyclicity within 10 to 30 days (Abbott and Hearn, 1978), whereas removal of the mother from the group enables the daughter to become pregnant (Epple, 1967). The mechanisms by which the dominant female marmoset inhibits ovulation in her subordinates are unknown but could involve pheromones, as assessed from frequent scent markings (Epple, 1973).

III. THE COMMUNICATIVE SIGNIFICANCE OF ODOR CUES IN REPRODUCTIVE BEHAVIOR

There is a wealth of behavioral data indicating that olfactory cues play a significant part in the reproductive life of many primate species, regardless of their habitat or social organization (see reviews by Epple and Moulton, 1978; Michael *et al.,* 1976; Keverne, 1976). However, this topic has received significant investigation in only one laboratory species, the rhesus monkey, and here opinions have been somewhat divided as to the importance of olfactory mechanisms. However, everyone is agreed that a fundamental requirement for the sexual interest of male primates is the presence of attractive females. There are three major variables to be considered as part of female attractiveness: behavioral cues (sexual invitations or refusals of male-initiated interest); nonbehavioral cues (odor, sexual skin swellings, and coloration; tactile information); and female social status, which in turn is dependent on a wide variety of behaviors, particularly aggression. Many of these factors come under the influence of endocrine secretions, and in the laboratory it has been possible to determine not only which hormones influence female attractiveness, but the sites of hormone action and how they may differentially influence these various components of female attractiveness.

IV. HORMONES AND THE BEHAVIOR OF HETEROSEXUAL PAIRS OF RHESUS MONKEYS

The usual approach to understanding the effects of a given hormone is to measure changes in its secretion rate and correlate this with the behavioral interaction or, alternatively, to remove its secreting gland and then replace the hormone. Thus, when heterosexual pairs of rhesus monkeys are allowed to interact in a laboratory situation, a striking feature of their sexual interaction is the cyclicity in male sexual behavior with respect to the ovarian secretory activity in the female (Ball and Hartman, 1935; Michael and Herbert, 1963), an observation also reported for free-living monkeys (Southwick et al., 1965; Loy, 1970). Hence, the endocrine changes occurring in the female at this time are being communicated to the male partner and are in turn influencing his sexual behavior, a view also supported by experiments with free-ranging rhesus monkeys (Vandenbergh, 1969; Vandenbergh and Drickamer, 1974). During the follicular phase of the menstrual cycle, when estrogen secretion predominates, there is a gradual increase in sexual interactions, reaching a peak just before ovulation (Michael and Zumpe, 1970). In the luteal phase of the cycle, when progesterone predominates, sexual interactions decline as the females become progressively less attractive (Michael et al., 1977). Of course, there are a number of sensory channels other than olfaction by which a female can communicate changes in her attractiveness to the male, not the least of which are the visual displays of females directed at soliciting male attention or their ability to actively refuse the advances of an overmotivated sexually enthusiastic male. Nevertheless, female rhesus monkeys seem prepared to receive the male at all times during their menstrual cycle, and rarely does one observe unreceptive behavior (Keverne, 1976; Baum et al., 1976a). Moreover, females do not show obvious increases in sexual invitations around their ovulatory period, when male sexual behavior is highest (Czaja and Bielert, 1975). In fact, paradoxically they may show decreases (Michael and Welegalla, 1968). Such is the interest of the male at this time that females have little opportunity to make sexual invitations; the sexual initiative is firmly in the hands of the male.

Of course, there are immense problems in interpreting hormonal action during the menstrual cycle, since more than one hormone is changing simultaneously, and each is acting both peripherally and centrally. In order to ascertain which female behaviors are affected by which hormones acting on the central nervous system or on the periphery to influence female attractiveness, the endogenous source of these hormones must be removed. Thus, removal of the ovaries, and hence estrogen and progesterone, makes the female rhesus monkey less attractive, which in the laboratory may be characterized by a complete sexual disinterest in the female by males. Replacement of estrogen, but not progesterone, restores female attractiveness, whereas progesterone given to estrogen-treated females antagonizes this effect. Thus, the endocrine changes most relevant to enhancing female attractiveness appear to involve estrogen, since this hormone stimulates sexual behavior with either ovariectomized females (Herbert, 1970; Phoenix, 1973; Goldfoot *et al.,* 1976) or intact females out of the breeding season (Vandenbergh, 1969; Vandenbergh and Drickamer, 1974).

Since estrogen also has a central action, influencing the female's sexual invitations, it is necessary to evaluate how important sexual invitations are to female attractiveness. Experimental manipulations have been made which suggest that sexual invitations are not sufficient to induce male mounting in the absence of nonbehavioral cues signalling the female's attractiveness. Thus, ovariectomized females that have been administered testosterone display high levels of sexual invitations with little effect on male sexual interest (Trimble and Herbert, 1966; Michael, 1971). Conversely, females that are adrenalectomized and ovariectomized actively refuse to participate in sexual interactions but are still sexually stimulating and may be copulated with if their attractiveness is maintained with estrogen (Everitt *et al.,* 1972). Administration of progesterone to ovariectomized females given estrogen decreases the sexual interest of males in these females, despite marked and significant increases in sexual invitations (Baum *et al.,* 1976b). This increase in female sexual invitations is not due to a behavioral action of this hormone on the brain, since giving low doses of progesterone directly into the vagina produces exactly the same behavioral effect without reaching detectable levels in the plasma and hence the brain (Baum *et al.,* 1977). Here, then, not only do we see how a hormone can produce a behavioral change that is secondary to nonbehavioral aspects of attractiveness, but we can see how the female's attempts to sustain male interest by increasing her solicitations fail with the decline in the nonbehavioral aspects of her attractiveness. The converse is equally convincing, and administering very low doses of estrogen directly into the vagina markedly enhances the sexual interest of males in these females, compared with the same amount of estrogen given systemically. The sexual initiating behavior of the male is most stimulated by intravaginal estrogen, whereas the initiating behavior of the female is most stimulated by systemic estrogen administration (Michael and Saayman, 1968).

If one has to decide, therefore, which is most important in determining the male's sexual behavior, observations such as these lead to the inevitable conclusion that it is the nonbehavioral aspects of the female's attractiveness emanating from the vagina, at least within the confines of the laboratory cage. This is not to say that invitations are unimportant; indeed, one can envisage that such a behavioral backup is very important for arousing sexually sluggish males.

Of the nonbehavioral cues available to the male, vocalizations are rare and inconsistent in promoting sexual behavior and are certainly not governed by endocrine state. Although tactile cues may be important for the mounting and thrusting performance, clearly they are not what initiates male interest, since tactile feedback occurs only after the mounting sequence has started. Of the visual cues available, rhesus monkeys do not have a sexual skin swelling, but they do have a red skin coloration, the intensity of which changes with the menstrual cycle and is estrogen dependent (Hisaw and Hisaw, 1966). However, topical application of estrogen cream to the sex skin area promotes an intense red coloration with little or no effect on male sexual interest and behavior (Herbert, 1966; Michael and Keverne, 1970). Of course, this does not mean that such color changes have no communicatory significance; they may well act as signals over a distance, but within the laboratory context these color changes are not in themselves sufficient to stimulate male mounting behavior.

V. ODOR CUES AND COMMUNICATION OF SEXUAL STATUS

With this kind of information in mind it seemed appropriate to set up experiments that examined the role of olfactory cues in the initiation of male sexual interest and behavior with female partners. The following question was asked. Could female monkeys be made attractive to males by hormone treatments that did not influence either the sex skin color or proceptive behavior (sexual solicitations), and was this attractiveness communicated olfactorily? Since everyone is agreed that female attractiveness increases in the follicular phase of the cycle, when estrogens predominate, and that giving estrogen to ovariectomized females restores male sexual interest (Herbert, 1970; Phoenix, 1973), this was the hormonal manipulation selected. However, in order to avoid any actions of the hormone on the brain that enhance soliciting behavior, a very low dose of estrogen was administered directly into the female's vagina. In this way that part of the female's anatomy that most interests the male in a sexual context could be estrogenized without any effect on either sex skin coloration or sexual solicitations. Moreover, the imposition of a mesh barrier between the male and female provided a clearer assessment of the male's interest in the female since the male was obliged to work in order to gain access to the female. The work involved pressing a lever some 250 times to open a door providing access to the female (Michael and Keverne, 1968). At the time it seemed logical to assume that a male working with such dedication for access to a female had some interest in that female. Five males were trained on this schedule, and each had three ovariectomized partners, one of which received injections of estrogen to make her attractive. All males pressed for access to this female partner. Four showed little interest and rarely pressed for access to their ovariectomized partners receiving no hormone replacement. Nor did they show any sexual interest in these females when freely placed together in an open cage at a later time in the day. One male pressed for access to and mounted all his female partners and was therefore dropped from the study. There seemed little point in asking whether estrogen made the female partners of this male attractive when he already found them sufficiently attractive to initiate both his pressing for access and sexual behavior. However, of the remaining eight pairs, in which males showed no sexual interest, this idea could be tested. These ovariectomized females were now given intravaginal estradiol, and their male partners were made anosmic by the insertion of nasal plugs, which anesthetized the olfactory mucosa. In this condition these males failed to detect any change in the attractiveness of their female partners, although sexual behavior tests with normal control males clearly showed them to be attractive. On reversal of the anosmia following removal of the nasal plugs, the experimental males now pressed for access to these females for the first time and also showed mounting and ejaculation. The only novel sensory information available was olfactory, and therefore it seemed reasonable to conclude that these were the cues the males used. Hence, anosmia prevented the male from realizing that the females had become attractive. Anosmia did not, however, reduce male sexual behavior with those females made attractive by injections of estradiol, which also influences proceptive behavior and with which a great number of sexual experiences had already been obtained. It was therefore no surprise when experiments conducted some ten years later showed that anosmia in male rhesus monkeys does not alter copulatory activity (Goldfoot *et al.,* 1978), especially since these more recent studies consider only ejaculations and ejaculatory latencies. Anosmia did not alter the males' ejaculations in our studies, but it did prevent the males from recognizing the onset of female attractiveness.

Subsequent studies showed that the source of the odor cues that are attractive to males is the female vagina under the influence of estrogen (Michael and Keverne, 1970), and chemical analysis of the vaginal secretions further suggests that the odors responsible are a complex mixture of fatty acids and a number of other substances (Curtis *et al.,* 1971). It has also been stressed that the male response to applied olfactory attractants varies among individuals and is also dependent in part on the female partner with which the males are paired (Keverne, 1974, 1976).

All of these earlier studies suffered from a major methodological weakness, namely, the relatively small number of monkeys that were used and reused to demonstrate these effects. It is quite possible that these males became particularly adept at responding to odor cues and learned to attend to these particular sensory changes. However, in all studies in which females were made attractive, care was taken to avoid making such females receptive or proceptive, so that males frequently had their approaches actively refused. Since it is equally reasonable to expect males also to learn to respond appropriately to the behavioral cues of the female, their response to odor cues in this situation is all the more dramatic.

Studies involving the chemical analysis of the odors responsible for stimulating male sexual interest are generally in agreement that aliphatic acids form at least some of the constituents of vaginal secretions. However, some controversy exists as to the quantity and the capacity of a synthetic mixture of these acids to stimulate sexual behavior when a large number of males are used (Goldfoot *et al.,* 1976; Michael *et al.,* 1977). It is quite clear that this kind of detailed analysis of the chemical components of vaginal secretions will not give any indication of the perceptual qualities of the odor complex. The olfactory message is coded in terms of a patterning of neural input, each odor generating its own pattern with considerable receptor overlap among different odors. Hence, consideration of the chemical components of vaginal secretions will give no indication of the perceptual qualities of the secretion as a whole, because the neural pattern generated by each individual odor is lost in the total pattern produced by the odor complex.

VI. ODOR CUES AND BEHAVIOR IN THE SOCIAL GROUP

All of these studies using the rhesus monkey have been based on heterosexual pair tests, which do not take into account the complex social organization that plays an integral part in the mating of this species in its natural environment. Studies of this type do, however, have certain advantages, for in simplifying the social environment they maximize the conditions for demonstrating an effect. Ultimately, in order for these findings to have any biological meaning, the social context has to be broadened beyond heterosexual pair tests. This was achieved to some extent in an experiment conducted by the author on another Old World primate, the Talapoin monkey, in which members of the social group were made anosmic (Keverne, 1980). The taking away of specific sensory information has certain inherent weaknesses, and one is inevitably examining how the rest of the brain manages without this information rather than the significance of that particular sensory information itself (see Chapter 8 for a discussion of this issue). Thus, although one might not expect any remarkable change in sexual behavior as a result of anosmia, as our previous studies have already illustrated, the means by which this is achieved may well be different.

The testing situation employed for the Talapoins was somewhat different from that of the rhesus monkeys in that the cage was very much larger and could house a social group of four male and four female monkeys. For this study, however, each of the four males was initially considered alone with the group of females in the large cage, given access to them twice daily, behavioral interactions being scored from behind a one-way screen. The animals were caught and plasma samples taken twice weekly, following which behavioral interactions were not scored for at least 24 hr. All of the females were ovariectomized and given implants of estradiol, which enlarged their sexual skin swellings and made them attractive, enhancing sexual interactions. Each male's behavior with the females was compared under these hormonal conditions with the male first anosmic and then with the sense of smell normally intact. Temporary anosmia was induced for approximately 4 weeks by inserting two plugs, impregnated with bismuth iodoform paraffin paste, above the superior concha and in contact with the olfactory epithelium. The position of these plugs could be assessed radiographically and, when inserted correctly, they did not impair respiration but prevented air eddies from reaching the olfactory mucosa and also produced a local anesthetic effect. Simple olfactory discrimination tasks confirmed their effectiveness.

When each male was alone with the females, the effect of anosmia on that male's sexual behavior varied according to his previous social status. When we examine the effects of anosmia on the sexual interaction of the highest- and lowest-ranking males, we see marked changes in the females' contribution to the interaction, the differences in their behavior depending on the male. With the highest-ranking male, anosmia resulted in a reduction of ejaculations from a daily mean of six to four and, although the females increased their sexual invitations to the male when he was anosmic, they did not initiate more mounts. This would suggest that the stimulus value of female presentations had declined for this male when he was anosmic. The sexual behavior of the most subordinate male was more seriously impaired by the anosmia, with only 2 ejaculations occurring during the whole of this period compared with 24 in the same period before anosmia. Of course, this male was sexually less active than the dominant male, and the effects of anosmia were therefore more likely to influence his sexual behavior. It is interesting that the females were initiating all of this male's sexual behavior before anosmia and displaying extremely high levels of sexual invitations. With the virtual disappearance of ejaculations by this male when he became anosmic, female sexual invitations were also significantly reduced. Although the females were losing interest in this anosmic male, they were still initiating all of his mounting behavior and were displaying just as many sexual invitations as they had done to the high-ranking male.

With the social group reconstituted and now containing all four males together with the four females, sexual behavior became the prerogative of the highest-ranking male, and therefore in the social group the effects of anosmia on sexual behavior could be examined only for this male. In the presence of other males anosmia had no effect whatsoever on the ejaculatory scores of the highest-ranking male. Although there was a decrease in male-initiated mounts and an increase in those initiated by the females, this was not significant. However, the number of sexual invitations that the females made increased markedly at this time, whereas the success of these invitations in initiating a mount declined markedly. Once again, we see an increase in the females' contribution to the sexual interaction, presumably to compensate for the decrease in their stimulus value during the period that the male was anosmic.

Although there were no overall changes in sexual behavior of the alpha male when he was anosmic, it would be misleading to suggest that his behavior remained the same. His ejaculatory scores remained the same, but the manner in which he distributed them among the females changed even in this short period of anosmia. Among Talapoin monkeys most sexual behavior is observed with the higher-ranking females (Keverne *et al.*, 1978). During the period of anosmia male sexual behavior showed a tendency to decline with the high-ranking females and to increase significantly with the low-ranking females, and this trend was rapidly reversed following a return to olfactory acuity.

Anosmia in the Talapoin monkey could generally be described as having little effect on male sexual behavior. All males continued to mount and ejaculate with female partners when anosmic, although this behavior became rare in the lowest-ranking male, a result that was perhaps predictable considering the sexual sluggishness of this male. It could be argued that the presence of plugs up the nose is stressful and that any changes in sexual behavior are secondary to this discomfort. It could also be argued that the changes in male sexual performance that were observed were not directly due to a loss of olfactory sensory information influencing behavior, but indirectly caused via olfactory influences on gonadotropin release and testosterone secretion. However, in our hormone assays we found absolutely no effects of the anosmic condition on either luteinizing hormone or testosterone in either the dominant or subordinate male, and of the two stress hormones measured, prolactin and cortisol, no significant increases in concentration were seen.

Although anosmia can be described as having little effect on male sexual behavior, it would be quite misleading to relegate olfactory cues to a redundant role for sexual interaction. Sexual behavior is, after all, a social interaction, and these recent studies clearly show that, although the affliction was administered to the male, the behavior of the females in attempting to maintain the status quo cannot be overlooked. Therefore, although we see little change in the males' behavior, we witness a great deal of change in the females' behavior. They are now making a larger contribution to the sexual interaction by adopting the initiative and increasing sexual invitations. The fact that females need to increase their invitations and that the success of these invitations is decreased when the male is anosmic can be interpreted only as a loss in the stimulus value of the female. Moreover, the fact that females are increasing their proceptive behavior when their endocrine status remains unchanged illustrates the kind of plasticity in sexual behavior that is emancipated from endocrine influences.

The importance of the social dimension in the influence of olfactory cues on behavior was further illustrated with the top-ranking male. In the absence of other males, when this alpha male was not able to assert his dominance, his sexual performance was lower and the effects of anosmia produced a further decline in ejaculatory performance. In the social group, however, in the presence of competition from other males, there was no effect of anosmia on this male's ejaculation scores, and they were significantly higher than when he had been alone with the females. Moreover, although there was no overall decrease in this male's sexual behavior, the manner in which it was distributed among the females changed markedly with anosmia, the low-ranking females receiving male sexual attention for the first time. Exactly what this means is uncertain, unless it is assumed that the initial distribution of male sexual behavior to the high-ranking females is partly a result of the low-ranking females being unattractive and that this unattractiveness has something to do with their odor. Certainly, lower-ranking females are under some stress with higher levels of prolactin (Bowman *et al.,* 1978), which may affect both food and water intake and in turn gut cecotroph. Whether this affects their odor and in turn their attractiveness requires further investigation.

Taken together, these findings suggest that olfactory cues are important for sexual behavior. Although depriving the male of his sense of smell has little direct effect on ejaculation scores in the short term, the behavioral interactions that make these possible clearly change, with females having to take more of the initiative. There is no doubt, therefore, that olfactory cues tell the male something about changes in attractiveness that are dependent on endocrine status. How this information is used, however, depends on the male, presumably his past experiences, and certainly the social context in which it is perceived.

REFERENCES

Abbott, D. H., and Hearn, J. P. (1978). *J. Reprod. Fertil.* **53**, 155–166.
Abbott, D. H., McNeilly, A. S., Lunn, S. F., Hulme, M. J., and Burden, F. J. (1981). *J. Reprod. Fertil.* **63**, 335–345.
Altmann, S. A. (1959). *J. Mammal.* **40**, 317–330.
Ball, J., and Hartman, C. G. (1935). *Am. J. Obstet. Gynecol.* **29**, 117–119.
Baum, M. J., Everitt, B. J., Herbert, J., and Keverne, E. B. (1976a). *Arch. Sex. Behav.* **6**, 175–191.
Baum, M. J., Everitt, B. J., Herbert, J., and Keverne, E. B. (1976b). *Nature (London)* **263**, 606–608.
Baum, M. J., Keverne, E. B., Everitt, B. J., Herbert, J., and de Greef, W. J. (1977). *Physiol. Behav.* **18**, 659–670.
Bowman, L. A., Dilley, S. R., and Keverne, E. B. (1978). *Nature (London)* **275**, 56–59.
Charles-Dominque, P. (1977). *Z. Tierpsychol.* **43**, 113–138.
Clark, A. (1974). Ph.D. Thesis, University of Chicago.
Curtis, R. F., Ballantine, J. A., Keverne, E. B., Bonsall, R. W., and Michael, R. P. (1971). *Nature (London)* **232**, 396–398.
Czaja, J. A., and Bielert, C. (1975). *Arch. Sex. Behav.* **4**, 583–598.
Epple, G. (1967). *Folia Primatol.* **7**, 37–65.
Epple, G. (1973). *J. Reprod. Fertil., Suppl.* **19**, 447–454.
Epple, G. (1976). *In* "Mammalian Olfaction, Reproductive Processes, and Behavior" (R. L. Doty, ed.), pp. 257–282. Academic Press, New York.
Epple, G., and Moulton, D. (1978). *In* "Sensory Systems of Primates" (C. R. Noback, ed.), pp. 1–22. Plenum, New York.
Evans, C. S., and Goy, R. W. (1968). *J. Zool.* **156**, 181–197.
Everitt, B. J., Herbert, J., and Hamer, J. (1972). *Physiol. Behav.* **8**, 409–415.
Gesteland, R. C., Lettvin, J. Y., and Pitts, W. H. (1965). *J. Physiol. (London)* **181**, 525–559.
Goldfoot, D. A., Kravetz, M. A., Goy, R. W., and Freeman, S. K. (1976). *Horm. Behav.* **7**, 1–27.
Goldfoot, D. A., Essock-Vitale, S. M., Asa, C. S., Thornton, J. E., and Leshner, A. I. (1978). *Science* **199**, 1095–1096.
Harrington, J. (1974). *In* "Prosimian Biology" (R. D. Martin, G. A. Doyle, and A. C. Walker, eds.), pp. 331–346. Duckworth, Gloucester Crescent, London.
Hennessy, M. B., Coe, C. C., Mendoza, S. P., Lowe, E. L., and Levine, S. (1979). *Am. Soc. Primatol. Proc.* Seattle, Washington.
Herbert, J. (1966). *Int. Congr. Ser.—Excerpta Med.* **3**, 212.
Herbert, J. (1970). *J. Reprod. Fertil.* **11**, Suppl., 119–140.
Hisaw, F. L., and Hisaw, F. L. (1966). *Proc. Soc. Exp. Biol. Med.* **122**, 66–70.

Keverne, E. B. (1974). *New Sci.* **63**, 22–24.

Keverne, E. B. (1976). *Adv. Study Behav.* **7**, 155–200.

Keverne, E. B. (1980). *Symp. Zool. Soc. London* **45**, 313–327.

Keverne, E. B. (1982). *In* "Olfaction and Endocrine Regulations" (W. Breipohl, ed.), pp. 127–140. IRC Press, London.

Keverne, E. B., Meller, R. E., and Martinez-Arias, A. (1978). *Recent Adv. Primatol.* **1**, 533–548.

Klein, L. L. (1971). *Folia Primatol.* **15**, 233–248.

Latta, J., Hopf, S., and Ploog, D. (1967). *Primates* **8**, 229–246.

Loy, J. (1970). *Folia Primatol.* **13**, 286–296.

Michael, R. P. (1971). *In* "Frontiers in Neuroendocrinology" (L. Martini and W. F. Ganong, eds.), pp. 359–398. Oxford Univ. Press, London and New York.

Michael, R. P., and Herbert, J. H. (1963). *Science* **140**, 500–501.

Michael, R. P., and Keverne, E. B. (1968). *Nature (London)* **218**, 746–749.

Michael, R. P., and Keverne, E. B. (1970). *Nature (London)* **225**, 84–85.

Michael, R. P., and Saayman, G. (1968). *J. Endocrinol.* **41**, 231–246.

Michael, R. P., and Welegalla, J. (1968). *J. Endocrinol.* **41**, 407–420.

Michael, R. P., and Zumpe, D. (1970). *J. Reprod. Fertil.* **21**, 199–201.

Michael, R. P., Herbert, J., and Welegalla, J. (1967). *J. Endocrinol.* **39**, 81–98.

Michael, R. P., Bonsall, R. W., and Zumpe, D. (1976). *Vitam. Horm. (N.Y.)* **34**, 137–186.

Michael, R. P., Zumpe, D., Richter, M., and Bonsall, R. W. (1977). *Horm. Behav.* **9**, 296–308.

Moynihan, M. (1966). *J. Zool.* **150**, 77–127.

Phoenix, C. H. (1973). *Horm. Behav.* **4**, 365–370.

Powell, T. P. S., Cowan, W. M., and Raisman, G. (1965). *J. Anat.* **99**, 791–813.

Ravault, P.-P., and Ortavant, R. (1977). *Ann. Biol. Anim., Biochim., Biophys.* **17**, 459–473.

Schilling, A. (1970). *Mem. Mus. Natl. Hist. Nat. Ser. A, (Paris)* **61**, 203–208.

Schilling, A. (1980). *Symp. Zool. Soc. London* **45**, 165–193.

Smith, M. S., and Neill, J. D. (1976). *Endocrinology* **98**, 324–328.

Southwick, C. H., Beg, M. A., and Siddiqi, M. R. (1965). *In* "Primate Behaviour" (I. de Vore, ed.), pp. 111–159. Holt, Rinehart & Winston, New York.

Stephan, H. (1965). *Acta Anat.* **62**, 215–253.

Trimble, M. R., and Herbert, J. (1968). *J. Endocrinol.* **42**, 171–185.

Vandenbergh, J. G. (1969). *Physiol. Behav.* **4**, 261–264.

Vandenbergh, J. G., and Drickamer, L. C. (1974). *Physiol. Behav.* **13**, 373–376.

Part II

Priming Pheromones

4

Pheromonal Regulation of Puberty

John G. Vandenbergh

Department of Zoology
School of Agriculture and Life Sciences
North Carolina State University
Raleigh, North Carolina

I. INTRODUCTION

Biological systems are regulated by balancing stimulatory and inhibitory influences. For example, cellular synthesis of protein is controlled by the concerted effects of inducer and repressor molecules on DNA (Watson, 1976). At the level of the organism, motor function is achieved by balancing stimulatory signals to the target muscles with inhibitory signals, which gives form and coordination to the movement (Eccles, 1977). This chapter deals with the stimulatory and inhibitory pheromones that influence the onset of puberty and how such control over puberty can serve as a regulatory factor in the control of population density of small mammals.

Several studies have shown that the neural, endocrine, and urogenital components of the female reproductive system are present and can be activated before the spontaneous onset of puberty (Davidson, 1974; Ramaley,

PHEROMONES AND REPRODUCTION IN MAMMALS

Copyright © 1983 by Academic Press, Inc.
All rights of reproduction in any form reserved.
ISBN 0–12–710780–0

1979). The actual onset of puberty, as shown by studies using the rat, appears to be the result of hypothalamic or extrahypothalamic modulation of neural activity involving both excitatory and inhibitory pathways (Bogdanove and Schoen, 1959; Meijs-Roelofs, 1972). The notion that puberty could result as a release from inhibition grew from a series of studies showing that certain hypothalamic lesions resulted in precocial puberty in rats (Bogdanove and Schoen, 1959; Donovan and van der Werff ten Bosch, 1959; Gellert and Ganong, 1960). Excellent reviews of the neural control over puberty can be found in Davidson (1974), Donovan and van der Werff ten Bosch (1959), and Gorski (1974). For a discussion of the endocrine changes occurring during puberty and how tissue sensitivity to estradiol may be involved in its appearance, the reader should see Ramirez (1973), Ojeda *et al.* (1975), and Dudley (1981).

In this chapter I discuss the external factors acting both to stimulate and to inhibit the onset of puberty. In several cases these factors are known to be pheromones because chemical communication has been clearly identified as the mechanism influencing the timing of puberty. In other cases pheromones are only presumed to be involved by analogy or because some indirect evidence is available. I attempt to show how the interaction between stimulatory and inhibitory influences can control pubertal onset in natural populations and thus serve as a control mechanism in populations.

II. ACCELERATION OF PUBERTY IN FEMALES

Investigations of the factors causing acceleration of puberty in females have focused on the house mouse, *Mus musculus*. In this section I review these studies briefly and then discuss evidence relating to male acceleration of female puberty in other mammals.

The first evidence that the onset of puberty in the female mouse could be hastened by male stimuli was reported simultaneously by Castro (1967) and Vandenbergh (1967). These studies showed that vaginal opening and first estrus as detected by vaginal cornification occur earlier among females exposed to an adult male than among females reared in the absence of a male. For example, juvenile females exposed to an adult male reached first estrus 20 days sooner than females isolated from a male (Vandenbergh, 1967).

Soiled bedding material transferred from a male's cage to a cage housing females induces earlier puberty (Vandenbergh, 1969). Acceleration of puberty occurs to a similar degree following exposure to urine collected from adult males (Cowley and Wise, 1972; Colby and Vandenbergh, 1974; Drickamer and Murphy, 1978). Urine is remarkably effective at low levels of exposure. Solutions containing a 100-fold dilution of urine in water effectively stimulated earlier onset of puberty, but potency was lost at higher dilutions (Drickamer, 1982; Wilson *et al.,* 1980). Surprisingly, an enhanced effect was found at 10-fold dilutions of urine.

Attempts have been made to isolate from male urine the priming pheromone responsible for the acceleration of puberty. A reliable and efficient bioassay is a prerequisite to pheromone isolation attempts. The bioassay used in most of these studies is based on the uterine weight response to fractions isolated from urine or putative pheromones (Vandenbergh *et al.,* 1975). Small quantities of test substances are placed on the oronasal groove of juvenile females once per day for 8 days. On the ninth day the mice are killed and uterine weight is determined. This technique, with some modification, has been used as a reliable index of pubertal change in several studies (Bronson and Desjardins, 1974; Bronson, 1975; see Chapter 7 for a detailed review of the physiological responses of the female to priming pheromones). The uterine weight increase occurs as a consequence of estrogen production by the ovary in response to luteinizing hormone (LH) released by the pituitary. The release of LH occurs rapidly, within 20 min, after exposure to an adult male or his urine. A new and perhaps more efficient bioassay for determining pubertal onset could be developed on the basis of the finding that the subcutaneous aerolar layer of the skin rapidly increases in thickness at the onset of puberty in females (Bronson, 1979a).

The male's ability to hasten the onset of puberty in females is an androgen-dependent characteristic. Urine from juvenile males fails to accelerate puberty (Drickamer and Murphy, 1978). Within 10 to 15 days after castration the urine of the adult male loses its capacity to accelerate puberty in females. Replacement with testosterone propionate restores maximal potency within 60 hr after a single 1.0-mg dose, and a graded series of doses restores pheromonal activity in a dose-dependent fashion (Lombardi *et al.,* 1976). Similarly, urine from females, which is normally inactive, was active after the females were injected with testosterone propionate. The dependency of the urinary pheromone on androgen levels in the donor suggests that social factors having an effect on testosterone levels could control the presence of the puberty-accelerating pheromone in the donor's urine. To test this, adult males were exposed to trained fighter males for 1 week. Urine was then collected from the trained fighters (i.e., the dominant mice) and from the subordinate mice. When tested on juvenile females, only the urine of the dominant mice resulted in accelerated puberty (Lombardi and Vandenbergh, 1977). The dependence of the puberty-accelerating pheromone on social factors may be of significance in the regulation of rodent populations, a topic to be explored at greater length later in Section V.

Initial attempts to isolate active fractions of urine (Vandenbergh *et al.,*

1975) showed that the male donor has to be gonadally intact to produce the active material. The pheromone cannot withstand the heat of autoclaving and is not extractable in ether. It was present in the nondialyzable fraction after dialysis and could be precipitated by ammonium sulfate. Urine incubated with Pronase and then dialyzed loses its capacity to accelerate puberty. These results suggest that the pheromone is associated with the protein fraction of urine. This possibility is supported by the finding that the urine of mice and some other small rodents contains high levels of proteins (Parfentjev, 1932) the presence of which is androgen dependent (Thung, 1962). Subsequent chemical studies using column chromatography of male urine resulted in the isolation of an active fraction at a peak molecular weight of 860 which showed positive reactions for peptides (Vandenbergh *et al.,* 1976). Tests for the presence of steroids in this fraction were negative, suggesting that a direct catabolite of androgens is not involved but rather that androgens operate through a secondary pathway.

Attempts to purify the pheromone more precisely by using ion-exchange columns and high-performance liquid chromatography (HPLC) have been unsuccessful to date. No subfractions of the 860-dalton fraction have shown activity, and activity could not be restored after HPLC separation if all fractions were recombined. The tentative conclusion from these findings is that two or more substances may be involved and that one or more of the substances loses activity during separation. Although more progress has been made in characterizing the puberty-accelerating pheromone than any of the other priming pheromones, its identity still eludes us.

The acceleration of puberty following exposure to an adult male is only partly attributable to chemical signals from the male. Tactile cues from the male seem to contribute the remainder of the effect (Bronson and Maruniak, 1975). Exposing juvenile females to urine from a gonadally intact male results in an increase in uterine weight of approximately 50% after 54 hr, whereas exposing such females to a castrated male has no effect on uterine weight. When the treatments are combined and the juvenile females are exposed to male urine in the presence of castrated males, uterine weight increases over 100% above control weights. Drickamer (1974) exposed juvenile females to an adult male, male soiled bedding, a neonatally androgenized adult female, or a combination of these. The age of puberty was advanced most by an adult male, moderately by male soiled bedding, and not at all by a neonatally androgenized female. The combination of male soiled bedding and a neonatally androgenized female produced an effect equal to that of the adult male. These studies show that most of the acceleration of puberty seen as a result of the presence of a male can be attributed to chemical cues contained in his urine and the remainder to masculine tactile contact. In both studies it is possible that the presence of male urine could have altered the behavior of the castrated males or the androgenized females so that they delivered more potent tactile stimuli. The interpretation of the results may therefore be more complex than the investigators proposed.

Male stimuli accelerate the onset of puberty, and stimuli from other females typically inhibit rather than accelerate pubertal onset, as described in Section III. One exception to this was discovered by Drickamer and Hoover (1979). Urine from either pregnant or lactating females painted directly on the external nares of young females led to earlier puberty than did urine from isolated, nonpregnant, and nonlactating adult females. Drickamer and Hoover (1979) suggested that the presence of a puberty-accelerating pheromone in pregnant and lactating females may be due to altered hormone levels associated with these reproductive states. They speculated that the pheromone excretion may be a signal inducing other females to attain reproductive readiness at a time of favorable environmental conditions.

Although much of the initial work on puberty acceleration and inhibition was done on the house mouse, attention is now being devoted to factors influencing estrus onset and cyclicity in other taxa. Male stimulation of earlier puberty in females has been documented in a variety of mammalian species (Table I). In the first report suggesting that puberty may be accelerated by male stimuli in a primate, Epple and Katz (1980) described how juvenile female saddle-back tamarins reared with an adult male conceived at an average of 398 days compared with 631 days of age when reared with a male peer. The later maturation in the presence of the juvenile male could not be attributable entirely to his slower maturation because males reared with adult females were able to impregnate adult female cage mates at 444 days of age. It remains to be seen whether other primates more advanced on the phylogenetic scale than this relatively primitive South American primate show the male effect on female puberty.

Puberty in farm animals such as pigs and cows (Brooks and Cole, 1970; Izard and Vandenbergh, 1982) is also subject to acceleration by male stimuli. Control of pubertal onset in these species could be of considerable economic significance. In Chapter 9 Izard describes these studies in greater detail and reviews recent progress on the role of pheromones in many aspects of farm animal reproduction.

In the prairie vole, *Microtus ochrogaster,* the male provides a particularly potent stimulus for reproductive development in juvenile females (Carter *et al.,* 1980). The uteri of juvenile females doubled in weight within 2 days after only a 1-hr exposure to an adult male in comparison with the uteri of voles isolated from males. The uteri remained enlarged for at least 10 days after only such a brief experience with a male. A single drop of male urine applied once per day for 6 days to the upper lip of a female induced a

TABLE I

Mammals in Which the Onset of Puberty, as Measured by Age at First Estrus or Increases in Uterine Weight, Was Accelerated by Stimuli from an Adult Male

Species	Days advanced	Uterine weight	Male stimuli Presence	Male stimuli Urine	References
Mus musculus, house mouse	20	×2	×	×	Vandenbergh (1967), Vandenbergh, *et al.* (1975)
Rattus norvegicus, Norway rat	9	—	×	—	Vandenbergh *et al.* (1976)
Notomys alexis, hopping mouse	8	—	×	—	Breed (1976)
Peromyscus maniculatus, prairie deer mouse	—	×2	×	×	Teague and Bradley (1978)
Dicronstonyx groenlandicus, collard lemming	14	—	×	—	Hasler and Banks (1975)
Microtus orchrogaster, prairie vole	14	×2	×	×	Hasler and Nalbandov (1974), Carter *et al.* (1980)
Microtus pennsylvanicus, meadow vole	16	×4	×	×	Baddaloo and Clulow (1981)
Sus scrofa, pig	27	—	×	—	Brooks and Cole (1970)
Bos taurus, cow	—[a]	—	—	×	Izard and Vandenbergh (1982)
Saguinus fuscicollis, saddle-back tamarin	—[b]	—	×	—	Epple and Katz (1980)

[a] A higher proportion of heifers reached puberty after a fixed time of exposure to urine.
[b] Conceived 233 days earlier when reared with an adult male than when reared with a same-age male.

doubling of uterine weight. This increase is about the same as that produced by the presence of a male. Exposure to males behind a double wire mesh barrier does not accelerate puberty, indicating that direct physical contact with either the male or his urine is required.

It is possible that the accessory olfactory system is involved in the responses of the female vole to the male. A drop of urine placed on the upper lip of the juvenile female prairie vole results in remarkable neuroendocrine changes in the olfactory system (Dluzen *et al.*, 1981). The posterior half of the olfactory bulb, presumably consisting largely of the accessory olfactory bulb, shows a 54% depletion of norepinephrine and a 185% increase in LH-releasing factor within 1 hr after exposure to male urine in comparison with water-exposed controls. Associated with these neuroendocrine changes, LH levels in the blood increased significantly. Increased levels of LH were shortly followed by increased output of estrogens from the ovary and consequent uterine hypertrophy. The role of the accessory olfactory system as a receptor for priming pheromones is explored in Chapter 8.

III. INHIBITION OF PUBERTY IN FEMALES

Adaptive functioning within biological systems is often the result of a balance between stimulation and inhibition, as pointed out earlier in this chapter. The onset of puberty in many species seems to be subject to the same type of positive and negative control. We have seen how the onset of puberty can be stimulated at an early age in many species by social stimuli from the opposite sex. Often these stimuli have proved to be pheromones. In this section I examine our current knowledge of the social factors inhibiting puberty in female mice. As in studies of puberty acceleration the majority of the work has focused on house mice, but more recently several other species have come under examination (Table I).

Comparing the mean ages of pubertal onset when females are reared in groups of four to six with those of females reared in the absence of other females (Table II) reveals that the onset of puberty in females can be delayed by the presence of other females. The inhibitory effect of having female cage mates is clearly seen whether or not male stimuli are present.

Drickamer and colleagues conducted an extensive series of studies to determine the cues involved in puberty suppression. First, it was found that bedding material soiled by grouped female mice inhibits puberty in isolated juveniles (Drickamer, 1974). In a follow-up study McIntosh and Drickamer (1977) demonstrated that externally collected urine from females living in a group inhibits puberty, but urine from isolated females has no significant effect on the timing of puberty. Urine from grouped females results in a delay of 4 to 5 days in the onset of first estrus. The magnitude of the suppressive effect remains even at doses of urine as low as 0.001 ml/day applied to the external nares (Drickamer, 1982).

TABLE II

Effect of the Presence of a Male on the Mean Age of First Estrus of Females Housed Singly or in Groups of Six

	Age of first estrus (days ± SE)		
	Male present	Male absent	Reference
Single female	28.0 ± 0.6	35.9 ± 1.0	Vandenbergh et al. (1972)
Grouped females			
Replicate 1	35.7 ± 1.8	55.1 ± 1.7	Vandenbergh (1969)
Replicate 2	39.6 ± 0.6	54.6 ± 2.9	Vandenbergh (1969)

McIntosh and Drickamer (1977) also tested the effect of urine collected directly from the bladder of either grouped or isolated females. A comparison of results obtained from bladder versus externally collected urine would reveal whether an accessory organ downstream from the bladder was contributing the inhibitory substance. The results were quite clear but far from what was expected.

When collected from the bladders of either grouped or isolated females, urine was equally potent in suppressing puberty. However, when collected externally only the urine from grouped females was effective. This finding leads to the unexpected conclusion that the female mouse produces a puberty-inhibiting substance in her urine whether grouped or isolated. When the female is isolated, however, something downstream from the bladder either removes or inactivates the inhibitory substance or provides some chemical that blocks its action. The urethra is not known to resorb materials (Smith, 1956), so it seems most likely that something that blocks the action of the inhibitory pheromone is secreted into the urine as it flows through the urethra.

Experimental evidence has been provided by McIntosh and Drickamer (1977) that the urethra or its glandular structures could be secreting a blocking substance. They collected excreted urine from grouped and isolated female mice and mixed a portion of each kind of urine with homogenized urethras taken from either grouped or isolated females. The urethral homogenate blocked the puberty-inhibiting effect if the urethras were taken from isolated females but was without effect if the urethras were taken from grouped females. This finding suggests that some aspect of grouping prevents a presumed blocking agent from appearing in the urethra or alternatively that isolation induces the appearance of a blocking agent. A reasonable assumption to draw from these findings is that endocrine changes occurring as a result of grouping control the production of the putative blocking agent. The possible influence of the ovary was investigated first (Drickamer et al., 1978). The wall of the rodent urethra contains glands called Littre's glands, which are considered to be homologous to the prostate gland of the male (Shehata, 1974, 1980). Since prostate tissue is responsive to steroid hormones it is not unlikely that the urethral glandular tissue of the female also responds to steroid hormones. Ovariectomy did not affect the potency of either bladder or excreted urine in inhibiting puberty of juveniles if the donor females were grouped. If the donor females were isolated, only the bladder urine contained a puberty-inhibiting pheromone. These results are identical to those obtained from gonadally intact females.

After eliminating the ovary as a gland controlling the appearance of an inhibitory pheromone in the excreted urine of grouped females, Drickamer and McIntosh (1980) next examined the possible role of the adrenal glands. This set of experiments yielded more positive findings. Adrenalectomy abolished the inhibitory effect of excreted urine from grouped females, but it did not affect the capacity of the urethra to block the pheromone in isolated females. It seems that the production of the inhibitory pheromone is under adrenal control but that the adrenal does not influence the gating mechanism at the urethra.

The findings to date on how the puberty-inhibiting pheromone is controlled endocrinologically are as perplexing as they are fascinating. From the original finding that grouping was necessary to induce the appearance of an inhibitory pheromone in female urine, one could readily assume that the ovaries and adrenal glands are involved because of the relationship between the ovaries and the suppression of ovulation in groups (Whitten, 1959) and because of the known involvement of the adrenal glands in the response to social stress (Christian, 1971). Yet neither of these organs appear to be crucial since ovariectomy is without influence on puberty inhibition and adrenalectomy affects only the primary production of the inhibitory pheromone, not the gate that releases it at the urethral level. McIntosh and Drickamer (1977) opened an intriguing line of inquiry when they compared the effects of excreted urine and bladder urine on puberty in juvenile females. Although our understanding of the mechanism controlling the production and release of the inhibitory pheromone is not complete, at least we know that it involves a complex of interactions involving stimuli within a group, the adrenals, urine, and perhaps urethral glands.

Evidence that females can suppress the onset of puberty is available from other rodent species and two callitrichid primates (Table III). Abbott and Hearn (1978) showed that when the marmoset *Callithrix jacchus* was reared in peer groups, only the dominant female became pregnant. The onset of puberty (i.e., ovulation) was suppressed in the subordinate females. In the related saddle-back tamarin, young subordinate females living in a family group with their dominant mothers failed to show ovarian cyclicity for a 3-month period, as measured by excretion of urinary estrogen (Katz and Epple, 1980). The mothers showed a major peak of urinary estradiol levels at approximately 18-day intervals. When the subordinate females were removed from their family groups and paired with an adult, vasectomized male, their urinary estradiol levels rose rapidly and regular cyclicity appeared for the first time. Work is now in progress by Epple and associates to determine whether olfactory signals from dominant females contribute to the suppression of puberty in this species.

A similar suppression of sexual maturation and breeding activity occurs in gerbil females caged with their mothers (Payman and Swanson, 1980). In the case of the gerbil the suppressive effect of the mother is present only

TABLE III

Mammals in Which the Onset of Puberty Is Suppressed by Stimuli from Adult Females

| Species | Measure of puberty | Female | | References |
		Presence	Urine	
Mus musculus, house mouse	First estrus delayed 5 days	×	—	Vandenbergh *et al.* (1972), Cowley and Wise (1972) McIntosh and Drickamer (1977)
Peromyscus maniculatus, prairie deer mouse	Vaginal perforation delayed at 40 days of age	—	×	Lombardi and Whitsett (1980)
Notomys alexis, hopping mouse	First estrus delayed 25 days	×	—	Breed (1976)
Callithrix jacchus, common marmoset	Suppression of ovulation in subordinate females	×	—	Abbott and Hearn (1978)
Saguinus fuscicollis, saddle-back tamarin	Suppression of ovulation in daughters	×	—	Katz and Epple (1980)
Meriones unguiculatus, Mongolian gerbil	Suppression of breeding in daughters	×	—	Payman and Swanson (1980)

while she is lactating and rearing a second litter. A nonpregnant mother or a mother whose second litter is removed is without effect on sexual maturation of her daughters. This finding contrasts with the report of Drickamer and Hoover (1979) that urine from nonlactating or pregnant female house mice induces accelerated pubertal onset in juveniles. The two studies are not directly comparable since Drickamer and Hoover (1979) were not testing the effects of the adult female on her own offspring. Individual or familial recognition could be playing a role in the sexual maturation of gerbils and perhaps of the marmosets discussed earlier. Little work has been done on the interaction between chemical cues involved in individual recognition and those involved in priming effects.

IV. CONTROL OF PUBERTY IN MALES

Considerably less is known about the susceptibility of puberty in male mice to control by social stimuli. A few studies suggest, however, that stimuli from adults of either sex can influence the rate of sexual maturation in males. Male mice reared with a female show more rapid growth of the testes and epididymides at 37 days of age than mice reared in isolation or in a group of males (Fox, 1968). In comparing the effect of the presence of an adult male with the effect of the presence of an adult female on sexual maturation in male mice, Vandenbergh (1971) replicated the finding of Fox (1968) and further showed that the presence of an adult male inhibits testicular and accessory gland development. In more recent work cohabitation of adult female mice with juvenile males was shown to inhibit seminal vesicle growth in the young males (Svare et al., 1978). In this study the females were very aggressive toward the juvenile males; 23 of 30 males were severely wounded. This contrasts with the pacific nature of the interactions in the Vandenbergh (1971) study. Support for the importance of aggression in explaining this difference is provided by the study of Svare et al. (1978). When they confined the adult female stimulus animal behind a wire mesh barrier, the juvenile males showed accelerated growth of their seminal vesicles. This finding suggests that the cue causing accelerated puberty in males may be chemical.

In a study in which the effects of an adult female were contrasted with those of an adult male mouse, Vandenbergh (1971) found that female stimuli were generally acceleratory and male stimuli were generally inhibitory on the sexual development of juvenile males. The effect of adult male or female presence from weaning was measured at 36, 48, 60, and 78 days of age. The presence of a female stimulated more rapid testicular and seminal vesicle development. The stimulatory effect attributable to the female disappeared by 78 days. The presence of the adult male produced an inhibition of the development of these reproductive organs, but the effect was delayed, being most prominent at 78 days of age. The inhibitory effect of the male was also found by McKinney and Desjardins (1973). Exposing juvenile male mice to adult males from weaning to 48 days of age resulted in a reduction in spermatogenesis, reduced seminal vesicle and preputial gland weights, and reduced concentrations of seminal vesicle fructose and plasma androgens. Castration of adults eliminated their ability to suppress development of juvenile males.

As in the house mouse, puberty in male prairie deer mice can be inhibited by cohabitation with other males (Bediz and Whitsett, 1979). Groups of males of the same age showed lower seminal vesicle weights in comparison with isolated males or males reared with an adult female. The presence of a female did not have a statistically significant effect on the reproductive development of the male. Chemical communication may be involved in the inhibition observed with grouping of males (Lawton and Whitsett, 1979). The growth of seminal vesicles in juvenile prairie deer mice was retarded by exposure to bedding material soiled by adult males or by the direct application of urine collected from adult males. Fur·hermore, removal of the olfactory bulbs of the juvenile males blocked the inhibitory effect of male urine on sexual maturation. Olfactory stimuli may also be involved in the control of male sexual development in the common vole, *Microtus arvalis* (Lecyk, 1967). Voles reared for 40 days adjacent to cages containing dense groups of adult males showed inhibited testicular development.

V. INFLUENCES ON POPULATION DYNAMICS

The complex of factors controlling the density of animal populations has long fascinated investigators, and many aspects of the problem have received observational and experimental attention (Andewartha and Birch, 1954; Wynn-Edwards, 1965). Among mammals, population dynamics of small, rapidly breeding rodents have been scrutinized with greatest intensity (Bronson, 1979b; Chitty, 1967; Christian and Davis, 1964; Drickamer, 1981c). From these studies two explanations of how populations are regulated have emerged that are particularly relevant to this discussion of pheromonal control of puberty.

The first of these proposed explanations is that populations of small, rapidly breeding rodents are regulated through short-term genetic mechanisms. Selection over just a few generations can produce a behavioral phenotype showing higher levels of aggressive behavior (Chitty, 1967) or changes involving the spacing and dispersal patterns of animals (Krebs *et al.*, 1973).

Such rapid changes in genetic makeup within a population would have a powerful influence on population dynamics if they were shown to modify the onset of puberty in females or the susceptibility of pubertal mechanisms to environmental modification. That this may actually be the case is suggested by two studies.

Laboratory mice of the ICR strain were selected for early and late vaginal estrus (Drickamer, 1981b). Compared with a randomly bred control line, females selected for early sexual maturation reached puberty at 27 to 28 days of age after six generations. Females selected for slow sexual maturation attained puberty at 47 to 48 days of age. The rate of change for both early- and late-maturing lines was most rapid for the first three generations. Thus, short-term selection, perhaps in only three generations, can accelerate or slow sexual maturation significantly.

Mice from such early- and late-maturing lines were then used for experiments to test whether they retained their ability to respond to pheromonal or other social cues (Drickamer, 1981a). Among fast-maturing females the presence of an adult male or urine from adult males could not further accelerate puberty, but the presence of grouped females or urine from grouped females could inhibit the onset of puberty. Conversely, the onset of puberty in slow-maturing females could be accelerated by male stimuli, but these females were no longer susceptible to the inhibitory stimuli of grouped females. These results suggest that selection can produce females maturing at both ends of the range of pubertal onset for this species. Once at the genetic limit, either at the slow or rapid end of the spectrum, social factors cannot extend the range but can only bring the selected lines closer to the original time of puberty for the parent stock.

The second relevant explanation of how rodent populations are regulated posits that density-dependent social factors can accelerate or slow population growth through influences on reproductive functions (Christian *et al.,* 1965). As populations increase, agonistic interactions alter adrenal and gonadal activity, resulting in decreased reproductive performance (Christian, 1971). Chemical signals provide one means of communication among the individuals in a population. The priming pheromones I have discussed in this chapter and those discussed in Chapters 5 and 6 could serve important regulatory functions in populations. Several others have explored this notion (Bronson, 1979b; Drickamer, 1981c; Rogers and Beauchamp, 1976; Terman, 1968), but here I focus specifically on pheromonal control of puberty.

Stimulatory and inhibitory pheromonal influences on puberty in animals living in a population cannot be examined separately since undoubtedly all members of a population are exposed to urine deposited by both males and females. One signal could overwhelm the other, or the two could be balanced in their acceleratory and suppressive effects. Fortunately, a recent study helps to clarify the interaction between male and female urinary signals (Drickamer, 1982). Juvenile female mice exposed to urine from grouped adult females or to a mixture of urine from adult males and females all showed delayed onset of puberty in comparison with juvenile females exposed to male urine. Similarly, when test juveniles are exposed to urine of grouped adult females mixed with urine from pregnant and lactating females, which is an acceleratory signal (Drickamer and Hoover, 1979), the suppressive effect of the grouped female urine overpowers the acceleratory signal. Thus, in every test the inhibitory effect of the urine from grouped females takes precedence over urine sources that stimulate puberty.

The sensitivity of maturing female mice to an inhibitory pheromone from grouped females even in the presence of acceleratory signals from the male suggests that inhibition of puberty may play an important role in modulating population growth. A test of the possibility that puberty-modulating pheromones play a role in the regulation of natural populations was made by Massey and Vandenbergh (1980, 1981). Segments of highway cloverleafs, termed "highway islands," of about one-third hectare in size were populated with eight male–female pairs of wild house mice that had been born and reared in the laboratory. All mice were marked for individual identification. The number of mice on one highway island grew rapidly to reach about 75 individuals. The second population failed to increase even though some breeding did occur. Urine was collected from females trapped from both populations when the populations were at their seasonal high and low levels. The urine was then tested in the laboratory to determine whether it was capable of influencing the onset of puberty in juvenile albino mice (Massey and Vandenbergh, 1980). Only urine collected from females in the dense population when it was at its maximum density delayed puberty in test females. Urine collected when the population was at a low level or from females in the population that remained sparse failed to inhibit puberty.

Urine was also collected from male mice when the populations were at high and low densities (Massey and Vandenbergh, 1981). All urine collected from adult males in the populations induced accelerated pubertal onset among test females in the laboratory.

These results from studies of wild populations of house mice on highway islands suggest that the female's ability to inhibit the onset of puberty in juvenile females is density dependent, whereas the stimulatory effect of the male is independent of density. The fact that inhibitory influences of the female can override the stimulatory influences of the male (Drickamer, 1982) supports the suggestion that such density-dependent inhibitory influences can play an important role in the population dynamics of house mice and

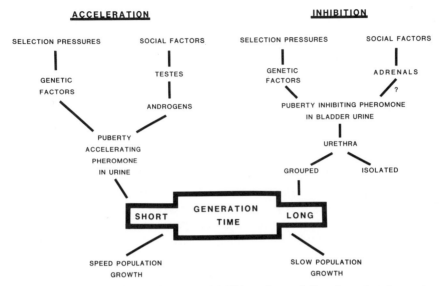

Fig. 1. Diagram of the acceleratory and inhibitory factors influencing pubertal onset in house mice. Early or late puberty can alter generation time, which can strongly influence population dynamics.

perhaps other species. A diagram showing how stimulatory and inhibitory influences on puberty can affect population growth and decline is presented in Fig. 1. Generation time is a very important parameter in the regulation of populations (Cole, 1954; Emlen, 1973; Pianka, 1974). As shown in Fig. 1 complex regulatory mechanisms exist involving pheromonal stimuli to influence this important parameter of population growth. An interaction between these pheromonal mechanisms and the known susceptibility of puberty in female mice to genetic manipulation (Drickamer, 1981b) provides a powerful control mechanism over generation time. Additional discussions of how pheromonal and other social factors can influence population regulation in house mice are given by Bronson (1979b) and Drickamer (1981c).

VI. CONCLUSIONS

Puberty, like many other biological functions, occurs as a result of stimulatory and inhibitory factors. Prominent among these factors in rodents and a few other animals are priming pheromones. Adult males excrete an androgen-dependent priming pheromone in their urine that accelerates the onset of puberty in females. Females, when housed in groups, produce a urinary pheromone that delays the onset of puberty in other females. These pheromones, particularly the puberty-inhibiting pheromone, may be important in the regulation of natural populations of small, rapidly breeding rodents. Both stimulatory and inhibitory pheromone systems involve complex interactions between behavior and hormones. Such complexity in the control system makes it susceptible to several checks and balances by environmental and genetic factors.

Although a considerable amount of information has been gathered on the pheromonal control of puberty since the male acceleratory effect was discovered in 1967, many important questions remain unanswered. As yet none of the priming pheromones involved has been specifically identified. Until this is achieved it will not be possible to determine whether the same or similar substances are involved with puberty acceleration, estrus synchronization, and pregnancy blockage. The possible supportive interactions between signalling and priming pheromones have not yet received experimental scrutiny. It seems reasonable to suppose that the attractants and repellants described in Chapter 1 and elsewhere can work in concert with priming pheromones to promote successful reproduction. Finally, considerably more work must be done to determine if priming pheromones play an important role in natural populations of mice and other species. To date only one study involving two populations has shown that puberty-controlling pheromones can be involved in population dynamics. That is hardly sufficient to provide the information we need to understand the role played by pheromones in the dynamics of mammalian populations.

REFERENCES

Abbott, D. H., and Hearn, J. P. (1978). *J. Reprod. Fertil.* **53**, 155–166.
Andrewartha, H. G., and Birch, L. C. (1954). "The Distribution and Abundance of Animals." Univ. of Chicago Press, Chicago, Illinois.
Baddaloo, E. G. Y., and Clulow, F. V. (1981). *Can. J. Zool.* **59**, 415–421.
Bediz, G. M., and Whitsett, J. M. (1979). *J. Comp. Physiol. Psychol.* **93**, 493–500.
Bogdanove, E. M., and Schoen, H. C. (1959). *Proc. Soc. Exp. Biol. Med.* **100**, 664–669.
Breed, W. G. (1976). *J. Reprod. Fertil.* **47**, 395–397.
Bronson, F. H. (1975). *Endocrinology* **96**, 511–514.
Bronson, F. H. (1979a). *Nature (London)* **281**, 301–302.
Bronson, F. H. (1979b). *Q. Rev. Biol.* **54**, 265–299.
Bronson, F. H., and Desjardins, C. (1974). *Endocrinology* **94**, 1658–1668.
Bronson, F. H., and Maruniak, J. A. (1975). *Biol. Reprod.* **13**, 94–98.
Brooks, P. H., and Cole, D. J. A. (1970). *J. Reprod. Fertil.* **23**, 435–440.
Carter, C. S., Getz, L. L., Gavish, L., McDermott, J. L., and Arnold, P. (1980). *Biol. Reprod.* **23**, 1038–1045.
Castro, B. M. (1967). *An. Acad. Bras. Cienc.* **39**, 289–291.
Chitty, D. (1967). *Proc. Ecol. Soc. Aust.* **2**, 51–78.

Christian, J. J. (1971). *Biol. Reprod.* **4**, 248–294.
Christian, J. J., and Davis, D. E. (1964). *Science* **146**, 1550–1560.
Christian J. J., Lloyd, J. A., and Davis, D. E. (1965). *Recent Prog. Horm. Res.* **21**, 501–578.
Colby, D. R., and Vandenbergh, J. G. (1974). *Biol. Reprod.* **11**, 268–279.
Cole, L. C. (1954). *Q. Rev. Biol.* **29**, 103–137.
Cowley, J. J., and Wise, D. R. (1972). *Anim. Behav.* **20**, 499–506.
Davidson, J. M. (1974). *In* "Control of the Onset of Puberty" (M. M. Grumbach, G. D. Grave, and F. E. Mayer, eds.), pp. 79–103. Wiley, New York.
Dulzen, D. E., Ramirez, V. D., Carter, C. S., and Getz, L. L. (1981). *Science* **212**, 573–575.
Donovan, B. T., and van der Werff ten Bosch, J. J. (1959). *J. Physiol. (London)* **147**, 78–92.
Drickamer, L. C. (1974). *Dev. Psychobiol.* **7**, 257–265.
Drickamer, L. C. (1981a). *Behav. Neural Biol.* **31**, 82–89.
Drickamer, L. C. (1981b). *J. Reprod. Fertil.* **63**, 325–329.
Drickamer, L. C. (1981c). *In* "Environmental Factors in Mammalian Reproduction" (D. Gilmore and B. Cook, eds.), pp. 100–111. Macmillan & Co., London.
Drickamer, L. C. (1982). *Anim. Behav.* **30**, 456–460.
Drickamer, L. C., and Hoover, J. E. (1979). *Dev. Psychobiol.* **12**, 545–551.
Drickamer, L. C., and McIntosh, T. K. (1980). *Horm. Behav.* **14**, 146–152.
Drickamer, L. C., and Murphy, R. X., Jr. (1978). *Dev. Psychobiol.* **11**, 63–72.
Drickamer, L. C., McIntosh, T. K., and Rose, E. A. (1978). *Horm. Behav.* **11**, 131–137.
Dudley, S. D. (1981). *Neurosci. Biobehav. Rev.* **5**, 421–435.
Eccles, J. C. (1977). "The Understanding of the Brain." McGraw-Hill, New York.
Emlen, J. M. (1973). "Ecology: An Evolutionary Approach." Addison-Wesley, Reading, Massachusetts.
Epple, G., and Katz, Y. (1980). *Int. Primatol.* **1**, 171–183.
Fox, K. A. (1968). *J. Reprod. Fertil.* **17**, 75–85.
Gellert, R. J., and Ganong, W. F. (1960). *Acta Endocrinol.* **33**, 569–576.
Gorski, R. A. (1974). *In* "Control of the Onset of Puberty" (M. M. Grumbach, G. D. Grave, and F. E. Mayer, eds.), pp. 182–207. Wiley, New York.
Hasler, J. F., and Banks, E. M. (1975). *J. Reprod. Fertil.* **42**, 583–586.
Hasler, M. J., and Nalbandov, A. V. (1974). *Gen. Comp. Endocrinol.* **23**, 237–238.
Izard, M. K., and Vandenbergh, J. G. (1982). *J. Anim. Sci.* **55**, 1160–1168.
Katz, Y., and Epple, G. (1980). *Proc. Int. Congr. Primatol., 8th, 1980* p. 219.
Krebs, C. J., Gaines, M. S., Keller, B. L., Myers, J. H., and Tamarin, R. H. (1973). *Science* **179**, 35–41.
Lawton, A. D., and Whitsett, J. M. (1979). *Horm. Behav.* **13**, 128–138.
Lecyk, M. (1967). *Acta Theriol.* **12**, 177–179.
Lombardi, J. R., and Vandenbergh, J. G. (1977). *Science* **196**, 545–546.
Lombardi, J. R., and Whitsett, J. M. (1980). *J. Mammal.* **61**, 766–768.
Lombardi, J. R., Vandenbergh, J. G., and Whitsett, J. M. (1976). *Biol. Reprod.* **15**, 179–186.
McIntosh, T. K., and Drickamer, L. C. (1977). *Anim. Behav.* **25**, 999–1004.
McKinney, T. D., and Desjardins, C. (1973) *Biol. Reprod.* **9**, 279–294.
Massey, A., and Vandenbergh, J. G. (1980). *Science* **209**, 821–822.
Massey, A., and Vandenbergh, J. G. (1981). *Biol. Reprod.* **24**, 523–527.
Meijs-Roelofs, H. M. A. (1972). *J. Endocrinol.* **54**, 277–284.
Ojeda, S. R., Kalra, P. S., and McCann, S. M. (1975). *Neuroendocrinology* **18**, 242–255.
Parfentjev, I. A. (1932). *Proc. Soc. Exp. Biol. Med.* **29**, 1285–1286.
Payman, B. C., and Swanson, H. H. (1980). *Anim. Behav.* **28**, 528–535.
Pianka, E. R. (1974). "Evolutionary Ecology." Harper & Row, New York.
Ramaley, J. A. (1979). *Biol. Reprod.* **20**, 1–39.
Ramirez, V. D. (1973). *In* "Handbook of Physiology, Sec. 7: Endocrinology" (R. O. Greep,

E. B. Astwood and S. R. Geiger, eds.), Vol. II, pp. 1–28. Amer. Physiol. Soc., Washington, D.C.

Rogers, J. G., and Beauchamp. G. K. (1976). *J. Mammal.* **57**, 320–330.

Shehata, R. (1974). *Acta Anat.* **90**, 381–387.

Shehata, R. (1980). *Acta Anat.* **107**, 286–288.

Smith, H. W. (1956). "Principles of Renal Physiology." Oxford Univ. Press, London and New York.

Svare, B., Bartke, A., and Macrides, F. (1978). *Physiol. Behav.* **21**, 1009–1013.

Teague, L. G., and Bradley, E. L. (1978). *Biol. Reprod.* **19**, 314–317.

Terman, C. R. (1968). *Ecology* **49**, 1169–1172.

Thung, P. J. (1962). *Acta Physiol. Pharmacol. Neerl.* **10**, 248–261.

Vandenbergh, J. G. (1967). *Endocrinology* **81**, 345–349.

Vandenbergh, J. G. (1969). *Endocrinology* **84**, 658–660.

Vandenbergh, J. G. (1971). *J. Reprod. Fertil.* **24**, 383–390.

Vandenbergh, J. G. (1976). *J. Reprod. Fert.* **46**, 451–453.

Vandenbergh, J. G., Drickamer, L. C., and Colby, D. R. (1972). *J. Reprod. Fertil.* **28**, 397–405.

Vandenbergh, J. G., Whitsett, J. M., and Lombardi, J. R. (1975). *J. Reprod. Fertil.* **43**, 515–523.

Vandenbergh, J. G., Finlayson, J. S., Dobrogosz, W. J., Dills, S. S., and Kost, T. A. (1976). *Biol. Reprod.* **15**, 260–265.

Watson, J. D. (1976). "Molecular Biology of the Gene," 3rd ed. Benjamin, Menlo Park, California.

Whitten, W. K. (1959). *J. Endocrinol.* **18**, 102–107.

Wilson, M. C., Beamer, W. G., and Whitten, W. K. (1980). *Biol. Reprod.* **22**, 864–872.

Wynne-Edwards, V. C. (1965). *Science* **147**, 1543–1547.

5

Pheromonal Regulation of the Ovarian Cycle: Enhancement, Suppression, and Synchrony

Martha K. McClintock

Department of Behavioral Sciences
University of Chicago
Chicago, Illinois

I. INTRODUCTION: THE PROBLEM

Timing is the essence of reproduction; the cost of mistimed reproductive events is often so high that a reproductive system cannot be described adequately without considering the factors that regulate its timing. This is particularly true for female mammals that ovulate spontaneously. If a female

113

PHEROMONES AND REPRODUCTION IN MAMMALS
Copyright © 1983 by Academic Press, Inc.
All rights of reproduction in any form reserved.
ISBN 0-12-710780-0

ovulates and becomes fertile at a time when she cannot conceive, she must wait at least one ovarian cycle before she will have a second opportunity for conception. The timing of conception is even more critical, since the cost of a mistimed pregnancy that results in the loss of offspring represents the waste of a substantially greater investment of energy and time.

Females can use signals from other females and from males to help them coordinate reproductive events with an appropriate social or physical environment. In some species it may be advantageous for a female to conceive and then to give birth in synchrony with other females because it can increase the opportunity for cooperative care of the young, as in the dwarf mongoose (*Helogale parvula*; Rood, 1978). It can also increase parental investment by males (Ralls, 1977; Knowlton, 1979). On the other hand, a female that is not in a social position to control limited resources may benefit by responding to cues from more dominant females and delaying or suppressing her own fertility until she has access to the resources that are necessary to support a full-term pregnancy, lactation, and care for her young. Using signals from reproductively active males ensures that fertile periods and mating will be coordinated with their presence and diminishes the chance of wasting energy by maintaining fertility when there is no opportunity for conception (Anderson, 1969).

Furthermore, social signals that reflect the reproductive state of other females and males can provide information about resources in the physical environment. Although each individual may respond to the physical environment directly, social signals can supplement individual information and provide a more accurate picture of the physical environment than any one individual could achieve alone (Emlen and Demong, 1975; Kiester and Slatkin, 1974).

This chapter focuses on pheromones as social signals that regulate the timing of fertility in females and is limited to mammalian species that have spontaneous ovarian cycles. Both female and male pheromones are evaluated as mechanisms for the enhancement, suppression, and synchronization of ovarian cycles. When data permit, the hormonal responses to these pheromones are discussed in an effort to identify the mechanisms by which pheromones regulate the timing of the ovarian cycle.

II. ENHANCEMENT AND SUPPRESSION
OF THE OVARIAN CYCLE

A. The Ovarian Cycle

The ovarian cycle represents a sequence of events that repeats itself spontaneously: follicular development, ovulation, and formation of the corpus luteum. Although the duration of each event in the sequence is not the same in each species, the sequence in the cycle is always the same (Fig. 1). Because this sequence repeats itself spontaneously and regularly, an ovarian cycle can be thought of as a simple clock or oscillator (as defined by Campbell, 1964). Ovulation marks the beginning of each cycle (phase $\phi° = 0$), and the length of the ovarian cycle or interval between successive ovulations corresponds to the period (τ) of the clock. Events that phase shift the cycle advance or delay the time of ovulation and thus change the length of the cycle in which the phase shift occurred.

Both social and physical events can alter the endogenous rhythm of the ovarian cycle. Nonetheless, by convention, the "normal" cycle length is considered to be that of a female living by herself in a laboratory, even though this is a highly artificial condition, far removed from the environments in which the ovarian cycle evolved.

It is possible to study pheromonal regulation of the ovarian cycle in the young adult rat by measuring the cyclic changes of the vaginal epithelium. Changes in the exfoliated cells found in a vaginal smear indicate changes in ovarian events and signify the occurrence of ovulation (Schwartz, 1964; Weick et al., 1971); these changes in the vaginal smear are rarely found during an anovulatory cycle (Bingel and Schwartz, 1969a). Estrogen produces a vaginal smear with cornified cells, indicating follicular activity (Nequin et al., 1979). The appearance of leukocytic cells in the smear is associated with progesterone, indicating luteal activity (Parkes, 1929). The transition between vaginal smears with these two types of cells is indicative of ovulation as well (Schwartz, 1973; Lamond, 1959). Therefore, a change in the proportion of smear types within a cycle can indicate which phase of the ovarian cycle is being lengthened or shortened by social odors.

Pheromones that modulate the length of the ovarian cycle by changing the timing of the endogenous oscillator are changing the timing of ovulation. This can be accomplished in three ways. (*a*) The time for follicular development can either be lengthened or shortened. (*b*) Once the follicles are mature, the time of ovulation itself can be delayed or advanced. (*c*) The life span of the corpus luteum can be lengthened or shortened. A social signal that can bring about any of these changes will alter the length of the ovarian cycle, phase shift the time of ovulation, and potentially serve to enhance, suppress, or synchronize the ovarian cycle.

B. Enhancement

There are several species in which the ovarian cycle is enhanced when a female lives in an all-female group; the cycle is consistently shortened and the rate of ovulation is thereby increased. However, many of the reported responses are weak and variable, probably because living in a group provides a mixture of signals that have different and opposing effects. For example, in the guinea pig (*Cavia porcellus;* Jesel and Aron, 1974), the net effect of living in a female group is a decrease in the time of vaginal closure (i.e., shorter luteal and early follicular phases; see Fig. 1); the estrous cycle is shorter. This effect of group living can be mimicked solely by exposing females to female urine, particularly urine that is collected at the time of vaginal opening (during the late follicular and ovulatory phases). Urine collected from the first 7 days of vaginal closure (during the functional luteal phase) does not affect cycle length (Jesel and Aron, 1974, 1976). It is not yet known whether the shortened cycle represents a shorter life span of the corpus luteum or a shortened time for follicular development, although there is a tendency for shorter estrous cycles to correlate with a smaller number of corpora lutea. This trend suggests that the net effect of late follicular and ovulatory urine is a reduction in corpus luteum function. In addition, urine from different phases of the cycle can have opposing effects on the number of ova that are ovulated. Urine from the late follicular and ovulatory phases decreases the number of ova shed, whereas urine from the luteal phase increases the number (Jesel and Aron, 1976). Thus, different estrous cycle odors may differentially affect both the life span of the corpus luteum and the probability of ovulation.

Female Wistar rats (*Rattus norvegicus*) that have been socially isolated

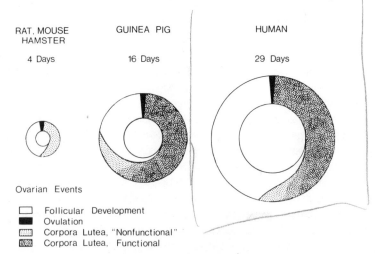

Fig. 1.   Species difference in ovarian cycle length is indicated by the diameter of the circle. The duration of each ovarian cycle event is indicated by the proportion of the circle occupied by that event. Proceeding clockwise, note that there are also species differences in the extent to which follicular development is concurrent with luteal function. Nonetheless, the follicular phase begins once the corpus luteum has regressed even though the onset of follicular development may occur during the luteal phase. These schematic cycles are drawn from data presented in Everett (1961), Nequin *et al.* (1979), Smith *et al.* (1975), and Yen and Jaffee (1978).

from weaning (1.5 months) to adulthood (4 months) usually have estrous cycles that are 5 days long (Aron, 1973). When such females live in all-female groups, 50% of them have shortened estrous cycles (Roser and Chateau, 1974), and the incidence of regular 4-day cycles is increased. This effect of group living can be mimicked by exposing females to female urine (Aron, 1973). However, female urine was reported to enhance only the estrous cycles of postpubescent females that had been isolated from conspecific female odors and not the cycles of females that had been raised in groups in the colony (Aron, 1979). Again, the female urine may have been a weak stimulus because it was collected from all phases of the estrous cycle and pooled, and may therefore have contained a mixture of different signals.

In the Sprague–Dawley rat, group living does shorten the estrous cycles of adult females that have always lived in a colony room (McClintock, 1981). Therefore, the effectiveness of a mixed signal is not restricted to females that have been isolated from conspecific odors. Even though odors from the follicular phase shorten the cycle and odors from the ovulatory phase lengthen it (McClintock, 1983a; see Section III,B,1), the net effect of group living in this species is biased toward a shortened cycle length. This is consistent with the observation that follicular odors produce a greater change in cycle length than ovulatory odors do (McClintock, 1983a; see Section III,B,1) and suggests that the cycles of adult Wistar rats might also be shortened if urine were collected only during the follicular phase.

In Wistar rats, the females that respond to social signals with a shortened, 4-day estrous cycle also have significantly lower ovarian progesterone secretion during the luteal phase (metestrus and diestrus I). Thus, while social signals in the rat enhance follicular growth and shorten the cycle (Chateau *et al.,* 1974), they do so by suppressing corpus luteum function and shortening its life span (Aron *et al.,* 1969; Roser and Chateau, 1974; Gay *et al.,* 1970). Although a functional corpus luteum is necessary for successful implantation of the blastula, the female rat can rely on the stimulation of mating to trigger the neuroendocrine events that support a corpus luteum of pregnancy (McClintock and Anisko, 1982).

In the Holstein dairy cow a mixture of periovulatory urine and cervical mucus advances the time of estrus and ovulation by augmenting the luteolytic effects of $PGF_{2\alpha}$ injections (Izard and Vandenbergh, 1979; see Chapter 9 for a detailed discussion). Whether this is also the predominant effect of living in a large herd on the length of spontaneous cycles is not yet known.

The effect of estrous cycle odors appears to vary among different species. The guinea pig seems to be similar to the cow and different from the rat in that periovulatory odors shorten rather than lengthen the cycle. However, these species differences should be interpreted cautiously until the neuroendocrine mechanisms and ovarian correlates of female pheromone production are known. For example, in the guinea pig, periovulatory urine was actually collected at the time of vaginal opening, which in this species corresponds to both late follicular development and ovulation. Therefore, it may have contained a mixture of compounds with different effects. This is probable because signals with opposing effects are likely to be produced in rapid succession (see Section III,A). Thus, even slight variation in collection times relative to ovarian events can confound a species comparison.

C. Suppression

1. The Phenomenon

When adult female mice live alone, ovulation occurs spontaneously and, in the absence of mating, is not spontaneously followed by a fully functional corpus luteum capable of supporting implantation. The female mouse, like the rat, relies instead on the stimulation of mating to trigger the neuroendocrine events that will support a corpus luteum. Thus, the mouse estrous cycle is relatively short (4–6 days), allowing a solitary female to return quickly to estrus if she does not mate successfully.

When adult female mice live together in a group, the most salient consequence is an increase in estrous cycle length. While cyclicity is usually maintained, and estrus is therefore only delayed, the phenomenon is usually called estrous suppression and is termed the Lee–Boot effect after those who first quantified the response (Andervont, 1944; van der Lee and Boot, 1955, 1956; Mühlbock, 1958). The following discussion focuses on estrous suppression in house mice (*Mus musculus*), on which the most work has been done. Similar effects have been reported in deer mice (*Peromyscus maniculatus* Bairdii; Lombardo and Terman, 1980), Indian field mice (*Mus booduga* Gray; Dominic and Pandey, 1979), and wild hopping mice (*Notomys alexis;* Breed, 1976).

The degree of estrous suppression in a group is partially determined by its size. The estrous cycles of mice living in pairs are lengthened only slightly; the maximum effect is obtained with 4 to 6 group members, depending on the strain (Champlin, 1971). The mechanism of this dose dependence on group size has not been identified. It could depend on the increase in social interactions or body contact found in larger groups. Alternatively, given a 4- to 6-day estrous cycle, a group size of 4 to 6 females may be just large enough to ensure that there is an estrous cycle dependent signal present whenever each female is maximally sensitive (see Section II,C,3).

Whitten (1959) reported complete suppression (anestrus) when all-female groups were very large ($N = 30$). However, others have reported that larger groups do not significantly increase the delay (Crowcroft and Rowe, 1957;

Ryan and Schwartz, 1977). The latter studies used different strains and were conducted at different seasons and with different light–dark cycles, which may have attenuated the magnitude of delay reported by Whitten.

The delay of estrus, or estrous suppression, has been regarded as a laboratory artifact in mice (Rogers and Beauchamp, 1976; Bronson, 1979), primarily because the strongest response occurs in the complete absence of males, a condition that is not likely in the field (Lloyd, 1975). However, the delay of estrus has been demonstrated in the presence of gonadally intact males and their odors (Lamond, 1959; Mody, 1963), albeit in an attenuated form. Furthermore, estrous suppression is found in confined populations of male and female wild house mice; when females are removed from their groups, they resume short cycles and become fertile (Crowcroft and Rowe, 1957). Thus, female signals can continue to modify the estrous cycles of other females even when males are present. The net effect of female signals may not be as dramatic as it is under the artificial conditions created in the laboratory, but this should not be taken to mean that female signals are not an integral part of the social mechanisms that regulate female fertility and reproductive cycles in a heterosexual population.

2. Nature of the Response

Because the variance of estrous cycle lengths is increased in all-female groups of mice, the effect of group living in this species is often reported simply as an increase in irregular cycles (Lamond, 1959). Nonetheless, a close inspection of the available distributions of cycle lengths reveals a negatively skewed and usually bimodal distribution (e.g., Fig. 2A) (bimodal distributions: Champlin, 1971; Lamond, 1959; Ryan and Schwartz, 1977; van der Lee and Boot, 1955; Whitten, 1959; unimodal distributions: Champlin, 1971; Clee et al., 1975).

No study indicates whether the bimodal distribution is the result of two different populations of individuals (i.e., those that have delayed and lengthened cycles and those that do not) or two different types of cycles within each individual. This is a particularly interesting question given the results of a log–survivor plot of the cycle lengths. Because this method has not been used to describe the timing of the ovarian cycle before, a short methodological digression may be helpful (for extended discussions of the method, see Gross and Clark, 1975; Fagen and Young, 1978; Lee, 1982).

The ovarian cycle is a temporal event defined by the interval between successive ovulations. Therefore, chemosignals that alter cycle length (i.e., repeatedly and consistently phase shift the cycle) will alter the rate of ovulation. It is possible to compare the rates of ovulation under different olfactory conditions by examining all cycle lengths in a log–survivor plot. This method provides a more informative picture of the temporal response to

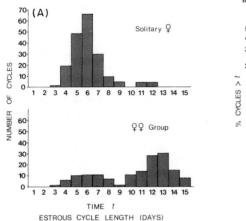

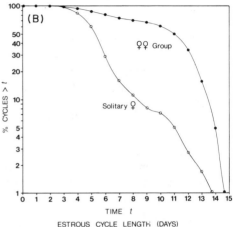

Fig. 2. Effect of grouping on the length of the estrous cycle in domestic house mice. (A) Frequency histogram; (B) log–survivor plot. (Analysis and figure based on data from Lamond, 1959.)

olfactory signals than the traditional methods that use only the mean cycle length.

Whenever ovarian cycles are measured, each individual is observed for a finite period of time and the number of cycles of each length is counted. However, a limited observation period biases the distribution of cycle lengths that can be observed; there is an inherently greater probability of observing a short cycle than a long cycle. This bias can be corrected, in part, by using the log of the number of cycles observed, so that greater weight is given to those long cycles that are actually observed. In addition, it is convenient to use the survivor distribution (plotting the percentage of cycles greater than length t) rather than the cumulative distribution because the steepness of the slope of a log–survivor plot at a given point is proportional to the rate of ovulation at that time since the previous ovulation. The steepness of the slope is also proportional to the probability of each cycle length.

A log–survivor plot reveals that the bimodal distribution of the cycles of grouped females is the result of two quite regular processes that are associated with significantly different rates of ovulation (Fig. 2B). First, the probability of cycles lasting between 4 and 9 days (approximately 60% of grouped-female cycles) is reduced. A striking feature of the plot is its constant slope between 4 and 10 days, indicating the equiprobability of cycles that are between 4 and 10 days long. This means, for example, that 9-day cycles are as likely as 5-day cycles even though fewer 9-day cycles are actually observed during the observation period. It also means that the rate of ovulation remains constant once 4 days have passed since the beginning of the cycle.

Second, there is another process, indicated by the "knee," or increase in the steepness of the slope, in Fig. 2B, which corresponds to a sharp increase in the probability of a cycle ending once 10 days have passed. This second process is more probable than the first and also occurs at a constant rate once it has begun. Thus, log–survivor analysis indicates that the most likely consequence of group living is cycle lengths between 11 and 14 days and that any variation among these cycle lengths is random.

The two processes inferred from the log–survivor plot of pooled data have, in some cases, been experimentally verified within individuals. The first process represents a lengthening of diestrus, the luteal phase of the estrous cycle (Champlin, 1971; Lamond, 1959; Mody, 1963; Clee et al., 1975), whereas the second process represents a spontaneous pseudopregnancy. Ryan and Schwartz (1977) have established that female odors lengthen the diestrous phase cycle by prolonging the life span of the corpus luteum (Ryan and Schwartz, 1977). This delays the next estrus, reducing the frequency of estrus in a given period of time. Thus, grouped female mice are more likely to have spontaneously functional corpora lutea than solitary females are. The corpora lutea produce a progesterone level that is comparable to that induced by mating with a male (Ryan and Schwartz, 1977), although they develop with a slightly different time course.

The second process corresponds to a pseudopregnancy, documented by the presence of corpora lutea (Mody, 1963), ova transfers (van der Lee and Boot, 1956), mammary development (Dewar, 1959; Mody, 1963), uterine endometriosis (Mody, 1963), weight gain (Dewar, 1959), and a decidual response (van der Lee and Boot, 1955; Ryan and Schwartz, 1977). Although these changes are comparable to the progestational state that is triggered by copulation, the response is more variable (Mody, 1963; Ryan and Schwartz, 1977). Whitten (1957, 1959) had suggested that anestrus, or complete suppression of cycles, is the result of living in very large groups ($N = 30$). However, in groups of comparable size, Ryan and Schwartz (1977) documented the existence of long cycles, 95–99% of which were in fact pseudopregnancies. Ryan and Schwartz suggested that Whitten may have missed the decidual cell response and cornification that indicate cyclic activity, because of the increased mucus in the vaginal smear and the temporal variability characteristic of socially induced pseudopregnancy.

Both processes, prolonged diestrus and pseudopregnancy, share maintenance of the corpus luteum as the final common path of the response. Van der Lee and Boot (1955) originally hypothesized that the increase in cycle length was mediated by an increase in prolactin secretion, whereas Whitten (1959) postulated an increase in secretion of follicle-stimulating hormone (FSH). Since then, it has been demonstrated that the corpus luteum is maintained by a combination of prolactin and FSH (Choudary and Greenwald, 1969). However, it is an increase in prolactin secretion that is more likely to be part of the primary response to group living in mice. The level of prolactin is increased in ovariectomized and low-dose estrogen-treated females that are living together (Bronson, 1976). In addition, treatment with a dopamine agonist that lowers prolactin levels (bromocriptine B154) interferes with the delay or suppression of estrus.

The effects of group living in mice are rapid and do not persist after separation from a group. A change in cycle length can occur within 4 days, or one cycle, after females are put in a group (van der Lee and Boot, 1955; Ryan and Schwartz, 1977). In addition, the effect can be reversed within 3 days after a female is removed from her group (Marsden and Bronson, 1964) or by presenting a male (Whitten, 1958).

The response to living in a female group appears to be highly variable when studies from different laboratories are compared. Much of this variability can be attributed to the use of different strains, ages, and lighting schedules, each of which affects the endogenous rhythm of the estrous cycle. Champlin (1971) reported a greater sensitivity in C57BL/6J mice than in the BALB/Ci strain. The Hall strain may also be more sensitive to female signals since it is the strain used by Whitten (1959) when he reported complete anestrus rather than pseudopregnancy in all-female groups. Older females are also more sensitive; the incidence of pseudopregnancy increases steadily, reaching a maximum at 7 to 10 months of age (van der Lee and Boot, 1955; Dewar, 1959).

Another important source of variation is the phase of the cycle at which the females are grouped. Not only is this an important point for resolving conflicting reports, but it is also a clue to the hormonal mechanisms of estrous delay and suppression. Ryan and Schwartz (1977) found that grouping females at estrus was most effective for delaying the subsequent ovulation and lengthening the cycle. Fresh corpora lutea are present at this time and can be maintained given the appropriate stimulus. In contrast, grouping females just before ovulation, at proestrus, does not alter the timing of the next estrous cycle.

These data can be conceptualized as forming a phase-resetting curve (Fig. 3; a general discussion of phase-resetting curves can be found in Winfree, 1980). In mice, grouping females consistently phase delays the next cycle. The strength of the response varies as a function of estrous cycle phase at the onset of group living. This variation in response may result from changes in the endocrine state and sensitivity of the recipient [e.g., during estrus, when fresh corpora lutea are developing and estrogen may have increased

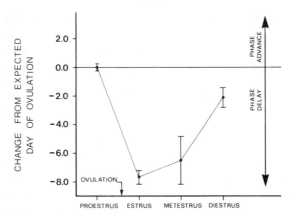

Fig. 3. Phase-resetting curve for the mouse estrous cycle by female social signals. (Analysis and figure based on data from Ryan and Schwartz, 1977.)

olfactory sensitivity (Pietras and Moulton, 1974)]. It could also result from changes in the endocrine state of the females that are producing the signal.

3. Signal and Receptors

Estrous suppression is produced by a specific signal and is not just part of a general stress response to crowding or group living. Corticosterone levels are not significantly elevated in grouped females. In fact, it is isolation, if anything, that is stressful for female mice; following isolation there is a transitory rise in corticosterone levels and a subsequent adrenal hypertrophy that depends on ovarian function (Bronson and Chapman, 1968; Brain and Nowell, 1970).

The initial attempts to identify the social signals that delay estrus focused on pheromones deposited in soiled bedding. Separating females from each other and from their bedding by a wire partition reduces the number of females with delayed cycles by half (Whitten, 1959). Contact with bedding soiled by grouped females partially reinstates the effect of group living (Champlin, 1971). It is presumed that pheromones are secreted in urine (Wolff and Powell, 1979). However, preputialectomy also attenuates estrous suppression (Chipman, 1967), suggesting that soiled bedding may also contain pheromones from the preputial glands (Hayashi, 1979).

In mice at least one of the pheromones is mediated by the vomeronasal system, since excision of the vomeronasal organ reduces the number of females with delayed estrous cycles (Reynolds and Keverne, 1979) and ablation of the olfactory bulbs prevents spontaneous pseudopregnancy in grouped females (Whitten, 1956; Mody, 1963).

In none of these studies that focused on putative pheromones was it possible to remove completely or to reinstate completely estrous suppression. Therefore, it is likely that these putative pheromones do not act alone. Because physical contact also seems to be necessary (Kimura, 1971; van der Lee and Boot, 1955; Whitten, 1959), social grooming may increase the effectiveness of chemosignals. Pheromones could also be distributed around the environment in different patterns throughout the estrous cycle through changes in marking behavior (Wolff and Powell, 1979). Other stimuli such as mounting (Dewar, 1959) or visual signals (Lamond, 1959; contra Whitten, 1959) may also lengthen the cycle and delay estrus.

Some of the social signals that delay estrus depend on ovarian function, although they are not necessarily pheromonal signals. Ovariectomy attenuates the ability to suppress estrous cycles in other females; a female living with a group of ovariectomized mice has shorter cycles than one living with intact females (Chipman, 1967; Clee et al., 1975). However, ovariectomy does not completely abolish the suppressive effect (Chipman, 1967; Kimura, 1971), indicating that there are other effective signals that are not dependent on ovarian hormones.

III. SYNCHRONY

A. A Model for Ovarian Synchrony

Synchronous ovarian cycles can occur among females that live together. Ovarian synchrony can result solely from the social interactions among females in groups of human beings (McClintock, 1971; Graham and McGrew, 1980; Russell et al., 1980; Quadagno et al., 1981), rats (Rattus norvegicus; McClintock, 1978), and golden hamsters (Mesocricetus auratus; Handelmann et al., 1980). It is striking that a similar phenomenon occurs in each of these species, even though their ovarian cycles are quite different. Human beings have a menstrual cycle that includes a functional corpus luteum, whereas rats and hamsters have an estrous cycle with only minimal luteal function. Nonetheless, the common feature of each type of ovarian cycle is ovulation that spontaneously occurs at regular intervals and is synchronized within a social group.

The process of ovarian synchrony can be conceptualized as the coupling, or mutual entrainment, of a set of oscillators. The mechanism that couples the oscillators depends on social communication. Neither rats, hamsters, nor human beings show synchrony among females that simply share the same physical environment; instead, the coupling mechanism for ovarian synchrony appears to rely on social signals from the other members of the group.

A coupled-oscillator model of synchrony suggests that there should be two types of signals that synchronize ovarian cycles: one that phase delays the cycle and one that phase advances it. This is a common feature of the synchronizing mechanisms underlying entrainment of neural rhythms (Sano *et al.,* 1978), cicada emergence cycles (Hoppensteadt and Keller, 1976), circadian activity rhythms (Aschoff, 1960), and fish fin movements (von Holst, 1969). In each of these instances synchrony is brought about by different mechanisms; even the synchronous flashing of fireflies is accomplished by different mechanisms in different species (Buck and Buck, 1968). Nonetheless, the functional equivalents of phase advance and phase delay are common to each process. Furthermore, synchronization is most rapid when these two opposing signals follow quickly one after the other (Winfree, 1980).

It is important to distinguish between the coupling of cycles and perfect synchrony, which is one manifestation of coupling and a specific form of entrainment. In perfect synchrony all cycles have the same cycle length and the same phase relationship. For example, in a completely synchronized group all females in the group ovulate on the same day at the same regular interval. However, if there is high variance in the length of the endogenous cycles, perfect synchrony is precluded (Winfree, 1980), even though the coupling between individual cycles may still be strong. Cycles are entrained if their lengths are similar as a result of being coupled but need not have a stable phase relationship. Thus, if a group is only partially synchronized, the pattern can reflect weak coupling between cycles, large variance in endogenous cycle lengths, or entrainment without synchrony.

Synchrony can result from the mutual entrainment of a group of oscillators (von Holst, 1969; Winfree, 1980). In this case each cycle is affected equally by the coupling. Alternatively, one of the individual oscillators can serve as an entrainer, or *zeitgeber,* and entrain the rest. If so, the periodicity of the entraining rhythm will remain relatively stable, while the other cycles phase shift to synchronize with it. Coupling mechanisms can also create a state that is intermediate between these two alternatives.

B. Estrous Synchrony in the Domestic Rat

1. The Phenomenon

When female rats live together, their estrous cycles synchronize (McClintock, 1978). Estrous synchrony can be measured in several ways. First, females in a synchronized group have a similar balance of cells in their vaginal smears on a given day. This indicates that they are at the same phase of the estrous cycle at the same time. However, this measure of synchrony is raised artificially if the females of a group all stopped cycling and remained in a similar acyclic condition (e.g., constant vaginal estrus; McClintock and Adler, 1978). Therefore, a second measure of synchrony is based on the percentage of females in the group that have regular cycles and are at a particular phase of the estrous cycle on the same day. A plot of this value against time graphically demonstrates the development and maintenance of synchrony in a group (Fig. 4).

Generally, 3 cycles are required for synchrony to develop (McClintock, 1978, 1983a), and it can be maintained for at least as long as 12 cycles (M. K. McClintock, unpublished data). Perfect synchrony is rare in the domestic rat. It is more common to find 50–75% of the group synchronized with fluctuations over time that result from individuals shifting to either lead or follow the rest of the group. This partial synchrony could well have had an adaptive advantage, reflecting the point at which the benefits of being synchronized are countered by the benefits of being asynchronous or overdispersed (Knowlton, 1979). Whether or not this level of synchrony has a function, it is probably the result of the endogenous variation that is characteristic of the rat's estrous cycle (4–6 days; Long and Evans, 1922; Nequin et al., 1979; Schwartz, 1969), a variation that is large enough to preclude perfect synchrony even when the cycles are coupled (Winfree, 1980).

Females that share a recirculated air supply have ovarian cycles that synchronize as quickly and to the same level as those of females that actually live together (McClintock, 1978). Therefore, airborne chemosignals provide a social coupling mechanism between individual ovarian cycles that is sufficient for estrous synchrony. Because a coupled-oscillator model of synchrony predicts that two opposing signals generate synchrony, I hypothesized that female rats produce at least two different odors that have opposing effects on the timing of ovulation and the estrous cycle: one that phase advances ovulation and shortens the cycle and one that phase delays ovulation and lengthens the cycle.

In order to test the model, each rat's ovarian cycle was partitioned into three different phases that were hormonally distinct: follicular, ovulatory, and "luteal" (the corpus luteum is nonfunctional in the rat) (Nequin et al., 1979; Smith et al., 1975). These phases were chosen because they represent distinct phases of the ovarian cycle and times when different odors are likely to be produced. Normally, these putative pheromones would be emitted as 1- or 2-day "pulses," and synchrony would result from the interaction of different and opposing signals. However, this process is sufficiently complex that I chose not to measure the end product, namely, synchrony, but chose instead to test the coupling mechanism directly and measure the effect of each different odor on the length of the cycle.

Therefore, odors from each part of the estrous cycle were presented continuously for 18 to 24 days. These constant odors were created by placing

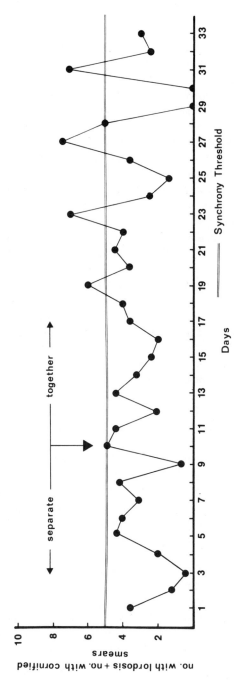

Fig. 4. Development of estrous synchrony in a group of domestic rats ($N = 5$) (McClintock, 1981).

females with normal spontaneous ovarian cycles in a source box when they were expected to enter a particular phase of the cycle. They were removed after 24 hr and replaced with another set of females that were just then entering the same phase. Thus, the females living downwind were exposed to constant odors characteristic of a particular phase of the estrous cycle, even though the females producing the odors had normal spontaneous estrous cycles.

This strategy is similar to that used to study the coupling mechanisms of other biological rhythms. The putative entraining stimulus is presented continuously at different intensities in order to assess its effect on the periodicity of the endogenous cycle. For example, depending on its intensity, constant light can either shorten or lengthen the period of the free-running circadian activity rhythm (Aschoff, 1960).

Odors from the follicular and ovulatory phases had opposite effects on the timing of the cycle. Constant follicular odors (lights-on diestrus to lights-on proestrus) shortened and regularized the cycle. All females had 4-day cycles instead of the range of cycle lengths (3–6 days) that is characteristic of the domestic strain living either in isolation or in a group. Constant ovulatory odors had the opposite effect. They increased both the length and the variance of the estrous cycle. Odors from the luteal phase (lights-on metestrus to lights-on diestrus) did not alter the timing of the estrous cycle significantly. The distribution of cycle lengths was indistinguishable from that of the control females.

Thus, females that are in their follicular phase and about to ovulate emit an airborne signal that phase advances and shortens the cycle of other females in the group. However, once they are in the ovulatory phase, they emit a signal that phase delays and lengthens the cycle of other females. Then there is a period when the odors are relatively neutral. This juxtaposition of opposing signals is exactly what the coupled-oscillator model predicts and is in fact one of the more effective coupling mechanisms for generating synchrony between oscillators (Winfree, 1980).

Odors from females in other reproductive states can interfere with synchrony by disrupting the ovarian cycle. For example, females that live in constant light are in a pathological state called constant vaginal estrus. Their ovarian cycles are suppressed (Campbell and Schwartz, 1980), and ovulation occurs only sporadically, if at all. Odors from these acyclic females disrupt the ovarian cycles of females living downwind from them by "jamming" the ovarian cycle and inducing persistent estrus (McClintock and Adler, 1978). As soon as the odors are removed, vaginal cyclicity resumes immediately, indicating that the coupling with an acyclic female produces a pathological state only temporarily.

2. Nature of the Response

Because estrous cycle odors affect the timing of the estrous cycle, a log–survivor plot was used to examine their effect on the rate of ovulation (Fig. 5). Each line represents the distribution of the cycles of 12 females observed for 20 days. Each individual responded in the same way as the population (McClintock, 1983b).

There are several striking features of this log–survivor plot. The middle line, representing the cycles of females exposed to luteal phase odors, is a straight line (once a threshold value of 3 days has passed). This indicates that the underlying distribution of cycle lengths is close to a Poisson distribution; ovulation occurs at a constant rate, and 4-, 5-, and 6-day cycles are equally likely in the population even though 4-day cycles are actually observed more frequently. The cycles of females exposed to background odors (McClintock, 1983a) form a distribution similar to those of females living in a colony room (M. K. McClintock, unpublished data). This forces an important conceptual change. Often variability in estrous cycle length is assumed to reflect an irregular process. These data indicate that this is not always the case. Variability can result when ovulation occurs at a constant rate that does not fluctuate with the passage of time.

Follicular odors increase both the rate and the time dependence of ovulation. The almost vertical slope of the log–survivor plot (Fig. 5) indicates that it is virtually certain that each cycle will be 4 days long. The follicular odors, however, do not advance ovulation beyond the 4-day lower limit that is presumably imposed by the sequence of ovarian events (Everett, 1948;

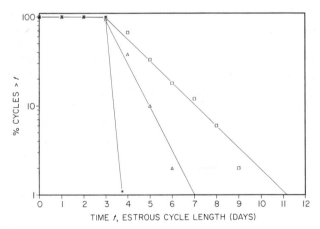

Fig. 5. Effect of estrous cycle odors on the length of the domestic rat's estrous cycle; log–survivor plot. Odors: □, ovulatory; △, luteal; *, follicular.

Krey *et al.,* 1973). Ovulatory odors have the opposite effect and reduce the rate of ovulation (indicated by the more shallow slope of the log–survivor plot in Fig. 5). Once the lower limit is passed, the probability of ovulation remains constant and is also relatively independent of the passage of time since the last ovulation.

The working hypothesis is that follicular and ovulatory odors exert opposing effects on ovulation by controlling the same event in the estrous cycle, namely, the life span of the corpus luteum. Follicular odors may well advance the time of ovulation by reducing the life span of the corpus luteum, and ovulatory odors may prolong it. This hypothesis is based on the fact that two mechanisms control the timing of ovulation in the rat. The first controls follicular growth, and the second controls the gonadotropin surge that immediately precedes ovulation from the ripened follicle (Schwartz, 1969). Both of these mechanisms are affected by progesterone levels; progesterone can retard follicular growth (Buffler and Roser, 1974) and, by acting centrally, it can delay the gonadotropin surge (Blake, 1977; Everett, 1961; Nequin *et al.,* 1979). The amount of progesterone secreted by the corpora lutea is enough to delay ovulation and control cycle length, even though it is not sufficient to support implantation (Everett, 1963; Naftolin *et al.,* 1972; Freeman *et al.,* 1976, Nequin *et al.,* 1979).

3. Signals and Receptors

The amount and composition of urine (Bellamy and Davies, 1971; Carr *et al.,* 1962), saliva (Block *et al.,* 1981), and sebaceous and preputial gland secretions (Ebling, 1972; Stoddart, 1976; Thody *et al.,* 1979) vary during the estrous cycle. Any of these substances, therefore, is a potential source of the airborne odors that couple the estrous cycles of female rats living in a group. In addition, the female rat's marking behavior changes during the estrous cycle. As a female approaches estrus, she moves about her environment, rubbing herself on stones and rocks (Calhoun, 1961, 1962). Around ovulation, estrous females are particularly active, leaving a trail of urine and sebaceous secretions (Birke, 1978). Although this behavior undoubtedly attracts males (Carr and Caul, 1962), it may also affect the estrous cycles of females that encounter the markings.

There are currently no data to indicate whether female pheromones in the rat are mediated by the main olfactory system or by the vomeronasal system (see Chapter 8). Olfactory bulbectomy, which impairs both systems, increases the length of the estrous cycle of group-housed female rats (Aron, 1973; Rosen *et al.,* 1940). However, bulbectomy does not affect the cycle length of females that live alone (Moss, 1971). Thus, the olfactory system mediates signals that change the length of the estrous cycle but is not necessary for the maintenance of the endogenous ovarian cycle itself. The fact that the signals are airborne and do not require body contact points to the main olfactory system (Johns, 1980). However, the direct projections between the accessory olfactory system and hypothalamus favor the vomeronasal system, particularly because the ventromedial nucleus is involved in the control of the rate of ovarian progesterone secretion during the luteal phase of the estrous cycle (Plas-Roser *et al.,* 1977; see Chapter 8 for an extended discussion of the olfactory and vomeronasal systems).

Olfactory acuity is highest around the time of ovulation (Pietras and Moulton, 1974; Curry, 1971). This is just prior to the point in the cycle when the corpus luteum develops (Nikitovitch-Winer and Everett, 1958). Thus, although more research is needed to determine exactly when females are responsive to estrous cycle pheromones, estrus is a likely candidate.

C. Ovarian Synchrony in Other Species

Ovarian synchrony has been documented in human beings and hamsters, although the female social signals that generate the phenomenon are less well understood. In human beings ovarian synchrony is manifested by menstrual synchrony; women who live together are more likely to menstruate at the same time (McClintock, 1971). This phenomenon has been documented by several investigators in predominantly female populations (McClintock, 1971) and in heterosexual populations (Graham and McGrew, 1980; Russell *et al.,* 1980; Quadagno *et al.,* 1981). It occurs whether or not women are aware of each other's menstrual cycles. In each of these studies synchrony developed among women who spent time together, not only between pairs of close friends or roommates, but among members of larger social groups as well. The parameters of menstrual synchrony are remarkably stable across the different studies, and all are consistent with a coupled-oscillator model of the phenomenon. First, synchrony is rarely perfect; instead, there is an increase above the random synchrony level, usually by a factor of 2. The absence of perfect synchrony could represent coupling between cycles with different periodicities. Second, a similar percentage of groups fail to synchronize (range 17–31%). Third, synchronization requires three to four cycles to develop.

Using the same physical space does not provide sufficient coupling for synchronization, for example, simply being neighbors (McClintock, 1971; Graham and McGrew, 1980); it is necessary to be at the same place at the same time, sharing a social environment.

Anthropological accounts have also documented menstrual synchrony among the Yurok Indians (Buckley, 1982; Spott and Kroeber, 1942) and the Karok Indians (Harrington, 1931), both aboriginal groups that lived in the Pacific Northwest. In these cultures it was expected that the women of a household would enter the menstrual hut at the same time. If a woman was not synchronized with the group, she was advised to talk to the moon in order to reinstate a normal cycle and her position with the menstrual group (Buckley, 1982). Thus, the coupling mechanism was partially attributed to light in this culture. Other factors that stem from a shared social environment could also be important, for example, a tendency to share strenuous physical activities (Shangold *et al.,* 1979; Quadagno *et al.,* 1981).

Some of the most promising preliminary data suggest that human female sweat may carry enough information for menstrual synchrony to develop (Russell *et al.,* 1980). This would be consistent with synchrony among the Yurok in that women spent one-third of each cycle close together in a structure similar to the males' sweat house.

Ovarian synchrony is also found between pairs of female golden hamsters (*Mesocrecitus auratus*; Handelmann *et al.,* 1980), although not among female hamsters that simply live in the same colony room (Laubscher and Magalhaes, 1962). This is particularly informative because the ovarian cycle of this species is relatively invariant. Nonetheless, when females with stable 4-day cycles live in pairs, they have both phase advances (short cycles) and phase delays (long cycles) until they are synchronized. Females that are 180° out of phase take four cycles to entrain, whereas those that are 90° out of phase take only one cycle. A similar pattern of phase shifts and synchrony can be obtained artificially with steroid injections (Gross, 1977), suggesting that social signals may act through a similar hormonal mechanism. Once synchronized, the pair retains 4-day cycles and remains synchronized for at least 1 month (seven cycles). The remarkably high level of synchrony in this species supports the hypothesis that large variation in cycle length may obscure a social coupling mechanism. For example, 100% of the groups of hamsters become synchronized when only females with stable 4-day cycles are used (Handelmann *et al.,* 1980). In our studies rats were selected for having 4- or 5-day cycles; we found that 80% of the groups become synchronized. Finally, among women the menstrual cycle ranges in length from 25 to 45 days, and synchrony develops in only 69 to 83% of the groups. Thus, there may be coupling or entrainment between cycles which is not expressed as synchrony because of variation in the cycle length.

In contrast with the rat the rate of synchronization is greatly enhanced by physical contact between hamsters. Furthermore, it is the behaviorally submissive female that entrains to the dominant female (Handelmann *et al.,* 1980). This supports both the hypothesis that socially dominant females can serve as *zeitgebern* for the cycles of other females in the group (McClintock, 1978; see also Section V) and the hypothesis that the vomeronasal system mediates olfactory signals (Johns, 1980).

D. Male-Generated Synchrony

In several rodent species, estrous synchrony can be generated by olfactory signals from a male if the females have estrous cycles that have been delayed or suppressed by living in all-female groups (laboratory house mouse, *Mus musculus*: Whitten, 1957, 1958; wild house mouse: Chipman and Fox, 1966; Indian field mouse, *Mus boonduga* Gray: Dominic and Pandy, 1979; deer mouse, *Peromyscus maniculatus*, Bronson and Marsden, 1964). Male-generated synchrony in these rodents is different from the synchrony found among groups of female rats, because it is triggered by an external signal and is not solely the result of coupling among spontaneous cycles. Nonetheless, male-generated synchrony is not wholly independent of this coupling, because the degree of synchrony depends on the degree of mutual suppression of cycles within the female group.

If a male is introduced into a cage with a group of female mice, the majority of them will be in heat 3 days later (Whitten, 1958). However, the effectiveness of the male as a synchronizer is markedly attenuated if the females are not living in a group (Whitten, 1959) or are not exposed to urine of grouped females before the male is introduced (Marsden and Bronson, 1964; see Fig. 6). This is because the grouped females maintain each other at a similar phase of the estrous cycle, delay each other's cycles, and can therefore respond to the male's phase-advancing signal in the same way at the same time. Thus, female signals accentuate the impact of male phase-advancing signals and enhance synchrony within a group. In this respect male-generated synchrony is similar to female synchrony in the rat. They

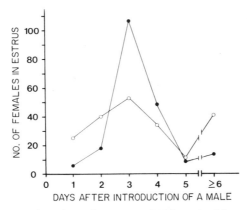

Fig. 6. Male-generated synchrony is attentuated without the delay or suppression that is produced by female social signals (*Mus musculus*). Key: ●—●, grouped females; ○—○, solitary female. (Figure redrawn from data presented in Whitten, 1959.)

both rely on two opposing signals: one that lengthens or phase delays the cycle and a second that shortens or phase advances it.

In the mouse the effect of male stimulation is limited to those cycles in which male signals are present (Whitten, 1958). The male has a luteolytic effect, which releases the gonadotropin surges and eventually results in estrus and ovulation (Ryan and Schwartz, 1976; Bronson, 1975). Male-induced estrus is similar to spontaneous estrus in terms of reproductive organ weights and pituitary luteinizing hormone (LH) content (Bingel and Schwartz, 1969b).

A short exposure to the male does not produce a luteolytic effect; a full 48 hr is usually required to permit ovulation (Whitten and Champlin, 1973). Furthermore, although male mouse urine (Marsden and Bronson, 1964; Monder et al., 1978) or even air from a male's cage (Whitten et al., 1968) can induce synchrony, neither stimulus is as effective as the male himself (Marsden and Bronson, 1965). Thus, male pheromones may be augmented by other social signals in order to override the female pheromones that sustain the corpus luteum.

Simply separating the females and isolating them from the female odors of their group generates a greater degree of synchrony than does the introduction of a male pheromone (Marsden and Bronson, 1965). This indicates that male signals produce synchrony by counteracting the suppression or phase delay that is maintained by female signals. The result is a phase advance of all females in the group at the same time.

In other species, males can also modulate the estrous cycle but without necessarily generating synchrony or overriding the effect of the female signals. Urine from male rats can induce reflex ovulation in females that are not cycling because of environmental factors such as inadequate food (Cooper and Hayes, 1967) or constant light (Johns et al., 1978). Male rat urine can also shorten a 5-day cycle to a 4-day cycle in female rats (Hughes, 1964; Chateau et al., 1972; Aron and Chateau, 1971). In the guinea pig, male urine shortens the cycle by shortening the duration of vaginal closure but does not alter the number of ova shed (Jesel and Aron, 1974).

It is likely that responses to male urine are mediated by the vomeronasal system in each of these species. In each case direct contact with male urine or soiled bedding is required for the response, in contrast with female signals, which can be airborne (McClintock, 1978; except Whitten et al., 1968). Furthermore, ablation of the vomeronasal system prevents reflex ovulation in light-induced persistent estrous rats (Johns et al., 1978), and peripheral (Mora and Gallego, 1977) or central vomeronasal deafferentation (Sánchez-Criado, 1979; Sánchez-Criado and Gallego, 1979) blocks shortening of the estrous cycle by male odors.

Women who live in predominantly female communities have shortened and regularized menstrual cycles when they associate with males (Mc-Clintock, 1971). However, this correlation is not significant in heterosexual communities (Quadagno et al., 1981; Graham and McGrew, 1980), although menstrual synchrony still occurs (Quadagno et al., 1981; Graham and McGrew, 1980; Buckley, 1982). It is not yet established whether this correlation results from a pheromonal signal. It could also be the result of regular, as opposed to sporadic, sexual activity (Cutler et al., 1979), although other investigators have failed to find such a correlation (Graham and McGrew, 1980).

IV. SOURCE AND FUNCTION OF INDIVIDUAL DIFFERENCES

In groups of female mice there are usually individuals whose estrous cycles are not completely suppressed (Clee et al., 1975; Dewar, 1959; Lamond, 1959; Ryan and Schwartz, 1977; van der Lee and Boot, 1956; Whitten, 1959; contra Reynolds and Keverne, 1979). Identifying the source of these individual differences is potentially of great importance for interpreting the social and ecological significance of female pheromones in mice. In some species, only the dominant females of the group have reproductive cycles (e.g., dwarf mongoose; Rood, 1974). Therefore, it is hypothesized that it is socially dominant female mice that are not completely suppressed. Whitten (1959) briefly considered this hypothesis but rejected it without actually measuring social dominance. Therefore, the hypothesis still must be tested.

The estrous cycle and fertility of subordinate females may also be suppressed in species in which the net effect of group living is an enhancement of cyclicity. In rhesus monkeys seasonally acyclic females resume cyclicity sooner if they are placed in a group with estrogen-treated females than they do in groups without such females, demonstrating that estrogen-treated females can enhance cyclicity (Vandenbergh and Drickamer, 1974; Vandenbergh, 1977) In this same species subordinate females are less likely to conceive than are dominant females (Keverne and Michael, 1970). Similarly, in Talapoin monkeys, LH is suppressed by the presence of a dominant female (Keverne, 1979; see Table I for a summary of social suppression of reproductive cycles).

In the hamster socially subordinate females are entrained by dominant females (Handelmann et al., 1980). This supports the hypothesis that socially dominant females can serve as zeitgebern for the cycles of other females in the group (McClintock, 1978). However, in the rat a social relationship is not essential for synchronization, given that synchrony develops among isolated females that have simply shared an air supply. This suggests that social relationships among rats may modulate the production

TABLE I

Documentation of Reproductive Synchrony, Suppression, and Enhancement within Female Groups of a Variety of Mammals

136

Mammal	Group synchrony[a]	Individual Female suppression	Individual Female enhancement	Putative signals	Putative functions	Reference[b]
Marsupialia						
Didelphidae						
Opossum, *Didelphis virginiana virginiana*	♀♀	—	—	Sisters, season	?	Reynold (1952), C
Chiroptera						
Phyllostomatidae						
Spear-nosed bat, *Phyllostomus hastatus*	♀♀ or ♀♂	—	—	Social and/or environmental	?	McCracken and Bradbury (1981), F
Primates						
Lemuridae						
Lemur, *Lemur fulvus*	♀♀ or ♀♂	—	—	Dominance	?	Jolly (1967), Harrington (1976), van Horn (1975), F and C
Lemur, *Lemur catta*	♀♀ or ♀♂	—	—	Day length, temperature	?	
Callithricidae						
Marmoset, *Callithrix jacchus*	♀♂	×	—	Dominance	Access to resources	Epple (1973), Rothe, (1975), Abbott and Hearn (1978), Katz and Epple (1980), C
Tamarin, *Saguinus fuscicollis*	—	×	—	Dominance, social	?	Kleiman (1980, 1982), Epple (1981), C
Tamarin, *Leontopithecus rosalia rosalia*	—	×	—	Dominance, social	?	

Species				Dominance	Access to resources	References
Cercopithecidae						
Rhesus monkey, *Macaca mulatta*	—	×	×	Dominance	Access to resources	Conoway and Koford (1965), Rowell (1972), Drickamer (1974), Vandenbergh and Post (1976), F and C
Talapoin monkey, *Miopithecus talapoin*	♀♀ or ♀♂	×	—	Social, dominance	Variable resources	Rowell (1977), Keverne (1979), C
Vervet monkey, *Cercopithecus aethiops*	♀♀	—	—	Social, rainfall	Social attention, nutrition	Lancaster (1971), Klein (1978), Rowell and Richards (1979), C
Gelada baboon, *Theropithecus gelada*	♀♀ or ♀♂	×	—	Social, dominance	Access to resources	Dunbar and Dunbar (1977), Dunbar (1980), F
Yellow baboon, *Papio cyanocephalus*	—	×	—	Dominance	Access to resources	Hausfater (1975), F
Hamadryas baboon, *Papio anubis*	♀♀ or ♀♂	—	—	♂ takeover	?	Abegglen (1976), F
Patas monkey, *Erythrocebus patas*	♀♀ or ♀♂	×	×	Social ?	Social coordination	Rowell and Hartwell (1978), C
Langur, *Presbytis entellus*	♀♂	×	—	Social ?	?	Sugiyama *et al.* (1965), Hrdy (1974), F
Mangabey, *Cercocebus albegena*	—	×	×	Social, dominance	?	Rowell and Chalmers (1970), C

(continued)

137

TABLE I (*continued*)

Mammal	Group synchrony[a]	Individual		Putative signals	Putative functions	Reference[b]
		Female suppression	Female enhancement			
Pongidae						
Chimpanzee, *Chimpanzee troglodytes*	♀♀	—	—	Social ?	?	Nishida (1979), Wallis (1982) (in litt.), F and C
Hominidae						
Human, *Homo sapiens*	♀♀	—	—	Sweat pheromone?	Coordinate fertility with resources	McClintock (1971), Graham and McGrew (1980), Russell *et al.* (1980), Quadagno *et al.* (1981), Buckley (1982)
Rodentia						
Cricetidae						
Deer mouse, *Peromyscus maniculatus*	♀♂	×	—	Pheromone	?	Lombardo and Terman (1980), C
Golden hamster, *Mesocricetus auratus*	♀♀	—	—	Pheromone, dominance	?	Handelmann *et al.* (1980), C
Mongolian gerbil, *Meriones unguiculatus*	—	×	—	Dominance	Variable resources?	Ågren (1976), Payman and Swanson (1980), C
Vole, *Microtus ochrogaster*	—	×	—	Urine	?	Milligan (1974), Baddaloo and Clulow (1981), Getz *et al.* (1982), F

Muridae						
Hopping mouse, *Notomys alexis*	♀ ♂	×	—	Pheromone	Variable resources	Breed (1976), C
House mouse, *Mus musculus*	♀ ♂	×	—	Pheromone	?	Crowcroft and Rowe (1957), C
Indian fieldmouse, *Mus booduga*	♀ ♂	×	—	Pheromone	?	Dominic and Pandey (1979), C
Norway rat, *Rattus norvegicus*	♀ ♀	×	×	Pheromone	?	Miller (1911), C
Bathyergidae						
Naked mole rat, *Heterocephalus glaber*	—	×	—	Pheromone ? dominance	?	Jarvis (1981), C
Carnivora						
Canidae						
Wild dog, *Lycaon pictus*	♀♀ or ♀♂	×	—	Cannibalism ?	Limited resources; reduce loss of foraging time	Frame *et al.* (1979), F
Wolf, *Canis lupus*	—	×	—	Inadequate mating	?	Zimen (1976), C
Procyonidae						
Coati, *Nasua narica*	♀♀ or ♀♂	—	—	Social	Variable food supply	Russell (1982), F
Viverridae						
Banded mongoose, *Mungos mungo*	♀♀ or ♀♂	—	—	Musk odor, common defecating grounds	Share nursing; increase ♂ parental care	Neal (1970), Rood (1974, 1975), F

(*continued*)

TABLE I (*continued*)

| Mammal | Group synchrony[a] | Individual | | Putative signals | Putative functions | Reference[b] |
		Female suppression	Female enhancement			
Dwarf mongoose, *Helogale parvula*	♀♀ or ♀♂	×	—	Infanticide	Subordinate aids with nursing	Rasa (1973), Rood (1978, 1980), F
Felidae						
Lion, *Panthera leo*	♀♂	×	—	♂ takeover	Decrease infanticide	Bertram (1975), Packer and Pusey (1983), F
Hyracoidea						
Procaviidae						
Bush hyrax, *Heterohyrax brucei*	♀♀ or ♀♂	—	—	Social, rainfall	?	Hoek (1981), F
Artiodactyla						
Bovidae						
Feral goats, *Capra hircus*	♀♂	—	—	Urinary pheromone	Sexual selection on ♀ and ♂	Coblentz (1976), F
Wildebeeste, *Connochaetes taurinus*	♀♀ or ♀♂	—	—	Rainfall, nutrition, social, ? moonlight	Migratory habits	Fraser (1968), Estes (1976), Sinclair (1977), F

[a] ♀♀, Synchrony from interactions among females alone; ♀♂, synchrony from interactions among females and males.

[b] F, Field population; C, captive population.

of or sensitivity to pheromones. For example, behavioral submission is mediated by adrenal steroids (Leshner, 1975), which can alter the timing of the ovarian cycle (Mann and Baraclough, 1973) and may, in turn, increase olfactory sensitivity (Henkin and Bartter, 1966).

In mice there is also evidence that intrauterine location of the fetus affects production of and sensitivity to pheromones during adulthood. Females that have been exposed to testosterone from their brothers *in utero* are more aggressive and also relatively insensitive to the effects of female grouping during adolescence [the age group used by Clee *et al.* (1975) and Ryan and Schwartz (1977)]. Females that have developed *in utero* between other females are more sensitive. This may be because they have shorter endogenous cycles, produce more cues, are more sensitive to cues, or are more socially subordinate (vom Saal *et al.*, 1981).

Female mice that have been reared together since weaning do not have delayed or suppressed estrous cycles when they live in all-female groups (Lamond, 1959). However, if these females are separated briefly for 4 weeks and then regrouped, suppression does occur. This suggests that familiarity and individual recognition (Halpin, 1980; Yamazaki *et al.*, 1979) may be an important component or modifier of pheromonal signals.

V. FUNCTION OF REPRODUCTIVE SYNCHRONY, SUPPRESSION, AND ENHANCEMENT

Because there is such a paucity of information about the social structure and ecology of the species from which laboratory strains were derived, the incidence of synchrony, suppression, and enhancement in wild populations of these species has yet to be determined. It has been suggested that some of the phenomena may be laboratory artifacts or epiphenomena (Bronson, 1979; McClintock, 1981; Rogers and Beauchamp, 1976), even though the pheromonal mechanisms have been well documented in the laboratory. Thus, the problem of the functions of synchrony, suppression, and enhancement still requires documentation of their social and ecological correlates in wild populations and testable models of their evolutionary mechanisms (e.g., Knowlton, 1979).

Both synchrony and the more general patterns of suppression and enhancement have been documented in wild populations of a variety of nonlaboratory mammalian species with spontaneous ovarian cycles. Table I presents a list of species in which one or more of these reproductive patterns have been found and in which there is also some indication that pheromones could be part of their mechanisms. However, olfactory involvement is putative in most cases.

It is premature to generalize about the advantages of males or females as synchronizers. Nonetheless, a few methodological generalities can be made on the basis of species comparisons. First, in each case of synchrony there is a greater degree of social coupling within a female social unit, such as a family (Rood, 1975, 1980), troop (Kummer, 1968), or pride (Bertram, 1975), than there is across the population as a whole. Second, synchrony is rarely perfect. This suggests that there are selective advantages to being asynchronous (or overdispersed in time) as well as synchronous. This balance between selective factors has been modeled by Knowlton (1979). Under the assumptions of her model the benefits of being synchronous reach an asymptotic value at 50 to 60% synchrony. Thus, the absence of perfect synchrony is not sufficient to discount synchrony as an important factor timing the ovarian cycles in a wild population. Third, it is necessary to interpret the function of coupling in the temporal context of the entire reproductive life span. From this perspective suppression is transitory; fertility is only delayed. A female may be temporarily suppressed and thus delay her cycle until conditions are more optimal for undertaking a pregnancy and raising young. For example, she could emmigrate to another social group (Jarvis, 1981), or the dominant female in her group might die or become reproductively inactive (Payman and Swanson, 1980), making the resources within her own group more accessible.

In the laboratory rat, estrous synchrony can result in group mating, a mating system in which behavior is better coordinated with the neuroendocrine mechanisms of sperm transport and implantation than it is during pair mating (McClintock, 1981; McClintock and Anisko, 1982; McClintock et al., 1982). Furthermore, there is interesting correlative evidence that social coupling may also have evolved as a timing mechanism for reproductive cycles in the wild strain. Wild female rats do form stable social groups, living in groups of 10 to 11, even when there is space for dispersal (Calhoun, 1961, 1962; Davis, 1955). They huddle together in a single sleeping site (Timmermans, 1978; M.K. McClintock, unpublished data). Urination and marking behavior vary with the ovarian cycle (Bellamy and Davies, 1971; Calhoun, 1962), indicating that a female's behavior would differentially broadcast the variety of chemosignals that are produced throughout the estrous cycle (McClintock, 1983a). This correlative evidence is given weight by its parallel with synchrony in wild populations of other species (see Table I).

In addition, environmental variables, such as light, are relatively weak modulators of reproductive state in the rat. The olfactory bulbs inhibit or mask the photoperiodic control of fertility (Nelson and Zucker, 1981). Thus, olfactory signals may be more prepotent than day length as cues for coordinating and regulating reproductive events in this species.

A life-span perspective also leads one to consider the possibility that coupling mechanisms may have evolved because of their consequences at other points in the reproductive life span, when achieving a fertile state requires a substantial energy investment. For example, in the rat a female mating at postpartum estrus must make the decision whether to undertake the enormous energy expenditure required to become pregnant again and carry a second litter to term while she is still nursing her first litter (Woodside et al., 1981; see Chapter 2 for a detailed discussion). Information about her social and physical environment is of particular importance during postpartum estrus, and she may therefore be even more sensitive to social information that can modulate her fertility than she is during a cycling estrus.

Puberty is another time when a high energy investment is required to achieve a fertile state, and female social signals could be a source of information about the suitability of the physical and social environment. In the yellow baboon (Papio cynocephalus), the absence of many consecutive cycles precludes the development of synchrony among adult females. However, menarche is accelerated and synchronized within cohorts of pubescent females (J. Altmann, personal communication). Although other environmental cues may be partly responsible, the high degree of synchrony that is correlated with a stable social group suggests that social signals could be part of the coupling mechanism.

It has been suggested that estrous suppression in mice is simply a holdover from the puberty-delaying pheromone, which does have a selective advantage in wild populations (Bronson, 1979; Drickamer, 1977; Massey and Vandenbergh, 1980; see also Chapter 4). However, the hormonal basis of these two signals is not the same. The puberty-delaying pheromone is dependent on adrenal and not on gonadal function (Drickamer and McIntosh, 1980; Drickamer et al., 1978), whereas suppression in the adult is dependent on ovarian function (Chipman, 1967; Clee et al., 1975) and is not part of an adrenal response to group size (Bronson and Chapman, 1968). Thus, in this case there may be at least two different signals that modulate fertility at different points of the reproductive life span.

Alternatively, pheromones produced during the ovarian cycle may have been selected because they share hormonal mechanisms with other reproductive states (McClintock, 1981, 1983b). The signals could be stronger at this time than those generated during a spontaneous estrous cycle. For example, in gerbils (Meriones unquiculatus; Payman and Swanson, 1980), pregnant or lactating mothers suppress the fertility of their daughters completely. Kin selection makes this an adaptive strategy when resources are limited. However, when the mothers are not pregnant and they resume spontaneous estrous cycles, only some of their daughters remain suppressed. Others resume estrous cycles and conceive. It is not known whether pheromones mediate this system. Nonetheless, the pattern suggests that pheromones could serve a similar function.

Data that document enhancement are notably sparse (see Table I). This is because few studies have considered the possibility of its existence, and therefore the limited number of findings should not be taken as an accurate indication of the incidence of reproductive enhancement among females.

VI. SUMMARY

Different pheromones are produced at different phases of the ovarian cycle. These pheromones can either shorten or lengthen the ovarian cycle and could do so by changing the length of follicular development, the time of gonadotropin surges, or the life span of the corpus luteum. These changes can either enhance or suppress the ovarian cycles of other females in a social group.

The synchronization of ovarian cycles is the special case when both types of signals are present and timed in a way that leads to the development of synchrony within a social group. In the rat, females produce signals that phase advance and signals that phase delay. On the other hand, female mice appear to produce only signals that phase delay the cycle, and it is the males that produce the phase-advance signal. Thus, the social mechanisms of synchrony are different in the two species, even though each is consistent with a coupled-oscillator model. In order to test this model of synchrony further, future studies will have to determine the phase-resetting curves for each of the pheromones, ideally in reference to the different functional phases of the cycle: follicular development, ovulation, and maintenance of the corpus luteum.

Similar coupling mechanisms can produce very different effects on the timing of reproduction, ranging from complete suppression to enhancement and creating either synchrony or overdispersal of ovulation within the group. Several of these phenomena are known to have selective advantages, each specific to a particular ecology and social structure. However, these advantages have been documented only in species for which pheromonal coupling has yet to be established. Therefore, the development of a complete model of the evolution of pheromonal coupling mechanisms of synchrony awaits information about both the mechanisms and the function of pheromonal coupling within the same species.

ACKNOWLEDGMENTS

The author's research is supported by grants from the National Science Foundation (BNS 80–19496) and National Institute of Aging (PHS 5 R23AG02408). The invaluable assistance of Terri Butler is gratefully acknowledged, as is the bibliographic work of Sheryl Schumacher and the editorial insight of Terra Ziporyn.

REFERENCES

Abbott, D. H., and Hearn, J. P. (1978). *J. Reprod. Fertil* **53**, 155–166.
Abegglen, J. J. (1976). Ph.D. Dissertation, pp. 166–169. University of Zurich, Switzerland (unpublished).
Ågren, G. (1976). *Biol. Behav.* **1**, 267–285.
Anderson, L. L. (1969). *In* "Reproduction in Domestic Animals" (H. H. Cole and P. T. Cupps, eds.), pp. 541–568. Academic Press, New York.
Andervont, H. B. (1944). *J. Natl. Cancer Inst. (U.S.)* **4**, 579–581.
Aron, C. (1973). *Arch. Anat. Embryol. Norm. Exp.* **56**, 209–216.
Aron, C. (1979). *Physiol. Rev.* **59**, 229–282.
Aron, C., and Chateau, D. (1971). *Horm. Behav.* **2**, 315–323.
Aron, C., Roos, J., Asch, G., and Roos, M. (1969). *C. R. Seances Soc. Biol. Ses Fil.* **163**, 2691–2694.
Aschoff, J. (1960). *Cold Spring Harbor Symp. Quant. Biol.* **25**, 11–28.
Baddaloo, E. G. Y., and Clulow, F. V. (1981). *Can. J. Zool.* **59**, 415–421.
Bellamy, D., and Davies, U. J. (1971). *J. Endocrinol.* **51**, xix.
Bertram, B. C. R. (1975). *J. Zool.* **177**, 463–482.
Bingel, A. S., and Schwartz, N. B. (1969a). *J. Reprod. Fertil.* **19**, 215–222.
Bingel, A. S., and Schwartz, N. B. (1969b). *J. Reprod. Fertil.* **19**, 223–229.
Birke, L. J. A. (1978). *Anim. Behav.* **26**, 1165–1166.
Blake, C. A. (1977). *Endocrinology* **101**, 1122–1129.
Block, M. L., Volpe, L. C., and Hayes, M. J. (1981). *Science* **211**, 1062–1064.
Brain, P. F., and Nowell, N. W. (1970). *J. Endocrinol.* **46**, xvi–xvii.
Breed, W. G. (1976). *J. Reprod. Fertil.* **47**, 395–397.
Bronson, F. H. (1975). *Endocrinology* **96**, 511–514.
Bronson, F. H. (1976). *Biol. Reprod.* **15**, 147–152.
Bronson, F. H. (1979). *Rev. Biol.* **54**, 265–299.
Bronson, F. J., and Chapman, V. M. (1968). *Nature (London)* **218**, 483–484.
Bronson, F. H., and Marsden, H. M. (1964). *Gen. Comp. Endocrinol.* **4**, 634–637.
Buck, J., and Buck, E. (1968). *Science* **159**, 1319–1327.
Buckley, T. (1982). *Am. Ethnol.* **9**, 47–60.
Buffler, G., and Roser, S. (1974). *Acta Endocrinol. (Copenhagen)* **75**, 569–578.
Calhoun, J. B. (1961). *Trans. N. Y. Acad. Sci.* [2] **23**, 437–442.
Calhoun, J. B. (1962). "The Ecology and Sociology of the Norway Rat." U.S. Public Health Service Publication No. 1008, Washington, D.C.
Campbell, A. (1964). *In* "Synchrony in Cell Division and Growth" (E. Meuthen, ed.), pp. 469–484. Wiley, New York.
Campbell, C., and Schwartz, N. B. (1980). *Endocrinology* **106**, 1230–1238.
Carr, W. J., and Caul, W. F. (1962). *Anim. Behav.* **10**, 20–27.
Carr, W. J., Solberg, B., and Pfaffmann, C. (1962). *J. Comp. Physiol. Psychol.* **55**, 415–417.
Champlin, A. K. (1971). *J. Reprod. Fertil.* **27**, 233–241.
Chateau, D., Roos, J., and Aron, C. (1972). *C. R. Seances Soc. Biol. Ses Fil.* **166**, 1110–1113.
Chateau, D., Roos, J., Roos, M., and Aron, C. (1974). *C. R. Seances Soc. Biol. Ses Fil.* **168**, 1422–1427.
Chipman, R. K. (1967). *Am. Zool.* **7**, 713.
Chipman, R. K., and Fox, K. A. (1966). *J. Reprod. Fertil.* **12**, 233–236.
Choudary, J. B., and Greenwald, G. S. (1969). *Anat. Rec.* **163**, 373–388.
Clee, M. D., Humphreys, E. M, and Russell, J. A. (1975). *J. Reprod. Fertil.* **45**, 395–398.
Coblentz, B. E. (1976). *Am. Nat.* **110**, 549–557.
Conaway, C. H., and Koford, C. B. (1965). *J. Mammal.* **45**, 577–588.

146   Martha K. McClintock

Cooper, K. J., and Hayes, N. B. (1967). *J. Reprod. Fertil.* **14**, 317–324.
Crowcroft, P., and Rowe, F. P. (1957). *Proc. Zool. Soc. London* **192**, 359–370.
Curry, J. J. (1971). *In* "Influence of Hormones on the Nervous System" (D. H. Ford, ed.), pp. 255–268. Karger, Basel.
Cutler, W. B., Garcia, C. R., and Krieger, A. M. (1979). *Psychoneuroendocrinology* **4**, 297–309.
Davis, D. E. (1955). *Behaviour* **8**, 335–343.
Dewar, A. D. (1959). *J. Endocrinol.* **18**, 186–190.
Dominic, C. J., and Pandey, S. D. (1979). *Endokrinologie* **74**, 1–5.
Drickamer, L. C. (1974). *Folia Primatol.* **21**, 61–81.
Drickamer, L. C. (1977). *J. Reprod. Fertil.* **51**, 77–81.
Drickamer, L. C., and McIntosh, T. K. (1980). *Horm. Behav.* **14**, 146–152.
Drickamer, L. C., McIntosh, T. K, and Rose, E. A. (1978). *Horm. Behav.* **11**, 131–137.
Dunbar, R. I. M. (1980). *J. Anim. Ecol.* **49**, 485–506.
Dunbar, R. I. M., and Dunbar, E. P. (1977). *Nature (London)* **266**, 351–352.
Ebling, F. J. (1972). *Gen. Comp. Endocrinol., Suppl.* **3**, 228–237.
Emlen, S. T., and Demong, N. J. (1975). *Science* **188**, 1029–1031.
Epple, G. (1973). *J. Reprod. Fertil., Suppl.* **19**, 447–454.
Epple, G. (1981). *Behav. Ecol. Sociobiol.* **8**, 117–123.
Estes, R. D. (1976). *East Afr. Wildl. J.* **14**, 135–152.
Everett, J. W. (1948). *Endocrinology* **43**, 389–405.
Everett, J. W. (1961). *In* "Sex and Internal Secretions" (W. C. Young, ed.), Vol. 1, pp. 497–555. Williams & Wilkins, Baltimore, Maryland.
Everett, J. W. (1963). *Nature (London)* **198**, 695–696.
Fagen, R. M., and Young, D. Y. (1978). *In* "Quantitative Ethology" (P. N. Colgan, ed.), pp. 79–114. Wiley, New York.
Frame, L. H., Malcolm, J. R., Frame, G. W., and van Lawick, H. (1979). *Z. Tierpsychol.* **50**, 225–249.
Fraser, A. F. (1968). "Reproductive Behavior in Ungulates." Academic Press, New York.
Freeman, M. E., Dupke, K. C., and Croteau, C. M. (1976). *Endocrinology* **99**, 223–229.
Gay, V. L., Midgley, A. R., Jr., and Niswender, G. D. (1970). *Fed. Proc., Fed. Am. Soc. Exp. Biol.* **29**, 1880–1887.
Getz, L., Dluzen, D., and McDermott, J. L. (1982). *Behav. Processes* (in press).
Graham, C. A., and McGrew, W. C. (1980). *Psychoneuroendocrinology* **5**, 245–252.
Gross, A. J., and Clark, V. A. (1975). "Survival Distributions." Wiley, New York.
Gross, G. H. (1977). *Horm. Behav.* **9**, 23–31.
Halpin, Z. T. (1980). *Biol. Behav.* **5**, 233–248.
Handelmann, G., Ravizza, R., and Ray, W. J. (1980). *Horm. Behav.* **14**, 107–115.
Harrington, J. (1976). *In* "Prosimian Behaviour" (R. D. Martin, G. A. Doyle, and A. C. Walker, eds.), pp. 331–346. London, Duckworth.
Harrington, J. P. (1931). *Int. J. Ling.* **6**, 121–161, 194–226.
Hausfater, G. (1975). "Dominance and reproduction in baboons (*Papio cynocephalus*). A quantitative analysis. Contributions to Primatology, Vol. 7." Karger, Basel.
Hayashi, S. (1979). *Physiol. Behav.* **23**, 967–969.
Henkin, R. L., and Bartter, F. C. (1966). *J. Clin. Invest.* **45**, 1631.
Hoek, H. N. (1981). Abstract. XVIIth *Int. Ethol. Conf.*, Oxford, England.
Hoppensteadt, F., and Keller, J. B. (1976). *Science* **194**, 335–336.
Hrdy, S. B. (1974). *Folia Primatol.* **22**, 19–58.
Hughes, R. L. (1964). *CSIRO Wildl. Res.* **9**, 115–122.
Izard, K., and Vandenbergh, J. (1979). Abstract. *East. Reg. Conf. Reprod. Behav.*, Tulane University, New Orleans, La. 1979.

Jarvis, J. U. M. (1981). *Science* **212**, 571–573.

Jesel, L., and Aron, C. (1974). *C. R. Seances Soc. Biol. Ses Fil.* **168**, 819–823.

Jesel, L., and Aron, C. (1976). *Neuroendocrinology* **20**, 97–109.

Johns, M. A. (1980). *In* "Chemical Signals in Vertebrates and Aquatic Invertebrates" (D. Müller-Schwarze and R. M. Silverstein, eds.), pp. 314–364. Plenum, New York.

Johns, M. A., Feder, H. H., Komisaruk, B. R., and Mayer, A. D. (1978). *Nature (London)* **272**, 446.

Jolly, A. (1967). *In* "Social Communication among Primates" (S. Altmann, ed.), pp. 3–14. Univ. of Chicago Press, Chicago, Illinois.

Katz, Y., and Epple, G. (1980). *Primatol., 8th, 1980* p. 219.

Keverne, E. B. (1979). *Ciba Found. Symp.* **62**, 271–297.

Keverne, E. B., and Michael, R. P. (1970). *J. Endocrinol.* **48**, 669–670.

Kiester, A. R., and Slatkin, M. (1974). *Theor. Popul. Biol.* **6**, 1–20.

Kimura, T. (1971). *Tokyo Daigaku Kyoyo-Gakubu* **21**, 161–166.

Kleiman, D. G. (1980). *In* "Conservation Biology" (M. E. Soule and B. A. Wilcox, eds.), pp. 243–261. Sinauer Assoc., Sunderland, Massachusetts.

Kleiman, D. G. (1982). *In* "Laboratory and Field Approaches to Social Behavior in New World Primates" (D. M. Fragaszy and J. L. Vogt, eds.). Karger, Basel (in press).

Klein, D. (1978). Ph.D. Dissertation, New York University (unpublished).

Knowlton, N. (1979). *Anim. Behav.* **27**, 1022–1033.

Krey, L. C., Tyrey, L., and Everett, J. W. (1973). *Endocrinology* **93**, 385–390.

Kummer, H. (1968). *Bibl. Primatol.* **6**, 177–179.

Lamond, D. R. (1959). *J. Endocrinol.* **18**, 343–349.

Lancaster, J. B. (1971). *Folia Primatol.* **15**, 161–182.

Laubscher, J. A., and Magalhaes, H. (1962). *Am. Zool.* **2**, 423.

Lee, E. T. (1982). "Statistical Methods for Survival Data Analysis," Lifetime Learning Publications, Belmont, California.

Leshner, A. I. (1975). *Physiol. Behav.* **15**, 225–235.

Lloyd, J. A. (1975). *J. Mammal.* **50**, 49–59.

Lombardo, D. L., and Terman, C. R. (1980). *Res. Popul. Ecol.* (Kyoto) **22**, 93–100.

Long, J. A., and Evans, H. M. (1922). *Mem. Univ. Calif.* **6**, 1–148.

McClintock, M. K. (1971). *Nature (London)* **229**, 244–245.

McClintock, M. K. (1978). *Horm. Behav.* **10**, 264–276.

McClintock, M. K. (1981). *Am. Zool.* **21**, 243–256.

McClintock, M. K. (1983a). Submitted for publication.

McClintock, M. K. (1983b). *In* "Chemical Signals in Vertebrates III" (D. Müller-Schwarze and R. M. Silverstein, eds.), Plenum, New York.

McClintock, M. K., and Adler, N. T. (1978). *Horm. Behav.* **11**, 414–418.

McClintock, M. K., and Anisko, J. J. (1982). *Anim. Behav.* **30**(2), 398–409.

McClintock, M. K., Toner, J., Adler, N. T., and Anisko, J. J. (1982). *J. Comp. Physiol. Psychol.* **96**, 268–277.

McCracken, G. F., and Bradbury, J. W. (1981). *Behav. Ecol. Sociobiol.* **8**, 11–34.

Mann, D. R., and Barraclough, C. A. (1973). *Proc. Soc. Exp. Biol. Med.* **142**, 1226–1229.

Marsden, M. M., and Bronson, F. H. (1964). *Science* **144**, 1469.

Marsden, H. M., and Bronson, F. H. (1965). *J. Endocrinol.* **32**, 313–319.

Massey, A., and Vandenbergh, J. G. (1980). *Science* **209**, 821–822.

Miller, N. (1911). *Am. Nat.* **45**, 623–635.

Milligan, S. R. (1974). *J. Reprod. Fertil.* **41**, 34–47.

Mody, J. K. (1963). *Anat. Rec.* **145**, 439–447.

Monder, H., Lee, C. T., Donovick, P. J., and Burright, R. G. (1978). *Physiol. Behav.* **20**, 447–452.

Mora, O., and Gallego, A. (1977). *Proc. Int. Union Physiol. Sci.* **13**, 525, cited in Sánchez-Criado (1979).

Moss, R. L. (1971). *J. Comp. Physiol. Psychol.* **74**, 374–382.

Mühlbock, O. (1958). *J. Endocrinol.* **17**, vii–xv.

Naftolin, F., Brown-Grant, K., and Corker, C. S. (1972). *J. Endocrinol.* **53**, 17–30.

Neal, E. (1970). *East Afr. Wildl. J.* **8**, 63–71.

Nelson, R., and Zucker, I. (1981). *Neuroendocrinology* **32**, 178–183.

Nequin, L. G., Alvarez, J., and Schwartz, N. B. (1979). *Biol. Reprod.* **20**, 659–670.

Nikitovitch-Winer, M., and Everett, J. W. (1958). *Endocrinology* **62**, 522–532.

Nishida, T. (1979). *In* "The Great Ape" (D. A. Hamburg and E. R. McCowan, eds.), pp. 73–121. Benjamin/Cummings, Menlo Park, California.

Packer, C., and Pusey, A. E. (1983). *Anim. Behav.* **31** (in press).

Parkes, A. S. (1929). *Proc. R. Soc. London, Ser. B* **104**, 183–188.

Payman, B. C., and Swanson, H. H. (1980). *Anim. Behav.* **28**, 528–535.

Pietras, R. J., and Moulton, D. G. (1974). *Physiol. Behav.* **12**, 475–491.

Plas–Roser, S., Chateau, D., and Aron, C. (1977). *Biol. Reprod.* **17**, 386–389.

Quadagno, D. M., Shubeita, H. E., Deck, J., and Francoeur, D. (1981). *Psychoneuroendocrinology* **6**, 239–244.

Ralls, K. (1977). *Am. Nat.* **111**, 917–938.

Rasa, A. (1973). *Naturwissenchaften* **6**, 303–304.

Reynold, H. (1952). *Univ. Calif., Berkeley, Publ. Zool.* **52**, 223–283.

Reynolds, J., and Keverne, E. B. (1979). *J. Reprod. Fertil.* **57**, 31–35.

Rogers, J. G., and Beauchamp, G. K. (1976). *In* "Mammalian Olfaction, Reproductive Processes, and Behavior" (R. L. Doty, ed.), pp. 181–195. Academic Press, New York.

Rood, J. P. (1974). *Nature (London)* **248**, 176.

Rood, J. P. (1975). *East Afr. Wildl. J.* **13**, 89–111.

Rood, J. P. (1978). *Z. Tierpsychol.* **48**, 277–287.

Rood, J. P. (1980). *Anim. Behav.* **28**, 143–150.

Rosen, S., Shelesnyak, M. C., and Zacharias, L. R. (1940). *Endocrinology* **27**, 463–468.

Roser, S., and Chateau, D. (1974). *C. R. Seances Biol. Strasbourg* **168**, 829–834.

Rothe, H. (1975). *Z. Tierpsychol.* **37**, 255–273.

Rowell, T. E. (1972). *Adv. Study Behav.* **4**, 69–105.

Rowell, T. E. (1977). *Folia Primatol.* **28**, 188–202.

Rowell, T. E., and Chalmers, N. R. (1970). *Folia Primatol.* **12**, 264–272.

Rowell, T. E., and Hartwell, K. M. (1978). *Behav. Biol.* **24**, 141–167.

Rowell, T. E., and Richards, S. M. (1979). *J. Mammal.* **60**, 58–69.

Russell, J. K. (1982). *In* "Seasonal Rhythms and the Ecology of a Tropical Forest: Barro Colorado Island" (E. G. Leigh, ed). Smithsonian Press, Washington, D. C. (in press).

Russell, M. J., Switz, G. M., and Thompson, K. (1980). *Pharmacol., Biochem. Behav.* **13**, 737–738.

Ryan, K. D., and Schwartz, N. B. (1976). *Fed. Proc., Fed. Am. Soc. Exp. Biol.* **35**, 686.

Ryan, K. D., and Schwartz, N. B. (1977). *Biol. Reprod.* **17**, 578–583.

Sánchez-Criado, J. E. (1979). *Rev. Esp. Fisiol.* **35**, 137–142.

Sánchez-Criado, J. E., and Gallego, A. (1979). *Acta Endocrinol. (Copenhagen)* **225**, 255.

Sano, T., Sawanobori, T., and Adaniya, H. (1978). *Am. J. Physiol.* **235**, H379–H384.

Schwartz, N. B. (1964). *Am. J. Physiol.* **207**, 1251–1259.

Schwartz, N. B. (1969). *Recent Prog. Horm. Res.* **25**, 1–55.

Schwartz, N. B. (1973). *In* "Handbook of Physiology" (R.O. Greep and E. B. Astwood, eds.), Sect. 7, Vol. 11, pp. 125–141. Am. Physiol. Soc., Washington, D.C.

Shangold, M., Freeman, R., Thysen, B., and Gatz, M. (1979). *Fertil. Steril.* **31**, 130–133.

Sinclair, A. R. E. (1977). "The African Buffalo," pp. 177–183. Univ. of Chicago Press, Chicago, Illinois.

Smith, M. S., Freeman, M. E., and Neill, J. D. (1975). *Endocrinology* **96**, 219–225.

Spott, R., and Kroeber, A. L. (1942). *Univ. Calif. Publ. Am. Archeol. Ethol.* **35**, 143–256.

Stoddart, D. M. (1976). *Inst. Biol. Stud. Biol.* **73**.

Sugiyama, Y., Yoshiba, K., and Parthasarathy, M. D. (1965). *Primates* **6**, 73–106.

Thody, A. J., Donohoe, S. M., and Shuster, S. (1979). *Acta Endocrinol. (Copenhagen)* **225**, 254.

Timmermans, P. J. A. (1978). Doctoral Dissertation, Catholic University of Nijmegen, Nijmegen, Netherlands (unpublished).

Vandenbergh, J. G. (1977). *In* "Use of Non-human Primates in Biomedical Research" (M. R. N. Prasad and T. C. Anand Kumar, eds.), pp. 174–182. Indian Science Academy, New Delhi.

Vandenbergh, J. G., and Drickamer, L. C. (1974). *Physiol. Behav.* **13**, 373–376.

Vandenbergh, J. G., and Post, W. (1976). *Physiol. Behav.* **17**, 979–984.

van der Lee, S., and Boot, L. M. (1955). *Acta Physiol. Pharmacol. Neerl.* **4**, 442–444.

van der Lee, S., and Boot, L. M. (1956). *Acta Physiol. Pharmacol. Neerl.* **5**, 213–214.

van Horn, R. N. (1975). *Folia Primatol.* **24**, 203–222.

vom Saal, F. S., Pryor, S., and Bronson, F. H. (1981). *J. Reprod. Fertil.* **62**, 33–37.

von Holst, E. (1969). [Zur Verhaltenphysiologie bei Tieren und Menschen: Gesammelte Abhandlungen.] "The Behavioral Physiology of Animals and Man" (R. Martin, transl.) Univ. of Miami Press, Coral Gables, Florida.

Wallis, J. (1982). *Am. J. Primatol.* **2**(4) (in press).

Weick, R. F., Smith, E. R., Dominguez, R., Dhariwal, A. P. S., and Davidson, J. M. (1971). *Endocrinology* **88**, 293–301.

Whitten, W. K. (1956). *J. Endocrinol.* **14**, 160–163.

Whitten, W. K. (1957). *Nature (London)* **180**, 1436.

Whitten, W. K. (1958). *J. Endocrinol.* **17**, 307–313.

Whitten, W. K. (1959). *J. Endocrinol.* **18**, 102–107.

Whitten, W. K., Bronson, F. H., and Greenstein, J. A. (1968). *Science* **161**, 584–585.

Whitten, W. K., and Champlin, A. K. (1973). *In* "Handbook of Physiology" (R. O. Greep and E. B. Astwood, eds.), Sect. 7, Vol. II, pp. 109–123. Am. Physiol. Soc., Washington, D.C.

Winfree, A. T. (1980). "The Geometry of Biological Time." Springer-Verlag, Berlin and New York.

Wolff, P. R., and Powell, A. J. (1979). *Behav. Neural Biol.* **27**, 379–383.

Woodside, B., Wilson, R., Chee, P., and Leon, M. (1981). *Science* **211**, 76–77.

Yamazaki, K., Yamaguchi, M., Baranoski, L., Bard, J., Boyse, E. A., and Thomas, L. (1979). *J. Exp. Med.* **150**, 755–760.

Yen, S. D., and Jaffee, R. B. (1978). "Reproductive Endocrinology, Physiology, Pathophysiology, and Clinical Management," pp. 71–75. Saunders, Philadelphia, Pennsylvania.

Zimen, E. (1976). *Z. Tierpsychol.* **40**, 300–341.

6

Pregnancy Blocking by Pheromones

Anna Marchlewska-Koj

Department of Genetics
Institute of Zoology
Jogiellonian University
Krakow, Poland

I. INTRODUCTION

The term "pregnancy block" is generally considered to refer to pregnancy termination in the preimplantation period by olfactory stimulants delivered by the male. This phenomenon was first described by Bruce (1959; Parkes and Bruce, 1961). The authors reported that newly mated female mice separated from the stud males and exposed to other males may terminate pregnancy and return to estrus. Pregnancy fails in over 20% of females if the second male ("strange" male) belongs to the same strain as the stud male, but pregnancy may be blocked in 80% of females if the second male ("alien" male) belongs to a strain different from the stud male. Direct contact with the male is not necessary. The pregnancy block was also observed when females were exposed to fresh male urine (Dominic, 1971) or transferred to cages soiled by alien males. Frequency of the pregnancy block

PHEROMONES AND REPRODUCTION IN MAMMALS

Copyright © 1983 by Academic Press, Inc.
All rights of reproduction in any form reserved.
ISBN 0-12-710780-0

was not influenced by the number of alien males occupying the cage (Parkes and Bruce, 1962). However, Chipman and Fox (1966b) found a higher percentage of pregnancies blocked after exposure to six males (85%) than to one male (42%). The stronger effect observed in the former case may be the consequence of an accumulation of olfactory stimulants, or alternatively it may result from the fact that a female exposed to several males has a greater chance of meeting the producer of a proper chemical signal.

A long exposure to alien males is not necessary for the pregnancy block to occur. Chipman and co-workers (1966) were successful when females were in contact with a male for 15 min three times in 4 days.

In mice the pregnant female is sensitive to the male for only a short period of time. Females return to estrus when they are exposed to an alien male during the first 4 days. In some, pregnancy is blocked by an alien male only during the first 12 hr (Bruce, 1961). The presence of the stud male eliminates the reaction of the female to a second male. Similarly, the presence of other females decreases pregnancy block to a degree proportional to the size of the group (Bruce, 1963).

The main question that now arises is, How is a female able to discriminate between the stud and nonstud males? Lott and Hopwood (1972) investigated the correlation between the length of exposure to a male during copulation and frequency of the pregnancy block by alien males. The short-term exposed females showed a lower rate of pregnancy blockage than the long-term exposed females. The authors speculated that "the effect of exposure to the stud male during breeding is to 'sensitize' the female to stimulation by the alien males." However, in very simple experiments Bloch (1974) demonstrated that the female terminates pregnancy not because she recognizes the male that performed coitus but because she is accustomed to the male's odor after having been with him for a long period. It is possible that all males are potentially capable of blocking pregnancy, but the normal ineffectiveness of the stud male is due to the habituation of the female to this male during the period of stud mating. This hypothesis could be true when pregnancy block appears only under laboratory conditions, but not if this phenomenon exists in the feral population.

In rodents, odor plays an important role in sex recognition, so the ability of the female to differentiate between two males cannot be discounted. There is some experimental evidence that female mice can discriminate not only between sexes (Bowers and Alexander, 1967) but also between the genotypes of males (Gilder and Slater, 1978). Observations on the mating behavior of congenic strains differing only at the MHC/H-2 locus indicate that a male shows a preference toward a female with an H-2 type that is different from his own (Yamazaki et al., 1980). In lemmings, a species in which the Bruce effect also occurs (see Section III), females are able to discriminate between dominant and subordinate males by odor (Huck and

Banks, 1982). These results indicate that rodents are able to discriminate even between congenic individuals, so differentiation of males by a pregnant female cannot be ruled out.

The role of male-induced pregnancy termination by olfactory signals in feral populations is still discussed and criticized, but during the past 20 years many details about the occurrence of this phenomenon under laboratory conditions have been collected. In this chapter an attempt is made to summarize briefly information about the chemical nature of the pregnancy-blocking pheromone and its effect on hormonal excitation of pregnant rodent females and also to discuss a possible function of this phenomenon in the wild population.

II. PREGNANCY BLOCK IN MICE

A. Hormonal Excitation in the Preimplantation Period

Implantation in rodents occurs at a well-defined time soon after the arrival of the blastocysts in the uterus. Nidation in mice requires the presence of the ovaries, because their removal before the fourth day of pregnancy usually prevents implantation from taking place (Humphrey, 1967). Both ovarian hormones, progesterone and estrogen, are necessary for implantation in mice and rats (Amoroso and Finn, 1962). In preparation of the uterus for nidation three hormonal components participate: The tissues are primed by estrogen release during proestrus and then stimulated by progesterone and estrogen after copulation (Finn and Martin, 1970, 1972). In experiments carried out with ovariectomized mice Martin and Finn (1968) demonstrated that the uterine endometrium is gradually primed by progesterone during days 2 and 3 of pregnancy and that progesterone in combination with estrogen induces implantation on day 4. Changes in the plasma concentration of progesterone and estrogen during early pregnancy are consistent with these observations (McCormack and Greenwald, 1974; Murr *et al.,* 1974b).

The pituitary hormones are directly involved in the release of these ovarian steroids in the early stages of gestation. Pregnancy was terminated when hypophysectomy was performed during the first 10 days after coitus (Choudary and Greenwald, 1969). Bindon (1971), in his elegant experiments with hypophysectomized mice, demonstrated that a mixture of follicle-stimulating hormone (FSH) and luteinizing hormone (LH) is required for implantation. However, in normal females nidation was inhibited by treatment with only antiovine LH. Later, Murr *et al.* (1974a) directly measured plasma levels of gonadotropins in female mice and found that the concentration of LH rose steadily, whereas that of FSH remained relatively low. At the same time the number of large antral follicles in the mouse ovaries gradually increased (Bindon, 1969). The antral follicles are probably the consequence of tonic FSH secretion and significant elevation of the LH level (Rattner *et al.*, 1978). The postcoital surge of estrogen probably originates from these antral follicles.

The increase in plasma progesterone level occurs during the first 4 days of pregnancy, corresponding to the development of corpora lutea, which is influenced by prolactin (Choudary and Greenwald, 1969). The prolactin level also rises significantly in the same period. There is no doubt that this pituitary hormone plays an important role during the time of nidation (Bartke, 1971), but the function of prolactin is not quite clear. Prolactin could be luteotropic directly (MacDonald and Greep, 1968), or it may only enhance the sensitivity of luteal cells to LH by increasing the number of luteal LH receptors, as occurs in the corpus luteum in rats (Richards and Williams, 1976).

Our information about the hormonal excitation of female mice during the early stage of pregnancy is very fragmentary, but undoubtedly the first stage of gestation (when the uterus is prepared for nidation, which follows endometrium formation) is controlled by a complex hormonal system. Even a small deviation from the required proportion of circulating hormones can prevent nidation. This may explain why females are so sensitive to external stimulants. Noxious stimuli, such as noise (Zondek and Tamari, 1967), nutritional deprivation (McClure, 1959), and hypoxia (Rattner *et al.*, 1978), interfere with blastocyst implantation in rodents. The olfactory stimulants that are discussed in this chapter are also among the factors influencing pregnancy before nidation.

B. Female Reaction to Male Pheromones

Rodents, like many other mammals, possess a dual olfactory system: the sensory receptors in the olfactory epithelium in the nasal cavity and a second set of receptors localized in the epithelial lining of the vomeronasal organ. (This topic is reviewed in greater detail in Chapter 8.) The involvement of the accessory olfactory bulb projection in the mediation of endocrine changes associated with reproduction has been also demonstrated in mice. Ablation of both the main and accessory olfactory systems as performed by Bruce and Parrott (1960) eliminated the pregnancy block effect. More recently, Reynolds and Keverne (1979) have shown that ablation of only the vomeronasal system results in a similar loss of the pregnancy block effect in female mice.

Blockage of pregnancy after exposure of the female to an alien male during the first 4 days after copulation indicates that male olfactory stimulants affect the preimplantation hormonal excitation of females. Early reports

(Dominic, 1966a) indicated that depletion of the biogenic amine level by injection of reserpine completely inhibited the Bruce effect. More recently, Sahu and Dominic (1980a) found that stimulation of serotoninergic receptors by quipazine eliminated the Bruce effect in one stock of laboratory mice. In our experiments (Table I) the expected increase in serotonin level after injection of 5-hydroxytryptophan did not inhibit pregnancy blockage, but in females with blocked pregnancy the next estrus was significantly delayed when the treatment was prolonged to the fourth or fifth day of pregnancy. Selective blocking of dopaminergic neurons by pimozide prevented implantation failure in the presence of an alien male. This finding is in agreement with the observation of Sahu and Dominic (1980b), who inhibited the Bruce effect by using chloropromazine, a dopaminergic antagonist. Injection of propranolol, a blocker of β-adrenergic receptors, impaired implantation, and the new estrus appeared later than after exposure to males. Blocking of α-adrenergic receptors by phenoxybenzamine neither abolished the Bruce effect nor altered the course of pregnancy (Table I).

The block of dopaminergic neurons gave an effect similar to hyperprolactinemia evoked by injection of prolactin (Parkes and Bruce, 1961; Dominic, 1967a) or by a pituitary graft that served as a permanent source of the hormone (Dominic, 1966b, 1967b).

Hoppe and Whitten (1972) were able to interrupt pregnancy in mice by

TABLE I

Influence of Several Drugs on Pregnancy Blockage in CBA/kw Female Mice

Drug [a]	Daily dose (mg/female)	Male	No. nonpregnant/ No. treated	Estrus (days after coitus [b])
Oil	0.2 ml	Yes	9/10	5.5 ± 0.01
Pimozide	0.1	Yes	0/19	—
5-Hydroxytryptophan	10.0	Yes	8/10	5.4 ± 0.01 [c]
5-Hydroxytryptophan[d]	10.0	Yes	7/10	8.0 ± 0.03
Propranolol	0.2	No	8/10	9.6 ± 0.02 [e]
Propranolol	0.2	Yes	9/10	6.1 ± 0.02
Propranolol + pimozide	0.2 0.1	No	0/10	—
Phenoxybenzamine	0.2	No	0/8	—
Phenoxybenzamine	0.2	Yes	8/12	5.4 ± 0.01

[a] Injected subcutaneously on second and third days of pregnancy.

[b] Mean ± SEM.

[c] $p < 0.001$ versus treatment with 5-hydroxytryptophan from second to fifth day of pregnancy.

[d] Injected subcutaneously from second to fifth day of pregnancy.

[e] $p < 0.001$ versus propranolol treatment and exposure to the male.

administering the ovulating dose of pregnancy mare serum (PMS) on the first or second day after copulation. When the females were treated on the third day, the number of implantations was reduced, whereas no effect was observed following treatment on the fourth day. Hoppe and Whitten did not report the time course of the reaction or the characteristics of the pregnancy failure induced by PMS in comparison with male-induced blockage. Our data (Marchlewska-Koj and Jemiolo, 1978) indicate that the return to estrus is much delayed following treatment with PMS. Injection with prolactin for four consecutive days prevented a pregnancy block in the presence of alien males, but it did not abolish the PMS effect (Table II). An explanation for the termination of pregnancy by PMS treatment could be that the secretion of estrogen was reduced because of luteinization of the ovarian follicles as a result of gonadotropin secretion.

The presence of an alien male was not effective when females had a pituitary graft as a source of prolactin. However, newly mated females carrying the pituitary graft did not remain pregnant after treatment with ergocriptine (CB-154), a drug that inhibits prolactin production by a direct effect on pituitary cells. The next estrus occurred after an interval similar

TABLE II

Influence of Several Agents on Pregnancy Blockage in CBA/kw Female Mice

Treatment[a]	Dose per female	Male	No. nonpregnant/ No. treated	Estrus (days after coitus[b])
Physiological saline	0.2 m	Yes	16/20	5.8 ± 0.01
HCG[c]	10.0 IU	No	0/6	—
		Yes	7/10	6.2 ± 0.02
PMS[c]	5.0 IU	No	5/5	10.2 ± 0.03[d]
		Yes	5/6	5.8 ± 0.02
PRL[e]	0.1 mg	Yes	0/10	—
PRL[e] +PMS[c]	0.1 mg 5.0 IU	No	6/6	11.3 ± 0.02
Pituitary graft[f]	1	Yes	0/8	—
CB-154[c]	0.5 mg	No	8/8	6.0 ± 0.00
Pituitary graft[f] +CB-154	1 0.5 mg	No	7/7	6.2 ± 0.03

[a] Abbreviations: HCG, human chorionic gonadotropin; PMS, pregnant mare serum; Prl, prolactin; CB-154, ergocriptine CB-154.

[b] Mean ± SEM.

[c] Injected subcutaneously on second day of pregnancy.

[d] $p < 0.001$ versus physiological saline; $p < 0.001$ versus PMS injection and exposure to male.

[e] Injected subcutaneously from second to fifth day of pregnancy.

[f] Grafted 3–4 weeks earlier.

to that observed in females after exposure to alien males. The appearance of the new estrus in pregnant females after exposure to the alien male and after treatment with CB-154 at the same time suggests that in both cases the mechanism of ovulation is similar and prolactin is the pituitary hormone that responds first to olfactory stimulation. Using a bioassay, Chapman *et al.* (1970) found some evidence for an increase in prolactin concentration in the pituitary of mated females exposed to alien males. They also found a decrease in pituitary LH level during the first 24 hr. From this observation the authors suggested that gonadotropin release is the primary hormonal response in the Bruce effect. It is very likely that, as prolactin is depleted, LH is stimulated. However, a role for adrenocorticotropin (ACTH) cannot be ruled out. Snyder and Taggart (1967) found that adrenalectomy completely eliminated the Bruce effect in the CR strain of mice.

Brain catecholamines and indolamines have been postulated to be the neurotransmitters involved in the control of gonadotropins and prolactin secretion. We have practically no information about the mechanism involved in the neurohormonal regulation of the pituitary function in mice. Our considerations must be based on the results obtained for other species, mainly rats.

The dopaminergic system inhibits the release of prolactin from the pituitary gland. Blockage of dopaminergic receptors by pimozide increases prolactin discharge (Ojeda *et al.*, 1974). The noradrenergic system stimulates the release of this hormone, and blockage of α- or β-adrenergic receptors decreases serum prolactin levels in female rats. The serotoninergic system also has a stimulating effect on prolactin release in female rats (Subramanian and Gala, 1976) and female mice (Larson *et al.*, 1977). Inhibition of pheromonal influence by a selective blockage of the dopaminergic system indicates that only dopaminergic neurons are involved in the transmission of olfactory stimulants (Table I). Delayed ovulation after exposure to an alien male and injection of 5-hydroxytryptophan is probably due to the increase in prolactin release. A similar effect was evoked in regularly cycling female mice by the continuous administration of prolactin (Gupta *et al.,* 1978) or by the injection of haloperidol, which elevates prolactin level (Reynolds and Keverne, 1979). Hormonal suppression of the estrous cycle is similar to the effect evoked by grouped female mice. The lowering of prolactin level by the injection of CB-154 in grouped females (Reynolds and Keverne, 1979) or in recently mated females (Table II) evoked estrus on the fourth day after treatment. The results discussed above indicate that prolactin is the most sensitive hormone, responding immediately to olfaction stimulation. It is very likely that the female priming pheromones stimulate prolactin release and thus suppress estrous cyclicity, whereas male pheromones inhibit discharge of this hormone, allowing the ovary to cycle.

A pheromonally induced prolactin decrease in newly mated females leads to a failure to produce corpora lutea (Dominic, 1970) and consequent inhibition of progesterone release (Chapman *et al.*, 1970). Administration of exogenous progesterone completely eliminates male-induced blockage of pregnancy (Dominic, 1966b). The deficiency of this steroid hormone in an early stage of pregnancy makes the implantation impossible. In conclusion we can state that progesterone is the last link in the hormonal chain initiated by the male pregnancy-blocking pheromone.

C. Male Production of Pheromones

Despite very extensive studies during the past few years the chemical nature of pheromones is still unknown. In their pioneer works Bruce (1965) and Dominic (1964) demonstrated that the release of the pregnancy-blocking pheromone is dependent on circulating testosterone; this pheromone is produced only by mature males. Its release can be inhibited by castration and restored by testosterone treatment. Female mice injected with testosterone are able to evoke the typical Bruce effect (Dominic, 1969; Hoppe, 1975). Pheromone release was also stimulated by other androgens (Table III). The proportion of pregnancies blocked was significantly increased by the injection of epiandrosterone, androstenedione, and androsterone. Dehydroepiandrosterone increased the proportion of pregnancies blocked, but the value was not significantly different from that found in the control.

The capacity of males to prevent implantation in female mice disappears rather slowly after castration. We found that males retained pheromonal activity on the tenth day after castration. Injection of 1 mg testosterone propionate into the castrated male stimulated the release of pheromone. The maximum activity occurred during the second day after injection, when

TABLE III

Pregnancy Blockage in BALB/c Females after Exposure to Androgenized SJL Female Mice [a]

Treatment [b]	No. nonpregnant/ No. treated	Percentage of nonpregnant females
Oil	1/19	5.6
Dehydroepiandrosterone	2/10	20.0
Epiandrosterone	5/10	50.0
Androstenedione	14/18	77.8
Androsterone	17/19	89.5
Testosterone	16/17	94.1

[a] Modified from Hoppe (1975).

[b] Injection of 1 mg steroid in 0.1 ml sesame oil.

pregnancy was blocked in 8 of 12 females tested. The pregnancy-blocking pheromone continued to be released during the next 5 days (A. Marchlewska-Koj, unpublished data). A direct correlation between circulating testosterone level and synthesis of priming pheromones indicates that either these biologically active substances are the products of catabolism of androgens or their synthesis is stimulated by androgens.

Using gas chromatography, Hoppe (1975) analyzed highly volatile fractions of male urine and suggested that the pregnancy-blocking pheromone is a degradation product of androgens. However, separated fractions were not tested for biological activity. Monder and co-workers (1978) tried to establish whether the estrus-accelerating and pregnancy-blocking effects are caused by polar or nonpolar molecules in the urine. These authors reported that both effects could be induced in females by olfactory contact with a lipid fraction extracted from urine by dichloromethane.

The urine of male mice contains a high level of proteins. A major urinary protein complex synthesized in the liver depends on androgen hormones and occurs in mature males and androgen-treated females (Rümke and Thung, 1964; Finlayson et al., 1965). The proteins salted out with ammonium sulfate from male urine evoke the typical Bruce effect (Marchlewska-Koj, 1977). Pregnancy was blocked in 90% of the females exposed to these urinary proteins. The effect was similar to the reaction elicited by the presence of alien males (80%). When the protein fraction was dialyzed for 60 hr against phosphate buffer at pH 7.4, the biological activity disappeared and 12 females tested remained pregnant. However, the pheromonal activity could be detected in the dialyzate after the following treatment. The dialyzate was passed through a resin column (Amberlite XAD-4), the column was eluted with ethyl ether, and eluate was evaporated to dryness. When the residue was suspended in distilled water and used in the bioassay, pregnancy was blocked in all 10 females tested (Dworzański and Marchlewska-Koj, unpublished data).

Castration decreases the level of protein in urine and also leads to the loss of pheromonal activity. Testosterone treatment of castrated males and females results in the appearance of pheromonal activity in the protein fraction. The results of experiments described above indicate that the pheromone responsible for evoking the Bruce effect is associated with the protein components of urine.

Male urine was fractionated by chromatography on a Sephadex G-75 column (Fig. 1). Taking into account the elution pattern, the obtained fractions were suitably pooled (pools I–V) and evaporated to dryness at 38°C using a vacuum evaporator. The residue was dissolved in distilled water. Each pool was tested for biological activity. Pregnancies were blocked only after females were exposed to fraction IV, which contained low molecular

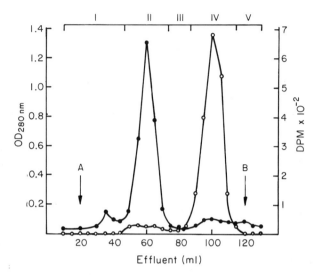

Fig. 1. Elution pattern and radioactivity of male mouse urine on a Sephadex G-75 column. The standards, (A) Blue Dextran (Pharmacia, Uppsala) and (B) L-α-alanine (Serva, Hei - delberg), were eluted at the positions shown by the arrows. A 3-ml sample of male urine collected during the 24 hr after injection of $1\mu Ci$ [1,2,6,7-³H]testosterone was dialyzed against 0.075 M NaCl/0.05 phosphate, pH 7.4, applied to a Sephadex column (18 × 450 mm), and eluted with the same solution. Absorption at 280 nm (●) and radioactivity (○) were measured in the effluent. The fractions bioassayed are indicated by roman numerals I–V.

weight peptides. Females exposed to other fractions remained pregnant (Marchlewska-Koj, 1981).

To investigate the chemical nature of the pregnancy-blocking pheromone further, mature males were injected intraperitoneally with 1 μCi of [1,2,6,7-³H]testosterone. The urine was collected in metabolic cages during the next 24 hr. After fractionation of the urine on a Sephadex G-75 column most of the radioactivity of the effluent was found in the peptide fraction co-inciding with the biological activity (Fig. 1).

In order to separate steroids and lipids the labeled or nonlabeled peptide fractions isolated by gel chromatography were extracted with dichloromethane. In the experiments with the nonlabeled peptide fraction both the water-soluble and the dichloromethane fractions were tested for biological activity. Twelve females were tested in each group. Pregnancy was blocked in 75% of the females exposed to the water-soluble fraction, whereas after contact with the chloromethane extract pregnancy was blocked in only 16%. This coincided with the distribution of radioactivity: After extraction of the peptide fraction from radio-labeled urine by dichloromethane, nearly all radioactivity remained in the water phase (92.1%), whereas the organic solvent contained only a small amount of the radioactivity (7.9%). These results suggest that the pregnancy-blocking pheromone is a product of testosterone catabolism bound to a peptide and in this form is excreted in male urine.

The source of male priming pheromones is still unknown. The pregnancy-blocking pheromone (Marchlewska-Koj, 1977), similar to the estrus-accelerating pheromone (Bronson and Whitten, 1968), is present in urine collected directly from the bladder and thus free of any accessory gland secretion. Also, hemizygous Tabby-J males with an inherited lack of preputial glands evoked the Bruce effect in a very high percentage of tested females (Gruneberg, 1971; Hoppe, 1975). Because several metabolic processes of the kidney are under androgen control (Pettengill and Fishman, 1962; Kochakian et al., 1963) this organ may represent the site of pheromone synthesis. As discussed above the biologically active substance appears to be strongly bound to the urinary protein fraction produced in the liver; the liver is therefore the next candidate for testing. However, the preputial glands cannot be definitely ruled out. These glands are known as the source of such androgen-dependent olfactory stimulants as the aggression-promoting pheromone (Mugford and Nowell, 1971, 1972) and the sex attractant pheromone (Bronson and Caroom, 1971, Caroom and Bronson, 1971). Also, the biologically active substances accelerating the estrous cycle (Gaunt, 1968; Chipman and Albrecht, 1974) and evoking the Bruce effect (Marchlewska-Koj, 1977) were found in these glands. From our present state of knowledge, it would seem quite possible that several organs are involved in the synthesis of the pheromone.

It is possible that the three priming effects associated with male urine—acceleration of puberty (Vandenbergh, 1967), acceleration of the estrous cycle (Whitten, 1956a), and blockage of pregnancy—are mediated by the same chemical messenger (or messengers) that evoke a different reaction depending on the hormonal status of the recipients. Chemical communication in mammals is an area explored mainly by physiologists, ethologists, and psychologists and only recently by chemists and biochemists. Probably for this reason we still have very little information about the chemical nature of these substances. We do not know the formulas of mouse pheromones, but some chemical properties of these substances have been described.

First, the Vandenbergh effect (Vandenbergh et al., 1975), similar to the Whitten effect and the Bruce effect (Marchlewska-Koj, 1977; Marchlewska-Koj and Biaty, 1978), can be evoked by a protein fraction of urine.

Second, the biologically active substances responsible for accelerating maturation and blocking pregnancy are present in the urinary peptide fraction (Vandenbergh et al., 1976; Marchlewska-Koj, 1981).

Finally, whether urinary pheromones are volatile is still in dispute. In the initial work of Whitten and co-workers (1968) it was demonstrated that the estrus-inducing pheromone can be transported in a tunnel if the airflow is 6 m/min. Moreover, on the basis of differences in the gas chromatographic pattern of urine from "blocking" and "nonblocking" male mice, Hoppe suggested that the Bruce effect is evoked by a volatile pheromone. In contrast, the persistence of pheromonal activity in the residue after evaporation of the urinary peptide fraction indicates that the puberty-accelerating pheromone (Vandenbergh *et al.*, 1976) and the pregnancy-blocking pheromone (Marchlewska-Koj, 1981) are nonvolatile substances.

Additional information indicating that the pregnancy-blocking pheromone is a low-volatile messenger comes from our laboratory. For more than 10 years mice from the outbred stock and CBA/kw strain were bred in the same animal room, and the typical Bruce effect was not observed. This was despite the fact that CBA/kw females are very sensitive to the male pheromone and terminate pregnancy in a very high percentage if directly exposed to outbred males or to male urine (Marchlewska-Koj, 1977).

Johns *et al.* (1978) suggest that the olfactory cues produced by male rats are nonvolatile substances. The reflex ovulation of female rats reared in constant light can be induced by male urine but only when the females have had direct contact with urine-soiled bedding. Lack of volatility is also a property of the aggression-reducing signal released by female mice (Evans *et al.*, 1978). One can hypothesize that quite different olfactory stimulants, the synthesis of which depends on steroid hormones, are all low-volatile compounds. The low-volatile substances from urine, after reaching vomeronasal epithelial cells, can be easily transposed into the organ undoubtedly involved in the transmission of chemical signals (Wysocki *et al.*, 1980; Beauchamp *et al.*, 1980).

D. Genetic Aspects of the Pregnancy Block Effect

Soon after Bruce described the pregnancy block effect in female mice Marsden and Bronson (1965) criticized her results because they were unable to evoke a similar effect using four different strains of mice. This could indicate that olfaction-dependent pregnancy termination is a characteristic only of albino Parkes stock females. Later, Godowicz (1968) and Chapman and Whitten (1969) confirmed Bruce's results, but they found a great variation among the strains of mice tested. These strain differences involved both the sensitivity of females and the ability of males to produce the pheromone.

The sensitivity or nonsensitivity of females to olfactory stimulants that evoke the pregnancy block effect appears to be strain specific. Marsden and

Bronson (1965) failed to reproduce the pregnancy block effect when using C57BL/6J females from the Jackson Laboratory (United States) colony. Also, Godowicz (1968) found the C57BL/kw females much less sensitive than CBA/kw females from a colony reared in Poland. The females of the CBA strain easily terminate pregnancy as a result of exposure to olfactory stimulants and were used in the bioassay of the Bruce effect by Dominic (1967a) (India) and in our laboratory.

The low susceptibility of C57BL females to male olfactory stimulants was also noted in another male effect. The presence of mature males facilitates ovulation in immature mice that have been treated with PMS. Among the strains tested, female C57BL/6J were the least sensitive to the presence of a mature male. (Zarrow et al., 1973; Ho and Wilson, 1980).

Variations among genotypes were found not only in sensitivity of female mice but also in pheromonal production by males. Males of the previously mentioned C57BL strain blocked pregnancy in a very low percentage of tested females (Chipman and Bronson, 1968; Hoppe, 1975; Marchlewska-Koj, 1977), whereas CBA males are known as producers of pheromones that frequently block pregnancy (Dominic, 1967; Godowicz, 1970). Eleftériou and co-workers (1972, 1973) found that the presence of C57BL/6J males did not result in a significant enhancement of the number of released ova. When females were exposed to SWR/J males, the number of ovulated eggs significantly increased. Taking into account the results of experiments with hybrids between C57BL/J and SWR/J males the authors suggested that pheromonal production is controlled by a single gene. They proposed to denote Ph^h as the gene determining high pheromonal production and Ph as its allele responsible for low production.

Long-term laboratory selection has produced different strains of mice that can be used as excellent subjects for pheromonal investigations. For instance, CBA mice represent typical animals for which olfactory stimulants play an important role in reproductive physiology. The females are sensitive—they easily terminate pregnancy—and the males produce the pheromone that is effective in blocking pregnancy. Mice from the C57BL strain belong to the opposite group. The females are not very sensitive, either as juveniles or during pregnancy. Also, the males from this strain do not produce strong pheromones. A correlation between the production of pheromones and the sensitivity to olfactory stimulants is not a general rule for all genotypes. Experiments on the KE/kw strain showed that males from this strain were able to block pregnancy in different genotype females (e.g., in CBA/kw), but they did not evoke any effect when tested with KE/kw pregnant females. However, these females were sensitive and easily terminated pregnancy when exposed to CBA/kw males (Godowicz, 1970). Lack of the stimulating effect of KE/kw males on the females of their own strain was also confirmed when the mice were tested for the Whitten effect (Krza-nowska, 1964).

The results summarized above point out that the reaction of female mice is strongly determined by an inherited feature concerning genetic variation in sensitivity of the olfactory system (Whitten, 1956b; Gandelman *et al.,* 1972; Vandenbergh, 1973) and responsiveness of the hormonal system (Hoppe and Whitten, 1972).

We have little information about genetic control of pheromone synthesis in males. Because the synthesis of the pregnancy-blocking pheromone depends directly on the presence of testosterone, all the loci that control the synthesis of this androgen have some influence on pheromonal production. This idea is supported by observations made on C57BL males. They are characterized by a low level of plasma testosterone (Bartke, 1974) and by low pheromonal activity (as described above). However, the lethal yellow (A^y) gene in the heterozygous state affects the reproductive function of male mice, probably due to the influence on cholesterol metabolism, but it does not decrease the ability to evoke the Bruce effect. The percentage of pregnancies blocked by yellow (A^ya) males was similar to that by nonyellow (*aa*) males (Bartke, 1968; Kakihana *et al.,* 1974).

Genetic aspects of pheromonal functions represent an underinvestigated area. Any information about the causes of inheritance responsible for the sensitivity and production of olfactory stimulants could be very helpful in further investigations of the role of pheromonal communication, in reproductive physiology, and in understanding the mechanisms involved in population selection.

III. PREGNANCY TERMINATION IN OTHER RODENTS

In rats, the other most commonly used member of the Muridae family, the influence of pheromones on the endocrine system is less pronounced than in mice. This species exhibited male-induced shortening of the estrous cycle (Aron, 1979; Sánchez-Criado, 1982), but the typical Bruce effect was not observed (Davis and deGroot, 1969). *Peromyscus maniculatus bairdii* females were very sensitive to male pheromones. Grouped mature females show prolonged estrous cycles, and after exposure to males or to male urine these cycles return to a normal interval (Bronson and Dezell, 1968). Pregnancy termination during the preimplantation period was also described when females were exposed to strange males or to urine cf deer mouse males (Eleuthériou *et al.,* 1962; Terman, 1969). Inhibition of the male effect by injection of prolactin into the female suggests that the initial action of the strange male on the endocrine system prevents prolactin release, which normally follows copulation in this species (Bronson *et al.,* 1969). This information indicates that the hormonal mechanism involved in the pregnancy block effect is similar in deer mouse and house mouse females.

Pregnant females of *P. m. bairdii* appear to be very sensitive to olfactory stimulants delivered by males from different species of rodents. The presence of male house mice prevented implantation in 56% of tested females, a value that is close to that obtained when male deer mice are used to induce the strange male effect (64%) (Bronson and Elefthériou, 1963; Bronson *et al.,* 1964). Until now the interspecific interaction has been described only in *P. m. bairdii* and probably is due to a different mechanism than the classical Bruce effect. The pregnancy block in this case cannot be explained by a stress effect acting through ACTH because these females did not interrupt pregnancy after being injected with a high dose of ACTH.

Merriones unguiculatus (Gerbillidae) females are next in the order of sensitivity to external stimulants, especially during the first day of pregnancy. They easily terminate pregnancy as a result of disturbances such as handling or being moved to a clean cage. However, there is no evidence of the alien male effect despite the fact that in this species olfactory communication may play an important role (Norris and Adams, 1979).

A number of Microtidae that are characterized by induced ovulation have been shown to be susceptible to male-induced pregnancy block: *Microtus agrestis* (Clulow and Clarke, 1968), *Microtus pennsylvanicus* (Clulow and Langford, 1971), *Microtus ochrogaster* (Stehn and Richmond, 1975), and *Dicrostonyx groenlandicus* (Mallory and Brooks, 1980). In addition, there is evidence suggesting that this phenomenon occurs in *Clethrionomys glareolus* (Clarke and Clulow, 1973).

The pregnancy block effect was investigated most extensively in the vole (*M. agrestis*). The termination of pregnancy, or hormonally induced pseudopregnancy, was observed in females exposed to a strange male between 48 and 72 hr after mating with stud males. The effect of the strange male was testosterone dependent. Castrated males did not interfere with pregnancy, but injection of testosterone restored the pregnancy block effect (Milligan, 1976a).

One hour's exposure of the female to the stud male during the time of mating is a sufficient period to allow the female to differentiate between the stud and the strange male. When females were reexposed to the stud male 48 hr later only 16% of the pregnancies were terminated. The time of exposure of a female to the stud male has no significant influence on the efficiency of pregnancy block caused by an alien male. When female voles were left with the stud male for 1 hr only at the time of mating and later exposed to a strange male, pregnancy was blocked in 65% of tested females. An increase in the time spent with the stud male to 48 hr did not signifi-

cantly affect the number of females blocked (Milligan, 1979). A direct contact between the female and male was necessary for pregnancy termination;
even a single-wire mesh barrier prevented the male effect from occurring.
Also, urine or feces of the male did not influence the pregnancy course
(Milligan, 1976a).

The information available for *M. agrestis* suggests that prolactin is an
important luteotropic hormone that controls the early stage of pregnancy.
The treatment of newly mated females with bromocriptine to suppress prolactin secretion results in a rapid failure of luteal function and pregnancy
termination (Charlton *et al.,* 1978). Milligan (1980) investigated the hormonal mechanism of pregnancy interruption by the strange male. Luteal
function was blocked 2 days after mating either by the injection of 1 mg
bromocriptine or by the exposure of the females to a strange male. After
48 hr new ovulations were induced by LH-releasing hormone. When the
pregnancies were blocked by the ergoalkaloid the majority of females (65%)
exhibited pseudopregnancies, but of females whose pregnancy was blocked
by the male only 28% showed such pseudopregnancy. The author suggests
that in voles the luteotropic effect of mating is mediated by a mnemonic
system. The strange male induces pregnancy failure by interfering with that
system, whereas the pregnancy termination caused by bromocriptine is due
to a short-term, direct inhibitory effect of this drug on the pituitary cells.
As in the mouse, pregnancy blocking in *M. agrestis* was associated with a
rapid degeneration of corpora lutea and the growth of Graafian follicles,
which appeared to be suppressed during pregnancy (Milligan, 1976b).

Evidence for pregnancy failure was also found in the meadow vole *M.
pennsylvanicus* (Clulow and Mallory, 1974). The females were able to pair
with a series of males. Each male, except the first, interrupted the pregnancy caused by the preceding male and initiated a further ovulation and
pregnancy. Examination of sections of ovaries revealed great differences in
the size and structure of corpora lutea. As a result of multiple consecutive
copulations the number of corpora lutea significantly increased (20.0 ± 1.3)
in comparison with the number produced by females that were mated only
once (5.6 ± 0.9). After four copulations three different generations of luteal
bodies were identified. When female meadow voles were paired with the
second males 24–48 hr after the first copulation, the first corpora lutea
degenerated rapidly in the next 24–96 hr (Mallory and Clulow, 1977). Ovaries of these females had two generations of corpora lutea. One set was
luteinized and increased in size, and the other set had cells with pycnotic
nuclei and vacuolated cytoplasm and was undergoing involution. Under experimental conditions, the repeated blocking treatment was the only treatment in which two generations of corpora lutea were found. This situation
was not observed in normal pregnancy or in postpartum copulation. This

appears to be a unique phenomenon associated with exposure to strange males.

Little is known about the mechanism involved in the control of preimplantation male-induced pregnancy termination. There is some evidence that pregnancy block is controlled by a similar mechanism both in spontaneous ovulators and in induced ovulators. For example, the implantation failure caused by the presence of a strange male is always accompanied by degeneration of corpora lutea. The other well-documented phenomenon is the inhibition of the strange male effect by an increase in the prolactin level, during lactation, for example. If prolactin has a luteotropic effect, then it is very likely that pregnancy blockage is due to the inhibition of the release of this hormone from the pituitary gland.

In contrast to the limited period when the pregnancy block can be elicited in *Mus musculus,* in some Microtidae the interruption of pregnancy by the introduction of a strange male is extended to nearly all stages of pregnancy. As described by Stehn and Richmond (1975) *M. ochrogaster* females produce litters about the twenty-fifth day after coitus. When the females were similarly paired but the stud males were replaced by unfamiliar (strange) males at intervals ranging from 5 to 15 days after the first pairing, the first pregnancy was interrupted. The termination of pregnancy was accompanied by a mucilaginous bloody discharge from the vaginal opening, usually within 36 hr after the introduction of the strange male. The females were fertilized by the new males. The intervals between insemination by the first male and delivery of litters are shown in Fig. 2.

The abortion response to the presence of a strange male was also observed in other species of microtine rodents. The introduction of the nonfamiliar male between 8 and 14 days of gestation terminated pregnancy in the females of *M. montanus* and *Pitymys pinetorum* (Stehn and Jannett, 1981). The strange male effect was not inhibited by lactation or by the presence of the stud male during the first period of pregnancy.

In the study of blockage in *M. pennsylvanicus* it was found that after exposure to the male on the fifth day after coitus the size of the corpora lutea decreased despite the fact that fetal swellings were still present on the uteri. Because the animals given this treatment showed blockage, it was concluded that the pregnancy block effect can occur even after implantation has been initiated (Mallory and Clulow, 1977). The postimplantation pregnancy disruption in *M. pennsylvanicus* was also observed after exposure to a male on the fourteenth day of pregnancy (Kenny *et al.,* 1977). Also, in the pine vole (*M. pinetorum*) male induction of abortion was described in a very high percentage of tested animals (Schadler, 1981). When they were paired after 10 days of pregnancy, 88% of the females were reinseminated. The presence of the strange male in the cage was not necessary for preg-

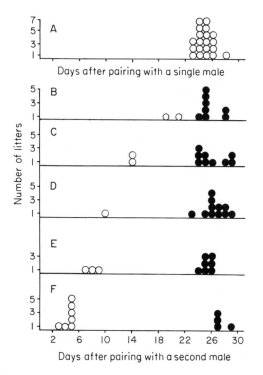

Fig. 2. Frequency of intervals from pairing until parturition in *Microtus ochrogaster* females after exposure to the stud male (A) or after replacement of the stud male by an alien male on the third to fourth day of pregnancy (B), eighth to ninth day of pregnancy (C), twelfth to thirteenth day of pregnancy (D), fourteenth to fifteenth day of pregnancy (E), or sixteenth to seventeenth day of pregnancy (F). Key: ○, the first litters maintained; ●, litters conceived after termination of the first pregnancy. (From Stehn and Richmond, 1975.)

nancy interruption. Of the females that were transferred to cages containing bedding soiled by nonstud males, 93% did not deliver litters, whereas among the control animals put in clean cages, nearly all delivered healthy pups on the twenty-fourth to the twenty-sixth day after copulation.

The abortion response to the strange male after the time of implantation is markedly different in mice and in microtines. The abortion response was recently described in a few species of rodents. The results of experiments with wild-caught Microtidae (Stehn and Jannett, 1981) point out that pregnancy termination during the postimplantation period is not a consequence of artificial selection in laboratory colonies, although the contribution of laboratory caging has not been investigated.

The possible function of pregnancy termination in the mechanism of population control is discussed in the next section.

IV. PREGNANCY BLOCK: LABORATORY ARTIFACT OR ADAPTIVE ADVANTAGE?

As a result of intensive investigations during the past few years some details are available about the hormonal and physiological background of the Bruce effect. The first information came from the experiments on house mice and deer mice. Now we have evidence for the existence of a similar phenomenon in a few species from the Microtidae family. Unfortunately, all these results have been obtained from experiments carried out in the laboratory. For this reason the question arises as to whether the pregnancy block effect evolved to serve an adaptive function in wild populations or whether it is the result of the artificial conditions of the animal room.

There is some evidence that female mice (Chipman and Fox, 1966a) and female meadow voles (Mallory and Clulow, 1977) from wild populations showed blocked pregnancy also, but the experiments with these animals were done in laboratories. However, in the ovaries of wild-trapped *M. pennsylvanicus* females two or three generations of corpora lutea were found. Similar luteal bodies were described by Mallory and Clulow (1977) in the laboratory when the females were blocked and remated. Corpora lutea were also found in the ovaries of females from wild populations of *M. californicus* (Greenwald, 1956), *C. glareolus* (Brambell and Rowlands, 1936), and *C. rutilis* (Hoyte, 1955) trapped during the breeding season. At first this was interpreted as evidence for spontaneous ovulation in Microtidae. While there is no doubt that microtines are induced ovulators, the presence of two or three sets of corpora lutea can indicate the number of copulations as a consequence of pregnancy blockage. This is the only observational evidence that the pregnancy block effect appears in wild populations, but several researchers have already attempted to explain the pregnancy block effect in terms of ecological concepts.

The Bruce effect can act on females at the peaks of density in populations. At these times, females can probably meet strange males easily and frequently. It may be that under such conditions the olfactory block of pregnancy reduces reproduction and suppresses population growth (Chipman *et al.*, 1966; Rogers and Beauchamp, 1976) or, as Bruce and Parrott (1960) suggested, this is a mechanism that prevents inbreeding in a small deme. If this adaptation can be explained only by group selection, it is still unknown how this feature is fixed in the course of natural selection.

According to Dawkins (1976) and Schwagmeyer (1979) pregnancy blockage functions to the advantage of a female deserted by her first mate, making it possible for her to remate with a male that will provide parental investment. This hypothesis would be true only for a species in which postcopulatory male parental care exists.

The pregnancy block may be a product of postcopulatory intermale competition. In reproduction one sex generally invests more than the other. In mammals this is usually the female, because she suffers the costs of gestation and lactation. Females cannot produce and rear offspring at the rate at which males can father them. Consequently, whereas the reproductive success of females is usually limited by the number of young they can produce and raise, males are often limited by factors affecting the number of females they can fertilize. In this relationship between the male and female, olfactory stimulants delivered at the appropriate time allow a male to inseminate a female even if she has already been fertilized. Some analogies exist between the prevention of pregnancy and the killing of unrelated young. Infanticide of unrelated neonates has been reported in lions (Bertram, 1975) and primates (Hrdy, 1977) and also in a few species of rodents: wild mice (Labov, 1980), several voles (Boonstra, 1980), and collared lemmings (Mallory and Brooks, 1980). Infanticide behavior may have selective advantage only for males, because females invest a large amount of time and energy. The interruption of pregnancy before implantation in mammals that produce microlecithal ova costs the female little in terms of energy. Even abortion in the late stages of pregnancy, which was described in Microtidae, is not a great waste of investment. For rodents the main problem is to cover the protein requirements. In that case at least part of the protein lost can be easily recovered by the pieces of embryo and placenta that the female eats (Stehn and Richmond, 1975). The evidence discussed above indicates that the olfactory pregnancy block does not cost females much energy. This may explain why selection did not avoid susceptibility to male stimulants. Labov (1981) minimizes the consequences of male infanticide and hypothesizes that the Bruce effect is a possible advantage for females because "those individuals which are capable of utilizing the process may actually produce more offspring which will survive past infancy and thus increase their potential individual fitness." The hypothesis that the pregnancy block effect is the infanticide of unborn offspring explains in a simple way the role of the Bruce effect in the mechanism of population control. However, this hypothesis will have to be confirmed by evidence showing that the male which interrupted pregnancy will have a chance to fertilize this particular female.

The role of the Bruce effect in modifying reproduction in feral populations remains unknown. Studies in the laboratory suggest a possible function, but only intensive joint experiments by ecologists and physiologists can offer an explanation for this intriguing phenomenon in the world of chemical communication.

REFERENCES

Amoroso, E. C., and Finn, C. A. (1962). *In* "The Ovary" (S. Zuckerman, ed.), Vol. 1, pp. 451–537. Academic Press, New York.

Aron, C. (1979). *Physiol. Rev.* **59**, 229–248.

Bartke, A. (1968). *Genetics* **60**, 161–163.

Bartke, A. (1971). *J. Reprod. Fertil.* **27**, 121–124.

Bartke, A. (1974). *J. Endocrinol.* **60**, 145–148.

Beauchamp, G. K., Wellington, J. L., Wysocki, C. J., Brand, J. G., Kubie, J. L., and Smith, A. B., III (1980). *In* "Chemical Signals in Vertebrates and Aquatic Invertebrates" (D. Müller-Schwarze and R. M. Silverstein, eds.), pp. 327–340. Plenum, New York.

Bertram, B. C. R. (1975). *J. Zool.* **177**, 463–482.

Bindon, B. M. (1969). *J. Endocrinol.* **45**, 543–548.

Bindon, B. M. (1971). *J. Endocrinol.* **50**, 19–27.

Bloch, S. (1974). *J. Reprod. Fertil.* **38**, 469–471.

Boonstra, R. (1980). *Oecologia* **46**, 262–265.

Bowers, J. M., and Alexander, B. K. (1967). *Science* **158**, 1208–1210.

Brambell, F. W. R., and Rowlands, I. W. (1936). *Philos. Trans. Br. Soc. London, Ser.* **116**, 71–181.

Bronson, F. H., and Caroom, D. (1971). *J. Reprod. Fertil.* **25**, 279–282.

Bronson, F. H., and Dezell, H. E. (1968). *Gen. Comp. Endocrinol.* **10**, 339–343.

Bronson, F. H., and Elefthériou, B. E. (1963). *Gen. Comp. Endocrinol.* **3**, 515–518.

Bronson, F. H., and Whitten, W. K. (1968). *J. Reprod. Fertil.* **15**, 131–134.

Bronson, F. H., Elefthériou, B. E., and Garick, E. J. (1964). *J. Reprod. Fertil.* **8**, 23–27.

Bronson, F. H., Elefthériou, B. E., and Dezell, H. E. (1969). *Biol. Reprod.* **1**, 302–306.

Bruce, H. M. (1959). *Nature (London)* **184**, 105.

Bruce, H. M. (1961). *J. Reprod. Fertil.* **2**, 138–142.

Bruce, H. M. (1963). *J. Reprod. Fertil.* **6**, 451–460.

Bruce, H. M. (1965). *J. Reprod. Fertil.* **10**, 141–143.

Bruce, H. M., and Parrott, D. M. V. (1960). *Science* **131**, 1526.

Caroom, D., and Bronson, F. H. (1971). *Physiol. Behav.* **7**, 659–662.

Chapman, V. M., and Whitten, W. K. (1969). *Genetics* **61**, Suppl. 9.

Chapman, V. M., Desjardins, C., and Whitten, W. K. (1970). *J. Reprod. Fertil.* **21**, 333–337.

Charlton, H. M., Milligan, S. R., and Versi, E. (1978). *J. Reprod. Fertil.* **52**, 283–288.

Chipman, R. K., and Albrecht, E. D. (1974). *J. Reprod. Fertil.* **38**, 91–96.

Chipman, R. K., and Bronson, F. H. (1968). *Experientia* **24**, 199–200.

Chipman, R. K., and Fox, K. A. (1966a). *J. Reprod. Fertil.* **12**, 233–236.

Chipman, R. K., and Fox, K. A. (1966b). *J. Reprod. Fertil.* **12**, 399–403.

Chipman, R. K., Holt, J. A., and Fox, K. A. (1966). *Nature (London)* **210**, 653.

Choudary, J. B., and Greenwald, G. S. (1969). *Anat. Rec.* **163**, 373–378.

Clarke, J. R., and Clulow, F. K. (1973). *In* "The Development and Maturation of the Ovary and Its Functions" (H. Peters, ed.), pp. 160–170. Excerpta Medica, Amsterdam.

Clulow, F. K., and Clarke, J. R. (1968). *Nature (London)* **219**, 511.

Clulow, F. K., and Langford, P. E. (1971). *J. Reprod. Fertil.* **24**, 275–277.

Clulow, F. K., and Mallory, F. F. (1974). *Can. J. Zool.* **52**, 265–267.

Davis, D. L., and deGroot, J. (1969). *Anat. Rec.* **148**, 366–369.

Dawkins, R. (1976). "The Selfish Gene." Oxford Univ. Press, London/New York.

Dominic, C. J. (1964). *J. Reprod. Fertil.* **8**, 266–267.

Dominic, C. J. (1966a). *Science* **152**, 1764–1765.

Dominic, C. J. (1966b). *J. Reprod. Fertil.* **11**, 415–421.

Dominic, C. J. (1967a). *Indian J. Exp. Biol.* **5**, 47–48.

Dominic, C. J. (1967b). *Nature (London)* **213**, 1242–1243.

Dominic, C. J. (1969). *Indian J. Zootomy* **10**, 88–92.

Dominic, C. J. (1970). *J. Anim. Morphol. Physiol.* **17**, 126–130.

Dominic, C. J. (1971). *Indian J. Exp. Biol.* **9**, 255–258.

Elefthériou, B. E., Bronson, F. H., and Zarrow, M. X. (1962). *Science* **137**, 764.

Elefthériou, B. E., Bailey, D. W., and Zarrow, M. X. (1972). *J. Reprod. Fertil.* **31**, 155–158.

Elefthériou, B. E., Christenson, C. M., and Zarrow, M. X. (1973). *J. Endocrinol.* **57**, 363–370.

Evans, C. M., Mackintosh, J. H., Kennedy, J. F., and Robertson, S. M. (1978). *Physiol. Behav.* **20**, 129–134.

Finlayson, J. S., Asofsky, R., Potter, M., and Runner, C. C. (1965). *Science* **149**, 981–982.

Finn, C. A., and Martin, L. (1970). *J. Endocrinol.* **47**, 431–438.

Finn, C. A., and Martin, L. (1972). *Biol. Reprod.* **7**, 82–86.

Gandelman, R., Zarrow, M. X., and Denenberg, V. H. (1972). *J. Reprod. Fertil.* **28**, 453–456.

Gaunt, S. L. (1968). Ph.D. Thesis, University of Vermont, Burlington.

Gilder, P. M., and Slater, P. J. B. (1978). *Nature (London)* **274**, 364–365.

Godowicz, B. (1968). *Folia Biol. (Krakow),* **16**, 199–206.

Godowicz, B. (1970). *J. Reprod. Fertil.* **23**, 237–241.

Greenwald, G. S. (1956). *J. Mammal.* **37**, 213–222.

Grüneberg, H. (1971). *J. Embryol. Exp. Morphol.* **25**, 1–19.

Gupta, S., Jailkhani, B., Gupta, C., and Talwar, G. (1978). *Indian J. Exp. Biol.* **16**, 1233–1235.

Ho, H., and Wilson, J. R. (1980). *J. Reprod. Fertil.* **59**, 57–61.

Hoppe, P. C. (1975). *J. Reprod. Fertil.* **45**, 109–115.

Hoppe, P. C., and Whitten, W. K. (1972). *Biol. Reprod.* **7**, 254–259.

Hoyte, H. M. D. (1955). *J. Anim. Ecol.* **24**, 412–426.

Hardy,S. B. (1977)."The Langurs Of Abu: Female and Male Strategies of Reproduction." Harvard Univ. Press, Cambridge, Massachusetts.

Huck, U. W., and Banks, E. M. (1982). *Anim. Behav.* **30**, 665–675.

Humphrey, K. W. (1967). *Steroids* **10**, 591–600.

Johns, M. A., Feder, H. H., Komisaruk, B. R., and Mayer, A. D. (1978). *Nature (London)* **272**, 446–447.

Kakihana, R., Ellis, L. B., Gerling, S. A., Blum, S. L., and Kessler, S. (1974). *J. Reprod. Fertil.* **40**, 483–487.

Kenny, A. McM., Evans, R. L., and Dewsbury, D. A. (1977). *J. Reprod. Fertil.* **49**, 365–367.

Kochakian, C. D., Hill, J., and Aonuma, S. (1963). *Endocrinology* **72**, 354–363.

Krzanowska, H. (1964). *Folia Biol. Krakow* **12**, 415–426.

Labov, J. B. (1980). *Behav. Ecol. Sociobiol.* **6**, 297–303.

Labov, J. B. (1981). *Am. Nat.* **118**, 361–371.

Larson, B. A., Sinha, J. N., and Vanderlaan, W. P. (1977). *J. Endocrinol.* **74**, 153–154.

Lott, D. F., and Hopwood, J. H. (1972). *Anim. Behav.* **20**, 263–266.

McClure, T. J. (1959). *J. Physiol. (London)* **147**, 221–224.

McCormack, J. T., and Greenwald, G. S. (1974). *J. Reprod. Fertil.* **41**, 297–301.

MacDonald, G. J., and Greep, R. O. (1968). *Perspect. Biol. Med.* **11**, 490–497.

Mallory, F. F., and Brooks, R. J. (1980). *Biol. Reprod.* **22**, 192–196.

Mallory, F. F., and Clulow, F. V. (1977). *Can. J. Zool.* **55**, 1–17.

Marchlewska-Koj, A. (1977). *Biol. Reprod.* **17**, 729–732.

Marchlewska-Koj, A. (1981). *J. Reprod. Fertil.* **61**, 221–224.

Marchlewska-Koj, A., and Bialy, E. (1978). *Folia Biol. (Krakow)* **26**, 311–314.

Marchlewska-Koj, A., and Jemiolo, B. (1978). *Neuroendocrinology* **26**, 186–192.

Marsden, H. H., and Bronson, F. H. (1965). *Nature (London)* **207**, 878.

Martin, L., and Finn, C. A. (1968). *J. Endocrinol.* **41**, 363–371.

Milligan, S. R. (1976a). *J. Reprod. Fertil.* **46**, 91–95.

Milligan, S. R. (1976b). *J. Reprod. Fertil.* **46**, 97–100.

Milligan, S. R. (1979). *J. Reprod. Fertil.* **57**, 223–225.

Milligan, S. R. (1980). *Symp. Zool. Soc. London* **45**, 251–275.

Monder, H., Lee, C.-T., Donovick, P. J., and Burright, R. G. (1978). *Physiol. Behav.* **20**, 447–452.

Mugford, R. A., and Nowell, N. W. (1971). *Physiol. Behav.* **6**, 247–249.

Mugford, R. A., and Nowell, N. W. (1972). *Horm. Behav.* **9**, 39–46.

Murr, S. M., Bradford, G. E., and Geschwind, I. I. (1974a). *Endocrinology* **94**, 112–116.

Murr, S. M., Stabeufeldt, G. H., Bradford, G. E., and Geschwind, I. I. (1974b). *Endocrinology* **94**, 1209–1211.

Norris, M. L., and Adams, C. E. (1979). *J. Reprod. Fertil.* **57**, 401–404.

Ojeda, S. R., Harms, P. G., and McCann, S. M. (1974). *Endocrinology* **94**, 1650–1657.

Parkes, A. S., and Bruce, H. M. (1961). *Science* **134**, 1046–1054.

Parkes, A. S., and Bruce, H. M. (1962). *J. Reprod. Fertil.* **4**, 303–308.

Pettingill, O. S., and Fishman, W. H. (1962). *Exp. Cell Res.* **28**, 218–253.

Rattner, B. A., Michael, S. D., and Brinkeley, H. J. (1978). *Biol. Reprod.* **19**, 558–565.

Reynolds, J., and Keverne, E. B. (1979). *J. Reprod. Fertil.* **57**, 31–35.

Richards, J. S., and Williams, J. J. (1976). *Endocrinology* **99**, 1571–1581.

Rogers, J. G., Jr., and Beauchamp, G. K. (1976). *In* "Mammalian Olfaction, Reproductive Processes, and Behavior" (R. L. Doty, ed.), pp. 181–195. Academic Press, New York.

Rümke, P. and Thung, P. J. (1964). *Acta Endocrinol. (Copenhagen)* **47**, 156–164.

Sahu, S. C., and Dominic, C. J. (1980a). *Ann. Endocrinol.* **41**, 425–429.

Sahu, S. C., and Dominic, C. J. (1980b). *Indian Exp. Biol.* **18**, 1025–1027.

Sánchez-Criado, J. E. (1982). *In* "Olfaction and Endocrine Regulation" (W. Breipohl, ed.), pp. 209–222. IRL Press, London.

Schadler, M. H. (1981). *Biol. Reprod.* **25**, 295–297.

Schwagmeyer, P. L. (1979). *Am. Nat.* **114**, 932–938.

Snyder, R. L., and Taggart, N. E. (1967). *J. Reprod. Fertil.* **14**, 451.

Stehn, R. A., and Jannett, F. J., Jr. (1981). *J. Mammal.* **62**, 369–372.

Stehn, R. A., and Richmond, M. E. (1975). *Science* **187**, 1211–1213.

Subramanian, M. G., and Gala, R. R. (1976). *Endocrinology* **98**, 842–848.

Terman, G. R. (1969). *Anim. Behav.* **17**, 104–108.

Vandenbergh, J. G. (1967). *Endocrinology* **81**, 345–349.

Vandenbergh, J. G. (1973). *Physiol. Behav.* **10**, 257–262.

Vandenbergh, J. G., Whitsett, J. M., and Lombardi, J. R. (1975). *J. Reprod. Fertil.* **43**, 515–523.

Vandenbergh, J. G., Finlayson, J. S., Dobrogosz, W. J., Dills, S. S., and Kost, T. A. (1976). *Biol. Reprod.* **15**, 260–265.

Whitten, W. K. (1956a). *J. Endocrinol.* **13**, 399–404.

Whitten, W. K. (1956b). *J. Endocrinol.* **14**, 160–163.

Whitten, W. K., Bronson, F. M., and Greenstein, J. H. (1968). *Science* **161**, 584–585.

Wysocki, C. J., Wellington, J. L., and Beauchamp, G. K. (1980). *Science* **207**, 781–783.

Yamazaki, K., Yamaguchi, H., Boyse, E. A., and Thomas, L. (1980). *In* "Chemical Signals in Vertebrates and Aquatic Invertebrates" (D. Müller-Schwartze and R. M. Silverstein, eds.), pp. 267–273. Plenum, New York.

Zarrow, M. X., Elefthériou, B. E., and Denenberg, V. H. (1973). *J. Reprod. Fertil.* **35,** 81–87.

Zondek, B., and Tamari, I. (1967). *In* "Effects of External Stimuli on Reproduction" (G. E. Wolstenholme and M. O'Connor, eds.), pp. 4–19. Little, Brown, Boston, Massachusetts.

7

Hormonal Responses to Primer Pheromones

F. H. Bronson and Bruce Macmillan

Department of Zoology
Institute of Reproductive Biology
University of Texas
Austin, Texas

I. INTRODUCTION

It is a biological truism that reproduction must be accomplished in accord with whatever demands are placed on an organism by its environment. To this end most higher organisms have evolved signalling systems that allow their reproduction to be modulated by relevant environmental variation. The ambient factors monitored by these systems originate in the physical, dietary, and social dimensions of the organism's environment. The crude environmental limits for mammalian reproduction, for example, are set by

175

PHEROMONES AND REPRODUCTION IN MAMMALS
Copyright © 1983 by Academic Press, Inc.
All rights of reproduction in any form reserved.
ISBN 0–12–710780–0

physical and/or dietary factors, whereas social stimuli function in the temporal regulation of specific reproductive events or processes. This chapter is concerned with one dimension of the latter phenomenon: the modulation of endocrine activity by sociochemical cues to regulate reproductive events temporally.

The importance of the chemoolfactory pathway to mammalian communication in general, and mammalian reproduction in particular, is indisputable. This book is testimony to that fact. Indeed, although mammalian communication almost always involves multiple cueing and simultaneous activity of more than one sensory modality, the liberation of a chemical cue by one individual and its perception by way of the primary or accessory olfactory pathways of another individual probably constitutes the dominant mode of communication under the widest variety of social circumstances. With specific regard to reproduction, chemical communication seems to serve three broad functions in mammalian populations. First, chemical cues are important in ensuring an appropriate dispersion of the social units that comprise the breeding population. From that perspective, one of the most common behaviors associated with foraging in mammals is the routine deposition of a time-delayed chemical signal that advertises the occupancy of a particular locale by an individual or a social group. Second, chemical cues often play important roles in the acute, short-range identifications that precede aggressive or sexual interactions. This function probably finds its greatest importance in nocturnal species, but it is relatively common in diurnal species as well. Third, chemical cues may evoke the stereotyped endocrine responses that are the major concern of this chapter.

The simple fact that chemical cues can elicit endocrine responses that culminate in changes in an individual's reproductive state is too well established and too well reviewed already to require detailed substantiation here (e.g., Whitten and Bronson, 1970; Vandenbergh, 1975; Bronson and Coquelin, 1980; Bronson, 1982). Worthy of comment, however, is the application of the term "primer pheromone" to such cues. The concept of a pheromone has had great utility in entomology, but its extension to mammals, first done by Whitten (1966) and later amended by Bronson (1968), has created considerable controversy (e.g., see Beauchamp et al., 1976). The basis for this controversy resides in a well-warranted concern about the potential implication of stereotypy for the more experience-dominated responses of the mammal. The position adopted in this chapter is as follows. First, in the absence of hard data demonstrating an effect of experience on a mammal's gonadotropic responses to sociochemical cues (and, indeed, with ample evidence to the contrary), there seems to be no good argument against using the term "priming pheromone" in relation to these particular responses. Second, however, as will be demonstrated later, the situation regarding nongonadotropic endocrine responses is more complicated and argues against the universal use of the term for all endocrine responses to all chemical cues in mammals.

The intent of this chapter is to develop a set of principles about the endocrine pathways activated by mammalian priming pheromones and about the reproductive benefits thereby gained. Unfortunately, endocrine data of a quality that allow one to do more than simply document a primer-induced change in a hormone titer have been collected in only one species, the house mouse. Thus, we have attempted to use this single species as a model for deriving generalities that can be tested later in other species. More specifically, this chapter has three goals, which are pursued in the following order. First, we attempt to organize our knowledge about priming phenomena in mice in an effort to identify the core endocrine pathways underlying these phenomena. Second, we discuss each such pathway in the context of its functional significance to the mouse's reproduction. Finally, we compare the mouse's priming system in its entirety with the other types of ambient modulating systems that are found in mammals.

II. PRIMING PHENOMENA IN LABORATORY MICE

Starting with the early observations of van der Lee and Boot (e.g., 1956) and, more significantly, with several papers published by Whitten between 1956 and 1959, interest in mouse priming phenomena has grown steadily. One result has been several recurring cycles of publication in which a reproductive effect of exposing one animal to another is first identified and then reproduced by exposure only to the animal's urine. This process has led directly to the conclusion that there are as many as six or seven priming phenomena in mice. Actually, as suggested in Table I, there probably are only three core phenomena: an accelerating action of male urine on the female ovulatory cycle, a decelerating action of female urine on the ovulatory cycle of other females, and the capacity of female urine to release luteinizing hormone (LH) in males to serve some unknown reproduction function.

There is an obvious danger of oversimplification in the reductionism evidenced in Table I and, indeed, there are bits and pieces of information suggesting that such a procedure may be misleading in one case. The weight of the evidence in regard to the number of hormonal pathways involved in primer effects in mice, however, supports the premise that there are only three basic phenomena. Using the presumably diverse effects of male urine on females as an example, there simply is no good reason to consider a

TABLE I

Effect of Urinary Priming Pheromones in Mice

Origin of primer	Responder	Effect	References[a]
Male	Female	Induce cycling and ovulation in both peripubertal and adult females, even if the latter are pregnant or pseudopregnant	Whitten (1956), Bruce (1959), Dominic (1964), Marsden and Bronson (1964), Vandenbergh (1967, 1969)
Female	Female	Inhibit cycling and ovulation in both adult and peripubertal females; antagonize male's action in young females	van der Lee and Boot (1955), Whitten (1959), Cowley and Wise (1972), Vandenbergh et al. (1972), McIntosh and Drickamer (1977)
Female	Male	Release LH and testosterone; reproductive effect unknown	Macrides et al. (1975), Maruniak and Bronson (1976)

[a] The references listed are the early papers that reported the reproductive effect itself, an important variation of that effect, or the fact that the effect could be elicited with urine alone.

male-induced ovulation in a progesterone-dominated, pseudopregnant female as being endocrinologically different from a strange-male-induced ovulation in a progesterone-dominated, early-pregnant female. Both effects can be elicited by exposure to urine collected as a pool from many males and, undoubtedly, the endocrine pathways underlying these two effects are the same also. Likewise, no good purpose seems served by maintaining as separate phenomena the induction of a female's first ovulation by exposure to a male or his urine and the induction of her second and later ovulations by the same stimuli. Thus, we attempt now to delineate the three core pathways suggested by Table I and to determine the endocrine variations that underly specific manifestations that are dependent on age or reproductive state.

A. Hormonal Responses of Females to Adult Male Stimuli

Our most comprehensive understanding of the endocrine responses of a female to a male stems from research done with peripubertal females. This section therefore begins with this variation. As first shown by Vandenbergh (1967; Vandenbergh et al., 1972) and as discussed in his chapter in this book (Chapter 4), puberty in a female mouse is a labile event that can be accelerated temporally by the presence of an adult male and delayed by the presence of other females. The two relevant cues emanating from the male are an androgen-dependent, urinary priming pheromone that has been partially isolated (Vandenbergh *et al.,* 1976) and an unidentified tactile stimulus (Drickamer, 1974). These two cues act in a truly synergistic manner, the urinary cue exerting a relatively small effect compared with the presence of the male itself, and the tactile cue yielding no discernible activity in the absence of the urinary primer (Bronson and Maruniak, 1975).

The most obvious result of exposing a young female to an adult male is an elicitation of the pubertal ovulation at an earlier age than would have occurred in the absence of the male. Therefore, the endocrine pathways activated by the male's cues are best examined functionally in the context of this first ovulation. By way of background, then, most of the endocrine changes that precede and evoke the pubertal ovulation remain only cursorily understood, regardless of the species in question. Indeed, there is general agreement among researchers only that developmental changes in two basic relationships are of central importance here: First, the negative feedback action by which the gonadal steroids tonically inhibit LH secretion and, second, the precise relationship between this tonic negative feedback action and the positive feedback elicitation of an ovulatory surge of LH release by the same steroids, particularly estradiol (reviewed by Ramirez, 1973; Davidson, 1974; Odell and Swerdloff, 1976; Ramaley, 1979).

Prevailing opinion, based mostly on studies done with rats and sheep, holds that one of the most important changes preceding the pubertal ovulation is a decrease in the sensitivity of the tonic negative feedback regulation of LH secretion by estradiol (the "gonadostat" concept of McCann and Ramirez, 1964). Thus, as development proceeds, the same amount of circulating estradiol is viewed as becoming progressively less capable of tonically inhibiting LH secretion. A decrease in negative feedback sensitivity then would allow progressively more and more LH to be secreted and, as a consequence, more and more estradiol would be secreted also. Continuing in this vein, the gradually increasing titer of estradiol eventually would exceed the critical threshold necessary for inducing an ovulatory release of LH via positive feedback. The data gathered so far on the mouse do not support all of this presumed sequence of events.

Indeed, blood levels of LH do rise slowly and gradually during development in the female mouse, starting at the juvenile stage (12–14 g in CF-1 females) and ending when full maturation is achieved, usually at 26–30 g (Bronson, 1981). This change, however, does not seem to reflect a decrease in the sensitivity of the negative feedback mechanism. On the contrary, the gradual increase in LH titer in the developing mouse seems to result from a change in the steroid-independent, direct drive by which the brain promotes tonic LH secretion (Bronson, 1981). Thus, in the absence of any social cues, male or female originating, ovulation will occur eventually in the mouse, presumably because of the progressive enhancement of estradiol secretion by LH. As noted earlier, however, social factors are of overriding importance in this species.

Turning first to the male's accelerating action on puberty, we find that exposure of a peripubertal female to a male results in an immediate elevation in LH secretion, a change that is followed shortly by a profound rise in serum estradiol levels (Fig. 1). The only effect of the male on serum levels of follicle-stimulating hormone (FSH) is to lower them on the second day of male exposure while, simultaneously, prolactin levels in the blood begin to rise (Bronson and Maruniak, 1976). Both of these actions probably are secondary reflections of a high estradiol titer because they do not occur in estradiol-implanted, ovariectomized adults that are exposed to males (Bronson, 1976). When the young female weighs 14 g, the sequential LH/estradiol response culminates in ovulation in 7 to 9 days, whereas at 17 to 18 g the ovulatory surge of LH occurs after only two daily elevations of estradiol (Fig. 1), and by 20 g only one such daily elevation is needed (Bronson, 1975a,b, 1981).

The endocrine bases underlying the decreasing time requirement for a male to induce ovulation in a developing female have been the subject of an extensive series of experiments (Bronson, 1981). All of these studies have involved comparisons of ovariectomized CF-1 females of various ages, and they have relied on a combination of encapsulated estradiol and injections of estradiol benzoate to mimic both the relatively stable estradiol background against which the male exerts its effect (mimicked by a slow-release capsule) and the action of the male to elevate acutely blood titers of this hormone (mimicked by an injection). These studies reveal the overriding importance of two developmental factors in determining the length of time required by a male to induce ovulation: (*a*) the immaturity of the LH-surging mechanism (positive feedback) before 15 to 17 g and (*b*) a continuous change between 14 g and full maturity in the flexibility of the relationship between the negative and positive feedback systems. Thus, although the male can elicit LH and estradiol release in the 14-g female, ovulation does not result until much later, when the LH-surging mechanism has matured. After this stage of development, however, the second factor comes into prominence.

One of the most important differences between females at 18 g and full maturity lies in the flexibility of the relationship between the negative and positive feedback systems. This relationship is extremely rigid in the younger animal and quite flexible in the adult. Stated in another way, it is relatively easy to induce experimentally an ovulatory-like surge of LH release in the ovariectomized adult with a variety of combinations of doses of encapsu-

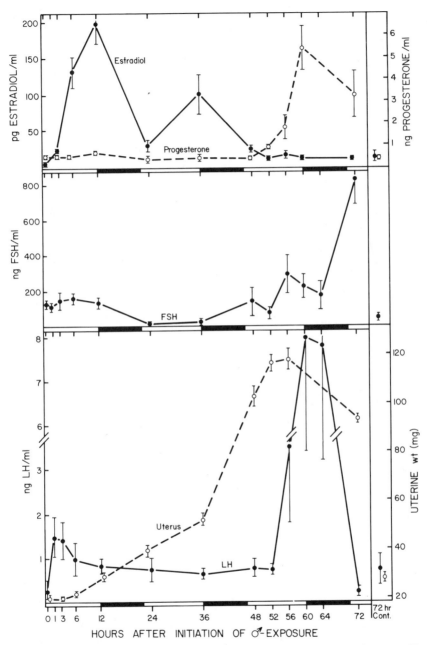

Fig. 1. Sequential changes in hormone titers in 17- to 18-g CF-1 female mice over a 72-hr period of male exposure. The "controls," which were killed at 72 hr, were held in isolation (Bronson and Desjardins, 1974).

lated and injected estradiol. This is not true in the ovariectomized immature female, particularly with regard to the background level of estradiol that is provided by a capsule. Background levels of circulating estradiol must be in a quite narrow, intermediate range if either the male or an injection is to induce an ovulating surge of LH release. Thus, in the 18-g female the male causes an abrupt elevation in estradiol on the first day of pairing (Fig. 1), which "resets" the base level of circulating estradiol in the intermediate range where the second day's elevation of estradiol will trigger an LH surge (Bronson, 1975a, 1981). Because background estradiol levels rise slowly throughout development (presumed in the mouse but not actually measured), the female requires only one such elevation of estradiol at 20 g and spontaneous ovulation may occur in a few individuals as early as 22 g. The relationship between the "resetting" process noted above and the concept of negative feedback is totally unclear at this time.

With only two physiological complications, there is no reason to believe that the ovulation-inducing action of a male, as described above, should be greatly different in adult females than it is in peripubertal females. Certainly the relevant male stimuli do not appear to change after the female has experienced her first ovulation (Bronson and Whitten, 1968). The two complications of concern here have both been mentioned earlier in passing. First, the relationship between the negative and positive feedback controls is much more flexible in the adult female. Theoretically, this should enhance the efficacy with which male stimuli induce ovulation. Countering this factor, however, is the second complication, namely, that adult females often have much higher circulating levels of progesterone, a steroid that antagonizes LH secretion. Specifically, males can induce ovulation in pseudopregnant and early-pregnant females, two conditions that are characterized by marked progesterone dominance. As noted earlier, the fact that ovulation can be induced in both situations with pooled male urine argues that the endocrine pathways modulated by the male are the same in the two conditions.

Not surprisingly, the LH/estradiol pathway activated by the male to induce ovulation in the young female remains functional in the adult. This fact was established in experiments with ovariectomized adults bearing slow-release, silastic implants of estradiol. Under these conditions the action of male urine is to enhance the release of LH markedly with no discernible effect on either FSH or prolactin (Bronson, 1976). The activity of the LH/estradiol pathway is partially obscured, however, if the female is pseudopregnant. Given the progesterone/prolactin dominance of pseudopregnancy, the significant effects of a male are to depress the female's high levels of progesterone progressively and, later, to enhance estradiol secretion (Ryan and Schwartz, 1980). The pituitary intermediaries of these two steroid effects were not well delineated by Ryan and Schwartz, but they seemed to include a progressive decline in circulating levels of prolactin with no change at all in LH. Injections of prolactin protect against the pregnancy-blocking action of a strange male (Bruce and Parkes, 1960), and injections of bromocriptine, a drug that lowers blood levels of prolactin, cause a return to cycling in females whose cycle is under progesterone dominance (Reynolds and Keverne, 1979).

Remembering that the end product of a male's action always must be an elevation in blood estradiol levels in order to trigger an LH surge, we can offer a theoretical model that encompasses all of the diverse endocrine responses that have been observed in both immature and mature females. The first element in this model is a neuroendocrine pathway that includes the potential for enhancing LH secretion while simultaneously depressing prolactin secretion. The second element is a threshold of some kind that allows the prolactin-suppressing dimension of the pathway to act only when blood levels of prolactin are high. Thus, blood prolactin levels are low in prepubertal animals and, as a consequence, only the LH-releasing action of the male is seen in these females. The third element of our model is a simple acknowledgment of the fact that the release of both prolactin and LH is dependent on the extant steroid milieu. Thus, prolactin and progesterone levels are high in pseudopregnancy and early pregnancy and, consequently, only the prolactin-suppressing action of the male would be seen here because LH secretion would be suppressed by progesterone. The fourth element of this model is a recognition that the steroid milieu changes dynamically during the 2- or 3-day period required by the male to induce ovulation, regardless of the female's age or reproductive state. Thus, FSH levels, which are not directly involved in the male's actions, are suppressed during the second day of male exposure, probably by estradiol. Furthermore, the low prolactin levels of the immature female are elevated on the second day of male exposure, again probably as a direct reflection of a high estradiol titer. Finally, the fifth element of this model concerns the ovary of the pseudopregnant and early-pregnant female. The steroidogenic nature of this ovary probably is such that greatly enhanced estradiol secretion will result more or less automatically when prolactin and progesterone secretion are depressed by a male.

To us the model presented here accounts for all of the observations made by the direct measurement of hormones or by injections given to mimic or counter the action of the male. Whether this model actually describes with accuracy the responses of females of all ages and reproductive states to the male's priming action remains to be seen.

B. Effects of Females on Other Females, and the Relative Impact of Male- and Female-Originating Cues on Ovulation

As shown in Table I, female-originating cues inhibit cycling and ovulation in other females. These cues also can effectively antagonize the ovulation-inducing action of a male, provided that the females in question are young enough. Thus, ovulation is inhibited by housing peripubertal females in groups regardless of whether a male is present, whereas the male's cues easily override the inhibitory effects of grouping adult females. The latter phenomenon, of course, was the basis for the first described effect of a priming pheromone in any mammal: the synchrony of ovulation that was observed by Whitten (1956) on the third day after grouped adult female mice were individually paired with males, and the verification that this synchrony could be elicited only with male urine (Marsden and Bronson, 1964).

The role of a urinary factor in female/female inhibitory interactions is well established now (e.g., McIntosh and Drickamer, 1977). Whether non-pheromonal stimuli add to this inhibition is not known, but this seems probable. Relatively little is known about the endocrine pathways involved in female/female suppression, but two types of experiment have shed a little light on these pathways. First, grouping of ovariectomized, estradiol-implanted adults depresses their LH secretion and dramatically elevates prolactin secretion relative to isolated controls (Bronson, 1976). Second, Ryan and Schwartz (1977, 1980) demonstrated that grouping females on the day of their estrus yields a true pseudopregnancy characterized by high levels of prolactin and progesterone.

Both types of data make physiological sense. It has long been established that adult female mice respond to grouping with a prolonged cycle that may adopt various forms ranging from a simple lengthening of the metestrous/early diestrous phase of the cycle to an actual pseudopregnancy. A decrease in circulating basal levels of LH would prolong the metestrous/early diestrous phase of a cycle, whereas a marked increase in prolactin would yield both a high progesterone titer and pseudopregnancy. Thus, again it would appear that the neuroendocrine pathways activated by priming pheromones in the female include the potential for simultaneous modulation of both LH and prolactin.

Returning now to the question of the male's accelerating actions in relation to female/female interactions, this relationship is best viewed from a developmental perspective. As shown in Table II and as noted earlier, ovulation is never seen in 14-g CF-1 females, but it is easily induced by a male in an 18-g female if the female is individually paired with the male. The presence of other females largely but not entirely blocks the ovulation-in-

TABLE II

Proportion of Female Mice Exhibiting Tubal Ova at Three Body Weights [a]

Weight (g)	Test females isolated from other females		Test females held in groups	
	Male absent	Male present	Male absent	Male present
14	0/24	0/24	0/24	0/24
18	0/24	19/24	0/24	5/24
22	2/24	20/24	2/24	18/24

[a] These females had been either isolated from other females or held in groups of four for 72 hr. Males had been either present or absent in both conditions for the same length of time (F. H. Bronson and B. Macmillan, unpublished data).

ducing actions of the male at this body weight (Table II). The capacity of female-originating cues to override the accelerating actions of a male is completely lost by 22 g in CF-1 females, and a few females begin to ovulate spontaneously at this body weight in the absence of stimulation by a male.

The changing relationship between male- and female-originating cues is equally obvious in Fig. 2, where uterine weight after 72 hr of male exposure is used as an index of the effect of the male on the LH/estradiol sequence. Uterine growth in response to a male is minimal among grouped females

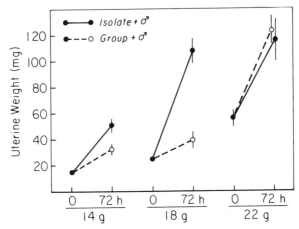

Fig. 2. Uterine weights (mean ± SE) of female mice at various body weights either before or after male exposure for 72 hr. Females were either grouped four per cage with a male present or singly housed with a male over the 72-hr experimental period (F. H. Bronson and B. Macmillan, unpublished data).

weighing 14 or 18 g, but grouping is totally without such male-antagonizing effects at 22 g.

C. Pheromonal Regulation of Ovulation in Female Mice—An Overview

To summarize the manner in which ovulation can be manipulated by primer pheromones in mice, the following can be stated. The capacity to release LH in response to a male is already present in the juvenile female, that is, as early as 12 g in CF-1 females (Bronson, 1975b). The capacity of female-originating cues to block the male's action must develop either concurrently or at an earlier time. After this stage of development both the separate and the interactive efficacies of the cues emanating from the two sexes depend on four physiological dimensions of the female, all of which vary independently in their rate of development: (a) the maturation of the LH-surging mechanism; (b) the slowly increasing strength of the direct drive of LH secretion; (c) the degree of flexibility in the relationship between positive and negative feedback, which changes from one of rigidity to one of marked flexibility at full maturation; and (d) the maturation of the neural and/or endocrine mechanisms that allow male-originating stimuli to override female-originating stimuli.

The development of all four of these factors seems to occur in complete independence of social cues; indeed, these factors seem to develop independently even of the pubertal ovulation itself (Bronson, 1981). Thus, as suggested in Fig. 3, there is an immense potential for variation in the timing of the first ovulation. In no case can ovulation occur in the CF-1 female before 15 to 17 g, when the LH-surging mechanism matures. After that, however, ovulation can occur at any time depending on the social milieu. Stated in another way, the pubertal ovulation can occur in the mouse at any of several different stages of sexual maturation and, for example, it is perfectly reasonable to speak about an adult female mouse (i.e., one that has ovulated and been inseminated) whose sexual development is still far from complete.

When all four of the factors noted above have matured, the female's responses to pheromonal (and tactile) cues encompass another important source of variation; that is, only after the first ovulation has occurred is there the potential for grouping to result in a prolactin-induced, progesterone-dominated pseudopregnancy. The speculative model we have presented to account for this additional source of variation may or may not be correct. In all probability, however, it is reasonably correct and, at the very least, it points out the direction that research must take if this problem is to be resolved.

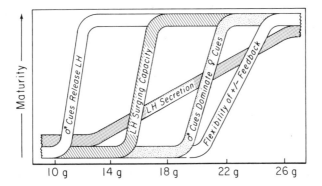

Fig. 3. Development of several factors that together determine the timing of pubertal ovulation in the female mouse. The horizontal scale is in terms of the body weight of CF-1 females.

D. Hormonal Responses of Males to Female Stimuli

The hormonal responses described above, although somewhat complex, nevertheless seem to encompass a relatively obvious adaptation involving a high degree of specificity. Specificity is defined here in terms of the discreteness of the relevant social cues, the discreteness of the reproductive events modulated by these cues, and the discreteness of the neural and hormonal pathways that link a cue to its response.

Not all hormonal responses to chemical cues exhibit the high degree of specificity shown by those leading to ovulation. This point is best made by examining another well-studied model, the manifold responses of an adult male mouse to stimuli associated with a female. This social interaction has been the focus of many experiments, most using cannulation procedures and microassay to allow simultaneous and almost continuous assessment of several blood hormone titers while a test male is interacting with a female. Starting first with the male's gonadotropic responses to female cues, it is important at the outset to acknowledge the normal episodic pattern of release of LH and testosterone in the male. A male's pituitary routinely releases a low and relatively steady level of LH. Set against this background, however, are periodic bursts or episodes of greatly enhanced release. These episodes occur every few hours in the mouse. They last only a few minutes, and they decay with a half-life of about 10 min, but each such episode can elevate the blood level of LH as much as 10-fold in a minute or two (Coquelin and Bronson, 1981). As a consequence of this pattern of LH release, the blood level of testosterone also displays episodic variation, but both the secretory and decay rates of this steroid are more prolonged than are those of LH (Coquelin and Desjardins, 1982).

Perception of a female can induce a reflexlike, sequential release of LH and testosterone whose characteristics are markedly similar to those of a normal, spontaneous episode of release (Macrides *et al.,* 1975; Maruniak and Bronson, 1976; Batty, 1978; Coquelin and Bronson, 1981). The female's cues of relevance here are at least twofold; one is a urinary primer and one is so far unidentified but probably tactile. Interestingly, these two cues act redundantly rather than synergistically. The basis for this conclusion is a comparison of the rates of habituation of the male's LH response to urine and to the female herself. The male habituates immediately to a single exposure to urine, but he habituates only slowly to repeated exposures to a female (Coquelin and Bronson, 1979). Thus, in male mice the release of LH that follows a single 10-μl spray of female urine is indistinguishable from that which accompanies a single exposure to a female, but this does not mean that the female's urinary factor is operating alone.

The reproductive function being served by a female-induced release of LH in a male remains obscure. More is said about possible functions of this response later but, because of this uncertainty, a concern has arisen that the response is simply a side effect of sexual arousal and, therefore, potentially unimportant in its own right. This possibility was examined in collaboration with Dr. Claude Desjardins in an experiment that compared the hormonal responses of sexually sated versus sexually rested males to receptive females. Some of the sexually rested males studied in this experiment were presented with receptive females whose vaginas were occluded in order to assess the effects of intromission separately. Six hormones were examined simultaneously. The major result of this experiment is best summarized, however, by looking at only two hormones: LH and norepinephrine.

As can be seen in Fig. 4, both sexually rested and sexually sated males release LH in response to a female, but only sexually rested males experience an elevation in norepinephrine. The somewhat lower peak LH values for sated males in Fig. 4 are due to a single male whose response was totally blocked by a spontaneous episode of LH release 10 min before the entrance of the female (Bronson and Desjardins, 1982). Thus, the female-induced release of LH in a male mouse clearly is independent of his potential for arousal. The female-induced release of norepinephrine, on the other hand, is completely dependent on arousal, and the fact that this hormonal response is independent even of intromission suggests that it is a direct reflection of the neurological activation that forms the core of arousal.

The extensive experiment mentioned above, when combined with the available literature, allows us to visualize the complex and dynamic relationship that exists between stimulus input and hormonal responses when a male mouse encounters a female. For convenience this behavioral sequence can be divided into three phases. In the first phase, that in which

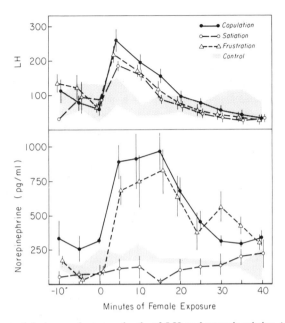

Fig. 4. Sequential changes in serum levels of LH and norepinephrine (mean ± SE) in male mice exposed to receptive females at time 0. Before this experiment the males had been exposed repeatedly to receptive females to sate them sexually ("satiation"), or they had been sexually rested. Either sexually rested males were allowed to copulate ("copulation"), or intromission was prevented by occluding the test female's vagina with cheesecloth ("frustration"). Control males were not exposed to a female at time 0 as a control for the blood collection procedure. (Redrawn from Bronson and Desjardins, 1982.)

the male first *perceives* the female, his determination of her species and her state of receptivity is heavily dependent on chemical cues and either primary or accessory olfactory mediation (reviewed by Bronson, 1979). Undoubtedly, other major communication modalities are contributing redundant information simultaneously. The first hormonal response experienced by the male is the immediate, reflexlike release of LH and the consequent rise in serum testosterone level described earlier. These responses are completely independent of both arousal and sexual experience, and they occur in response to any genetic female house mouse (Maruniak and Bronson, 1976).

The second phase of this sequence is that of *arousal,* a process that must find its initiation in the male's continuing multisensory recognition of the female. Chemical cues are important here but probably only as one more source of information about the female. Arousal has manifold behavioral manifestations and, as defined here, it exhibits endocrine manifestations as well. Adrenocorticotropin (ACTH) is released more or less continuously during arousal and, as a more direct reflection of the neural bases of arousal, blood levels of both epinephrine and norepinephrine also are markedly elevated. All three of these changes are relatively nonspecific responses that occur in a variety of socially stimulating circumstances such as fighting and/or subordination (Christian, 1970).

In the third phase, that of *preejaculation and ejaculation,* the primary sensory input maintaining arousal late in a normal copulatory sequence must be tactile feedback from the penis. There seem to be no hormonal correlates of this gradual shift from multisensory/olfactory-dominated input to tactile-dominated input, at least among the six hormones studied by Desjardins and Bronson (1982). Catecholamine and ACTH secretion remains high during this period, and this is independent of intromission. Prolactin is released in a surgelike manner at ejaculation, and LH may or may not be released at this time depending on a neural refractory period. Titers of FSH remain unaffected throughout an encounter with a female (Bronson and Desjardins, 1982).

When one visualizes the entire scheme presented above, it is obvious that some hormonal responses of the male are relatively specific and some are decidedly nonspecific. In the first category are the reflexlike episodes of LH release that are elicited by the male's initial perception of the female's pheromonal and tactile cues and, second, by ejaculation. Also in this category is the surgelike release of prolactin experienced by a male in response to ejaculation. In the nonspecific category are the ACTH and catecholamine responses, changes whose impetus is provided by arousal per se and probably, therefore, indirectly by multisensory input. Chemical information emanating from the female obviously is important in the elicitation of both types of responses, but the concept of a primer pheromone probably should be applied only to the LH response to the urinary factor. It must be emphasized, however, that even though the LH response is stereotyped and reflexlike in nature, it is a complex response with several known modulating factors, such as classic habituation and a neural refractory period that prevents the occurrence of two sequential releases that are separated by less than 25 to 40 min.

E. Adaptive Functions of Priming Pheromones in the Mouse

It is clear that mammals may experience a wide variety of hormonal changes when they interact with each other. In mice some of these changes seem to take the form of highly specific, reflexlike responses in which the secretion of LH and/or prolactin is stereotypically altered by the perception of chemical cues, usually acting in conjunction with tactile stimuli. Because of these neuroendocrine/pituitary responses, the pattern of gonadal steroid secretion is also altered in mice perceiving these cues. The receptors for the chemical stimuli of concern here seem to reside in the vomeronasal organ rather than in the primary olfactory tract itself (Keverne, 1978; see also Chapter 8). The sum of these stimulus–response systems can be conceptualized as the pheromonal priming system of mice, the reproductive actions of which are presented in Table I.

In considering the adaptive advantages associated with the mouse's priming system, it seems reasonable at the outset to draw a marked distinction between selective advantages and secondary effects of selection. As these terms are used here, a selective advantage can be inferred for a function only if it is reasonable to assume that selection could operate directly on that function. Secondary effects then refer to functions on which selection could not act directly. Stated in another way, secondary effects must result from selection for a primary selective advantage. For example, the capacity to modulate the time of ovulation in accord with prevailing social conditions would confer a decided selective advantage. Females showing this characteristic would be more fit, and selection could operate directly to promote this trait. On the other hand, it is known in at least one species, the deer mouse (*Peromyscus maniculatus*), that reproductive isolation is supported at the population level by priming incompatibilities between different populations; *P. m. palescens* males from Texas cannot induce uterine growth in immature *P. m. borealis* females from Alberta (Perrigo and Bronson, 1982). This type of incompatibility should be considered as a secondary effect because it would be difficult to select directly for a *failure* to reproduce when members of two different populations encounter each other. The distinction between selective advantages and secondary effects is of utmost importance in considering the house mouse's priming system because many of the individual actions that comprise this system result in a failure to reproduce.

The most obvious selective advantages of the mouse's priming system become apparent when this system is viewed in relation to the complete spectrum of environmental factors that regulate reproduction in mammals. As noted earlier, the ambient factors known to impinge importantly on mammalian reproduction originate in the physical, dietary, and social dimensions of the mammal's environment. Some of these factors exert their effects by altering gonadotropin secretion, and some act via nongonadotropic pathways (e.g., some dietary factors probably act in this manner, and some factors act in both ways). Table III presents the eight environmental factors known to influence mammalian reproduction by altering gonadotropin secretion; it should be noted again, however, that some of these factors also work via other pathways as well. These eight cues seem to serve two general classes of function. Most act as temporal regulators of one kind or another, but some may differentially enhance or depress the reproductive

TABLE III

Primary Effect(s) on Reproduction of Eight Environmental Factors Known to Alter Gonadotropin Secretion in Mammals

Environmental factor	Temporal regulation		Enhance or depress individuals
	Seasonal	Subseasonal	
Physical environment			
Day/night cycle	×	×	—
Temperature	×	—	—
Dietary environment			
Caloric intake	×	—	×
Nutritional factors	×	—	×
Social environment			
Specific auditory cues	—	×	—
Specific tactile cues	—	×	—
Primer pheromones	—	×	—
Multisensory cues	—	—	×

effort of individuals in a population. The temporal regulators may be divided for convenience into those that contribute to seasonality and those that time events or processes over shorter periods of time, recognizing that photoperiod regulates in both temporal dimensions.

In the context of Table III, then, one of the most important actions of physical and dietary factors is to promote interrupted breeding in variable environments. Depending on the location and the genetics of the population under consideration, most feral mammals breed either opportunistically or during distinct and predictable breeding seasons. Variation in a mammal's food supply always will set the temporal limits on such breeding. Dietary factors either will act alone to accomplish this objective or they will evoke genetic selection for an accurate predictor of dietary variation such as photoperiod. Availability of calories and nutrients also can act to depress reproduction in individuals that are excluded from prime food sources for behavioral reasons.

Physical and dietary factors typically exert their effects on reproduction in a decidedly nonspecific manner. Again, specificity is defined here in terms of discrete cues acting to regulate discrete reproductive processes via discrete neural and hormonal pathways. As an example of the typical nonspecificity of a physical factor, the circadian organization of a mammal by the day/night cycle ramifies throughout its neural and endocrine systems and, indeed, into most aspects of its physiology. Likewise, seasonal changes in photoperiod regulate a multitude of necessary adaptations for survival in addition to seasonal breeding, for example, molting, fat deposition, hibernation, and hoarding. As another example of nonspecificity, variation in caloric intake certainly alters patterns of gonadotropin secretion, but caloric variation affects other pituitary hormones as well, and its impact probably is felt at almost all tissue and cellular levels.

In sharp contrast to the typical characteristics of physical and dietary cues, most reproductively important social cues have a high degree of specificity as subseasonal, temporal regulators of particular reproductive events or processes. The classic examples here involve tactile cues. Cervical stimulation yields an ovulatory release of LH in reflex ovulators and prolactin release in spontaneous ovulators when the latter hormone is required for the formation of corpora. Suckling releases prolactin in many species, thereby increasing milk production. Similarly, there are well-known examples of such modulation by specific auditory cues, but we know of no instance in which specific visual cues act in this manner in a mammal. As detailed earlier, chemical cues may act within a broad range of specificity, but those of concern here act with great specificity on LH and prolactin secretion.

Different species and different populations of the same species face different environmental challenges. Reproductive solutions to these challenges must be compatible with the animal's other behavioral and physiological needs, which in turn are also subject to selection. Thus, there is an immense potential for variation in the evolution of ambient cueing systems in any group as diverse as the mammals. The house mouse has opted for a direct dependence on its food supply for its opportunistic seasonal breeding. This species also exhibits wide temperature limits on its reproduction, and it shows a heavy use of tactile and chemical cues to "fine tune" some of its reproductive processes (Bronson, 1979). In this sense, then, there is nothing particularly unique about the mouse's chemical priming system. Its evolution is simply a reflection of this species' need for specific social regulation of specific reproductive processes, as dictated and shaped by its combined ecological, sociological, and physiological requirements. How the mouse's priming system confers efficiency under natural conditions, however, is a much more difficult question.

It has been argued previously in great detail that all of the priming phenomena observed in mice probably constitute a single functional system designed to regulate the timing of ovulation (Bronson, 1979). This includes the hormonal reactions of the male to female cues, as well as the more obvious direct effects on ovulation of male- and female-originating cues. The detailed arguments supporting the concept of a functionally unified priming system are not presented again here. The crux of the matter, however, involves the reproductive importance of eliciting single episodes of LH and testosterone release in the male and the relationship between this response and a female's ovulation. The argument presented previously, and which still seems reasonable, is that the episodic pattern of LH release normally characteristic of the male under laboratory conditions may not occur at all under field conditions unless primed by a female. Thus, a male in the wild might not produce and disseminate his own primer pheromone unless first stimulated to do so by a female; both the synthesis of the male's primer and its dissemination by urinary marking are androgen-dependent phenomena. The single-system argument then visualizes a female as eliciting her own ovulation via her priming of a male to prime herself in turn.

A functional system in which the two sexes cooperate to promote ovulation while female/female interactions inhibit ovulation certainly would confer fitness. It would allow both sexes to remain more or less reproductively quiescent, engaging instead only in activity designed to promote survival, whenever dietary conditions were below the level required for successful reproduction. Such a system would be particularly beneficial when it prevented young females from becoming pregnant prior to dispersal. Indeed, this function may have played a key role in the house mouse's cockroach-like strategy of global colonization (Bronson, 1979).

Once a priming system such as that found in the mouse has evolved, a multitude of possibilities exist for secondary effects. Most of the secondary effects that have been postulated involve some benefit conferred on a population by a failure to reproduce. For example, the strange male pregnancy block could antagonize inbreeding and, simultaneously, act as a self-regulator for population density (see Chapter 6). Likewise, the loss of a male's capacity to stimulate a female could act as a density regulator, as could female/female inhibitory effects themselves. Little can be said about these possibilities except that they are both interesting and unsupported at this time by any evidence from field populations (Bronson, 1979, 1981). Indeed, in all probability there are many interesting secondary effects of the mouse's priming system, but our lack of detailed knowledge about the social organization of natural populations of wild house mice prevents us from gaining any real appreciation of these effects at this time.

As a final subject worth considering in regard to endocrine priming, it is unfortunate that so little progress has been made in determining how widespread the use of chemical priming actually is among mammals. This question and the issue of the "real functions" of chemical primers in natural populations probably are the two greatest challenges facing researchers in this field. There is good evidence now that chemical primers operate in cattle, pigs, and sheep, as well as in a variety of rodents (reviewed in Bronson, 1978; also see Chapters 4 and 9). Indeed, sufficient research has been accomplished to state that all of the priming phenomena found in *Mus* also occur in *Peromyscus maniculatus* and that the characteristics of these phenomena appear to be quite similar in the two species (Bronson, 1982). Thus, it is obvious that the use of chemical primers is not limited to one species, or even to a few closely related species. Undoubtedly, it is not universal among mammals either. What is needed now is the testing of a sufficient spectrum of species to establish the particular combinations of physiological, ecological, and sociological characteristics that optimize the use of chemical primers.

III. CONCLUSIONS

Chemical cues may elicit a variety of hormonal responses in mammals. In some cases these cues act with a high degree of specificity to alter the secretory patterns of LH and prolactin and the steroids whose secretion is regulated by these two tropic hormones. The reproductive consequences of these specific actions are obvious in the case of the female mouse—they regulate ovulation—but they are less obvious in the male. There is nothing particularly unique about the mouse's use of priming pheromones; other species use the same type of system to accomplish the same objectives, and still other species "fine tune" the same or similar reproductive events using other specific cues that act via other sensory modalities. In all cases the primary selective advantage of such systems is simply that they increase the efficiency of the organism's reproduction under a particular set of ecological, sociological, and physiological conditions. The important secondary effects of chemical primers in mice and in all other species remain largely speculative.

ACKNOWLEDGMENTS

Much of the research cited in this chapter was supported by NIH grants HD13155 and HD06158.

REFERENCES

Batty, J. (1978). *Anim. Behav.* **26,** 349–357.
Beauchamp, G., Doty, R. L., Moulton, D. G., and Mugford, R. A. (1976). *In* "Mammalian Olfaction, Reproductive Processes, and Behavior" (R. L. Doty, ed.), pp. 144–168. Academic Press, New York.
Bronson, F. H. (1968). *J. Reprod. Fertil.* **15,** 131–134.

Bronson, F. H. (1975a). *Endocrinology* **96**, 511-514.
Bronson, F. H. (1975b). *Biol. Reprod.* **12**, 431-437.
Bronson, F. H. (1976). *Biol. Reprod.* **15**, 147-152.
Bronson, F. H. (1978). *In* "Chemical Ecology: Odour Communication in Animals" (F. J. Ritter, ed.), pp. 97-104. Elsevier/North Holland Biomedical Press, Amsterdam.
Bronson, F. H. (1979). *Q. Rev. Biol.* **54**, 265-299.
Bronson, F. H. (1981). *Endocrinology* **108**, 506-516.
Bronson, F. H. (1982). *In* "Recent Advances in the Study of Mammalian Behavior" (J. F. Eisenberg and D. G. Kleiman, eds.), Spec. Publ. No. 7. Am. Soc. Mammal., Lawrence, Kansas (in press).
Bronson, F. H., and Coquelin, A. (1980). *In* "Chemical Signals in Vertebrates and Aquatic Invertebrates" (D. Müller-Schwarze and R. M. Silverstein, eds.), pp. 243-265. Plenum, New York.
Bronson, F. H., and Desjardins, C. (1974). *Endocrinology* **94**, 1658-1668.
Bronson, F. H., and Desjardins, C. (1982). *Endocrinology* **111**, 1286-1291.
Bronson, F. H., and Maruniak, J. A. (1975). *Biol. Reprod.* **13**, 94-98.
Bronson, F. H., and Maruniak, J. A. (1976). *Endocrinology* **98**, 1101-1108.
Bronson, F. H., and Whitten, W. K. (1968). *J. Reprod. Fertil.* **15**, 131-134.
Bruce, H. M. (1959). *Nature (London)* **184**, 105.
Bruce, H. M., and Parkes, A. S. (1960). *J. Endocrinol.* **20**, 29-30.
Christian, J. J. (1970). *Science* **168**, 84-90.
Coquelin, A., and Bronson, F. H. (1979). *Science* **206**, 1099.
Coquelin, A., and Bronson, F. H. (1981). *Endocrinology* **109**, 1605-1610.
Cowley, J. J., and Wise, D. R. (1972). *Anim. Behav.* **20**, 499-506.
Davidson, J. M. (1974). *In* "The Control of the Onset of Puberty" (M. M. Grumbach, G. D. Grave, and F. E. Mayer, eds.), p. 79. Wiley, New York.
Dominic, C. J. (1964). *J. Reprod. Fertil.* **8**, 265-266.
Drickamer, L. C. (1974). *Behav. Biol.* **12**, 101-110.
Keverne, E. B. (1978). *In* "Chemical Ecology: Odour Communication in Animals" (F. J. Ritter, ed.), pp. 75-84. Elsevier North Holland Biomedical Press, Amsterdam.
McCann, S. M., and Ramirez, V. S. (1964). *Recent Prog. Horm. Res.* **20**, 131.
McIntosh, T. K., and Drickamer, L. C. (1977). *Anim. Behav.* **25**, 999-1004.
Macrides, F., Bartke, A., and Dalterio, S. (1975). *Science* **189**, 1104.
Marsden, H. M., and Bronson, F. H. (1964). *Science* **144**, 3625.
Maruniak, J. A., and Bronson, F. H. (1976). *Endocrinology* **99**, 963-969.
Odell, W. D., and Swerdloff, R. S. (1976). *Recent Prog. Horm. Res.* **32**, 245.
Perrigo, G., and Bronson, F. H. (1982). *Behav. Ecol. Sociobiol.* **10**, 181-184.
Ramaley, J. A. (1979). *Biol. Reprod.* **20**, 1-28.
Ramirez, V. S. (1973). *In* "Handbook of Physiology" (R. O. Greep, ed.), Sect. 7, Vol. 2, Part I, pp. 1-28. Am. Physiol. Soc., Washington, D. C.
Reynolds, J., and Keverne, E. B. (1979). *J. Reprod. Fertil.* **57**, 31-35.
Ryan, K. D., and Schwartz, N. B. (1977). *Biol. Reprod.* **17**, 578-583.
Ryan, K. D., and Schwartz, N. B. (1980). *Endocrinology* **106**, 959-966.
Vandenbergh, J. G. (1967). *Endocrinology* **81**, 345-348.
Vandenbergh, J. G. (1975). *In* "Hormonal Correlates of Behavior" (B. E. Eleuthériou and R. L. Sprott, eds.), pp. 551-584. Plenum, New York.
Vandenbergh, J. G. (1969). *Endocrinology* **84**, 658-660.
Vandenbergh, J. G., Drickamer, L. C., and Colby, D. R. (1972). *J. Reprod. Fertil.* **28**, 397-405.
Vandenbergh, J. G., Finlayson, J. S., Dobrogosz, W. J., Dills, S. S., and Kost, T. A. (1976). *Biol. Reprod.* **15**, 260-265.

van der Lee, S., and Boot, L. M. (1956). *Acta Physiol. Pharmacol. Neerl.* **5**, 213–214.
Whitten, W. K. (1956). *J. Endocrinol.* **13**, 399–404.
Whitten, W. K. (1959). *J. Endocrinol.* **18**, 102–107.
Whitten, W. K. (1966). *Adv. Reprod. Physiol.* **1**, 155–177.
Whitten, W. K., and Bronson, F. H. (1970). *In* "Advances in Chemoreception" (J. W. Johnston, D. G. Moulton, and A. Turk, eds.), Vol. 1, pp. 309–322. Appleton, New York.

8

Sensory Physiology of Pheromone Communication

Michael Meredith

Department of Biological Science
The Florida State University
Tallahassee, Florida

PHEROMONES AND REPRODUCTION IN MAMMALS
Copyright © 1983 by Academic Press, Inc.
All rights of reproduction in any form reserved.
ISBN 0–12–710780–0

I. INTRODUCTION

Interest in the vomeronasal organ (VNO) has been renewed in recent years, especially following the report of Scalia and Winans (1970) that the mammalian VNO is connected via a single synapse in the accessory olfactory bulb to a region of the amygdala having direct connections with the hypothalamus. This observation suggested that the system might have some behavioral function distinct from that of the main olfactory system and this suggestion was supported by Powers and Winans's (1975) demonstration that the system is important in the induction of male mating behavior in the hamster. Since these studies, the speculation by Whitten (1963) that the VNO might be the sensory organ involved in responses to priming pheromones has been confirmed in a number of instances. This relatively sudden recognition that receptors other than those of the main olfactory system are important in chemical communication has also redirected interest to the other chemoreceptors and putative chemoreceptors of the nose: the trigeminal nerve endings, the septal organ, and the nervus terminalis endings (Tucker, 1971; Moulton, 1978). The history of discovery of nasal chemoreceptors has been concisely reviewed by Graziadei (1977).

In this chapter I intend to review briefly these chemoreceptor systems and their potential participation in chemical communication, to discuss the ways in which their influence might be revealed, and to evaluate those ex-

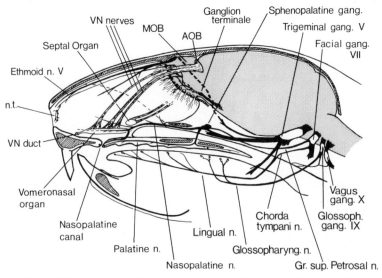

Fig. 1.   Diagram of the chemosensory nerves of the nasal and oral cavities.

periments that have attempted to separate the contributions of the vomeronasal and other systems to pheromone communication.

There have been many definitions and redefinitions of the word "pheromone" (Beauchamp et al., 1976). I shall use the word to mean chemicals emitted by one member of a species which when detected by another member result in behavioral or physiological changes that are likely to benefit both individuals.

Chemicals meeting this definition have many potential sources and conceivably could range from ions to macromolecules, making all known chemoreceptor systems possible pheromone detectors. The discussion here is restricted to vertebrates and concentrates on mammals.

Four to six different chemoreceptor systems (depending on species and classification) are found at the anterior end of the vertebrate body: the main olfactory system, the vomeronasal or accessory olfactory system, the septal organ, the trigeminal system, the nervus terminalis, and the taste system. These are diagramed in Fig. 1.

II. REVIEW OF CHEMOSENSORY SYSTEMS

A. Physiology and Anatomy

1. Main Olfactory System

The olfactory receptors are ciliated neurons with their apices in the mucus overlying the olfactory epithelium and with axons that pass back to the olfactory bulb in bundles running through the lamina propria below the epithelium. The bundles run through holes in the cribriform plate, which divides the nasal from the cranial cavity, and pass directly to all sides of the olfactory bulbs without forming a discrete nerve. This makes it difficult to cut all the olfactory nerves as an experimental means of cutting off olfactory input. Within the bulb, olfactory axons form synapses with second-order neurons, the mitral and tufted cells, and activate a complex synaptic network that must reencode the chemoreceptor information (Shepherd, 1972, 1974) and integrate it with the activity of centrifugal fibers from the higher levels in the brain (Moulton and Beidler, 1967).

The responses of olfactory receptors to particular odors do not appear to be very specific (Gesteland, 1978), although purified biologically significant odors have not often been tested. The current consensus is that the neural message characteristic of particular odors is carried mainly in the differential responses of different cells (Holley and Doving, 1977) and in the spatial pattern of activity across the olfactory mucosa (Moulton, 1976; Mackay-Sim, Shaman, and Moulton, 1982). At the bulbar level, the spatial pattern appears to be converted to a spatiotemporal pattern (Moulton and Beidler, 1967; Stewart *et al.*, 1979; Meredith and Marques, 1981) and may be further modified by centrifugal activity from the brain (Doving, 1966; Macrides, 1976; Pager, 1974). Bulbar response to biologically important odors has not been extensively investigated (Pfaff and Gregory, 1971; Macrides, 1976; Skeen, 1977). There is no obvious specificity in the responses to potential pheromone-containing materials, although highly specific responses could not be expected when unpurified materials are used (see Section V,C).

The olfactory system seems capable of responding to almost all molecules that can reach its receptors (except the smallest, e.g., nitrogen), including newly synthesized molecules that have never before been experienced. This all-embracing sensitivity argues that the main olfactory system exists as a general molecular analyzer rather than as a specific detector for particular chemical signals.

In mammals the receptors are located in a posterior–dorsal pocket off the main nasal respiratory airway. The distribution, concentration, and flow rate of odor stimuli across the olfactory mucosa are controlled by sniffing patterns (Marshall and Moulton, 1977), by vasodilation and constriction in the mucosa (Malcolmson, 1959; Bojsen-Moller and Fahrenkrug, 1971) or by secretion (Eccles and Lee, 1980). All of these can restrict or redirect airflow and, by the uptake of odor molecules into the nasal mucus, can localize and concentrate odors (Hornung and Mozell, 1977a,b). The partition of odors between air and mucus and their differential distribution in both media may be nearly as important in determining the pattern of afferent neural input as the specificity of individual receptor cells.

2. Septal Organ (Organ of Masera)

The septal organ consists of a patch of tissue located on either side of the nasal septum anterior and ventral to the main olfactory epithelium. It contains ciliated receptor neurons generally similar to the olfactory receptors (Graziadei, 1977). The septal organ has been identified in mice (Adams and MacFarland, 1971), rats (Bojsen-Moller, 1975), and hamsters (M. Meredith, unpublished observations) as well as in guinea pigs, rabbits, and the opossum fetus (Masera, 1943). The suggestion by Tucker (1963a) that it might exist in turtles was probably based on a misconception (Tucker, 1971). The distribution of the septal organ receptor axons to the glomeruli of the olfactory bulb and, indeed, whether they end there at all is unknown. It seems unlikely that they end in the accessory olfactory bulb because axon tracing materials taken up by receptor cells in the nasal cavity outside the VNO reach the accessory bulb sparingly if at all (Barber and Raisman, 1974;

Meredith *et al.,* 1980b). There are some ultrastructural differences between olfactory and septal organ receptors (Graziadei, 1977), but their significance is not clear. The sensitivity, selectivity, and central projections of the system are also unknown. The location of the septal organ receptors, more toward the main airflow through the nose, has led to the suggestion that the septal organ may detect odors during nonsniffing respiration (Bojsen-Moller, 1975; Moulton, 1978). The ventromedial region of the olfactory bulb appears to be active during the exposure of rats to room air to which no odors (that might have elicited sniffing) had been added (Stewart *et al.,* 1979). Because the septal organ nerves appear to project in this direction, it is tempting to speculate that the ventromedial bulb may be the terminal field of the septal organ, but there is no evidence to support this suggestion.

At the posterior end of the olfactory bulb is an area, possibly a single macroglomerulus, that has been shown by its uptake of a metabolic tracer (2-deoxyglucose) to be active during suckling in rat pups (Teicher *et al.,* 1980). Neither the peripheral nor central connections of this region are known.

3. Trigeminal System

The trigeminal is a somatic sensory nerve that has distributions to the epithelium inside the nasal cavity as well as to the skin of the head and cornea of the eye. The intranasal and corneal fibers are sensitive to airborne chemicals. The cell bodies of sensory trigeminal nerves are in the Gasserian ganglion near the entry of the nerve into the hindbrain. The peripheral fibers are myelinated and much larger than the unmyelinated olfactory nerves. The intranasal terminations appear to be free nerve endings insinuated between the epithelial cells of the olfactory and respiratory epithelia (Graziadei and Gagne, 1973). These endings may not reach the surface and, if so, are probably less affected by the physiological and chemical conditions in the mucus than are the olfactory receptors.

The system forms the chemosensory input for reflex changes in heart rate and respiration in response to strong irritating vapors (Allen, 1928; Stone *et al.,* 1968) and probably also for the reflex changes in autonomic activity (Tucker, 1963a) that produce changes in mucosal thickness and secretion (Blier, 1930; Eccles and Wilson, 1973) and modulate access of stimuli to various parts of the nasal cavity. This function has sometimes led to the presumption that strong irritating vapors such as ammonia and HCl are the only odors that can stimulate the system. Electrophysiological data (Tucker, 1963a,b, 1971; Silver and Moulton, 1982) suggest that, although it is less sensitive than the main olfactory system for many odors, the trigeminal system responds to some odors, phenylethanol for example, at concentrations that would not normally be considered irritating. It has been suggested that the system is sensitive to carbon dioxide, a substance that is said to be otherwise odorless (Cain and Murphy, 1980), although olfactory receptor cells do appear to respond to it (Getchell *et al.,* 1980). Trigeminal nerve bundles also give distinguishable electrophysiological responses to different odors at the same concentration (Tucker, 1963b), although it is not clear that this is a discrimination of different qualities or of different intensities of activation. Tucker, from electrophysiological data, and Stone *et al.* (1968), from nerve-blocking experiments, both concluded that no odorous substance can be considered to be purely an olfactory stimulant. All tested substances gave some evidence of trigeminal stimulation at high concentrations and many also at lower concentrations. Stone *et al.* (1968) also suggested that trigeminal input may modulate olfactory bulb activity via centrifugal fibers. Odor-elicited stimulation of the trigeminal system has also been shown to modify the activity of second-order taste neurons in the medulla (Van Buskirk and Erickson, 1977). This system cannot be dismissed as a pathway for pheromone detection per se or as a modifier of input through other systems. The interaction of trigeminal with olfactory and gustatory input has been reviewed by Silver and Maruniak (1982).

4. Vomeronasal System

a. **Structure.** The vomeronasal organ in mammals, also known as the Jacobson's organ (Negus, 1958; Wysocki, 1979), is an elaborate structure consisting of a crescent-section tubular cavity connected to the nasal cavity or nasopalatine canal via a narrow duct. One inner wall of the vomeronasal cavity is lined with sensory epithelium containing vomeronasal receptor neurons.

The vomeronasal receptor neurons lack cilia and have some other ultrastructural characteristics that differ from those of the olfactory receptors (Graziadei, 1977). The vomeronasal axons gather into rather larger and more discrete bundles than the olfactory axons and pass under the mucosa of the nasal septum to penetrate the cribriform plate as two or three bundles on each side of the midline. They pass between the main olfactory bulbs and enter the glomeruli of the accessory olfactory bulb at the posterior end of the main bulbs [except in the guinea pig, where the nerves pass around the lateral sides of the bulbs (McCotter, 1912)].

The entire vomeronasal lumen is continuously bathed in the secretions of the vomeronasal glands, which enter the lumen along the borders of the sensory epithelium (Bojsen-Moller, 1964). Presumably, this fluid has a net outflow through the vomeronasal duct because there is no other exit. As in the olfactory system, this fluid may be important for determining the response properties of the system.

b. Stimulus Access. Normal access of stimuli to the hamster VNO is controlled by an autonomically driven vascular pump (Meredith and O'Connell, 1979). Blood vessels surrounding the vomeronasal lumen constrict when sympathetic fibers, entering the VNO from the nasopalatine nerve, are stimulated. The reduction of volume within the vomeronasal capsule causes the lumen to open up, sucking fluid into the lumen from the nasal cavity. The suction can also be produced by injection of epinephrine into the carotid artery, which supplies the organ. Lumen compression and the expulsion of its contents is controlled independently by nonsympathetic fibers. The mechanism is capable of transporting a concentration of stimulus (delivered in vapor form and presumably dissolving in the mucus) sufficient to activate second-odor neurons in the accessory olfactory bulb (Meredith and O'Connell, 1979). Lesions of the nasopalatine nerves, which control the pump, result in deficits in male hamster sexual behavior that are similar to those produced by lesions of the vomeronasal nerves, suggesting that the pumping mechanism is important in delivering substances to the vomeronasal organ in behaving animals (Meredith *et al.,* 1980a). Similar arrangements of blood vessels within the vomeronasal capsule are found in many other species of mammals, and a similar pumping mechanism may exist in these (Negus, 1958; Wysocki, 1982; Ladewig and Hart, 1980; Eccles, 1982).

The lip curl, or flehmen behavior, of ungulates and certain other mammals was reported by Knappe (1964) to be associated with the presence of a well-developed VNO, especially where the vomeronasal duct opens into the nasopalatine canal. Various mechanisms by which flehmen or associated behaviors might assist stimulus access to the VNO have been proposed (Estes, 1972; Bailey, 1978; Jacobs *et al.,* 1980, 1981), but these have not been rigorously tested. Ladewig and Hart (1980) have shown in goats that tracer material added to female goat urine and/or placed in the mouth of males investigating the urine was delivered to the vomeronasal receptor epithelium in males that performed flehmen after contacting the urine. In those animals that did not perform flehmen the tracer penetrated only the anterior third of the vomeronasal lumen, where there are no receptor cells. The authors suggested that a vascular pumping mechanism may draw substances into the posterior part of the vomeronasal lumen. They did not demonstrate the mechanism by which flehmen assists stimulus access, and this remains unclear (Meredith, 1980). Ladewig *et al.* (1980) concluded that flehman in male goats was associated with detection of the approach of estrus and with maintaining copulatory behavior, because (*a*) it occurred much more frequently during than preceding copulation and (*b*) in contrast to the results of Verberne (1981) in cats, flehmen occurred more frequently in response to diestrous than to estrous female urine. Ladewig *et al.* also concluded that vomeronasal input stimulates flehmen because flehmen was reduced by bulbectomy. Better evidence that flehmen may be stimulated by vomeronasal (in addition to olfactory or other) input comes from Verberne (1976, 1981), who found reduced flehmen in cats following damage to the duct of the VNO or to its nerves.

The nasopalatine canal in rodents opens into the nasal cavity posterior to the VNO. It may or may not conduct vomeronasal stimuli in rodents (Wysocki *et al.*, 1980), but it does dilate synchronously with the suction phase of vomeronasal pump operation when the nasopalatine nerve is stimulated (M. Meredith, unpublished observation in the hamster). Whether this innervation is normally operated synchronously with the pump, whether it can produce the same effect in species where the vomeronasal duct opens into the nasopalatine canal, and whether it would assist vomeronasal stimulation is not known.

5. Nervus Terminalis

The nervus terminalis is present in all vertebrates so far studied, but no function has yet been definitely assigned to it. The system consists of a network of cells and unmyelinated nerve fibers strung out between the anterior–ventral end of the forebrain between the hemispheres (the lamina terminalis) and the anterior end of the nasal cavity. At several points there are accumulations of nerve cell bodies, especially in the ganglion terminale, medial to the olfactory peduncles in mammals (Schwanzel-Fukuda and Silverman, 1980), and in the mucosa of the vestibule, at the anterior end of the nasal cavity (Bojsen-Moller, 1975). Pearson (1941) and Larsell (1950) divided the nerve cells of the terminalis system into multipolar cells, whose axons end on glands and blood vessels of the nasal mucosa, and bipolar cells, whose processes enter the nasal epithelium (Larsell, 1950) without ending on specific structures and which are possibly sensory. Schwanzel-Fukuda and Silverman (1980) found high levels of luteinizing-hormone-releasing hormone (LHRH) immunoreactivity in nervus terminalis fibers and in cells that they concluded were probably bipolar sensory cells. Tracts of LHRH-positive fibers extend from the terminalis network between the bulbs and from the ganglion terminale to LHRH-positive cells in the olfactory tubercle, medial septum, and diagonal band. What proportion of these are the axons of LHRH cells in the peripheral ganglia and how many are afferent or efferent, regardless of soma position, is not clear. The putative vasomotor or secretomotor fibers ending on blood vessels or glands have been traced to nearby ganglion cells, but it is not known if these are activated by central nervous system (CNS) output, by local reflexes from afferent fibers, or by both. Several authors have suggested that some nervus terminalis components might be autonomic (Brookover, 1910; Pearson, 1941).

No electrophysiological or behavioral evidence exists for a chemoreceptive (or any other) function for the nervus terminalis, but the possibility is not negligible. The significance of the LHRH content of the nervus terminalis is discussed in Section III,B.

6. Taste System

The taste receptors consist of specialized epithelial cells contained in taste buds. These cells make synaptic contacts with gustatory nerve fibers whose cell bodies lie in cranial sensory ganglia and whose central processes enter the brain. In vertebrates above fish the taste buds are limited to (a) the anterior tongue (served by the facial nerve, cranial nerve VII), (b) the posterior tongue and pharynx (glossopharyngeal nerve, cranial nerve IX) and vagus nerve, cranial nerve X, and (c) the palate and nasopalatine canal. The latter area is served by branches of the trigeminal nerve (cranial nerve V), but palatal and nasopalatine taste buds are contacted by facial nerve afferents reaching the palatine nerves via the greater superficial petrosal nerve (Miller and Porcelli, 1976; Miller, 1982).

In many fish species there are external taste buds on the surface of the body; these are served by the seventh cranial nerves and are as sensitive to some stimuli as the olfactory system (Caprio, 1982). Social interaction, however, seems to depend on the olfactory system (Todd *et al.,* 1967; Atema, 1971).

In higher vertebrates the odorous secretions and excretions of other individuals are frequently licked or taken into the mouth as well as sniffed. In the hamster a conditioned aversion to female hamster vaginal secretion, which contains pheromones, can be induced in males that lick and ingest the secretion (Johnston *et al.,* 1978). Conditioned aversions of this type are generally easier to induce when the substance is detected with the gustatory rather than the olfactory system (Garcia and Rusiniak, 1980; see also Panhuber, 1982), but the pathway involved in this case and the significance of this finding for pheromone communication are not known. Potential sites of convergence of olfactory, gustatory, and oral trigeminal input have been described by Norgren (1977a). Possible functional interactions are discussed by Silver and Maruniak (1982).

The participation of the taste system in pheromone communication cannot be dismissed without experimental investigation. Beidler (1977) has noted the sensitivity of the human taste system to proteins and peptides. Such complex molecules have the potential for carrying much information, but if the system simply responds to them in a categorical fashion, for example, as sweet or not sweet, the potential is lost.

The simple elimination of contact should normally be sufficient to avoid the participation of the taste system in chemical detection because taste in air-breathing vertebrates is generally much less sensitive than the olfactory system and requires contact with reasonably concentrated sources of chemicals. Odorous materials might stimulate the taste system, however, and it is conceivable, although unlikely, that odor vapors might concentrate in oral or nasal fluids sufficiently to allow identification by this system.

7. Postingestional Chemosignal Detection

Many biological materials containing chemical cues such as urine and vaginal secretion are consumed by conspecifics that come into contact with them (Johnston, 1977; Ladewig and Hart, 1980). It is not inconceivable that substances contained in these materials could be taken up by the bloodstream and could act on internal receptors, either in the brain or at the periphery, to influence behavior or physiology.

B. Constraints on the Stimulus

1. Volatile Stimuli

Terrestrial distance chemoreception involves materials of significant vapor pressure, that is, volatile odors. The upper limit of molecular weight for reasonable volatility is generally placed somewhere around 300–400, but this is not an absolute figure because vapor phase concentration, although decreasing sharply with increasing molecular weight, never reaches zero; some numbers of molecules will be present in the vapor phase for substances of higher molecular weight and could be detected by sufficiently sensitive systems. Wilson and Bossert's (1963) prediction that insect pheromones would range in molecular weight from 80 to 300 was based on the notion that a single molecule must carry specific information. Too small a molecule would be insufficiently complex to allow a diversity of structure within the same molecular type and thus could not provide species-specific information; too large a molecule would involve metabolic cost in elaboration and transport. In mammals it is generally accepted that single species-specific pheromones with unique behavioral effects are not to be expected. The necessity for complexity in chemical structure is correspondingly less if mixtures of chemicals serve as pheromones.

The physical and chemical factors affecting the evaporation and dispersion of volatile odors have been analyzed by Bossert and Wilson (1963), Wilson and Bossert (1963), and Dravnieks (1975). The relative concentration of the components of a mixture in its vapor may be different from expectation because of intermolecular interactions between the components and with the substrate (Regnier and Goodwin, 1977; Guillot, 1967). This is especially important for biological secretions and biological substrates (Jellinek, 1964).

Extensive studies of the correlation between odor and molecular structure (Laffort and Dravnieks, 1974; Boelens, 1976) suggest that odor molecules fall into a range of moderate to high water solubility and low to moderate lipid solubility. These features are probably controlled by the necessity for the passage of stimulus molecules over and through the aqueous mucus layers in the nasal cavity before reaching the receptors and interacting with the lipid/protein receptor cell membrane. Hornung and Mozell (1977a,b) have shown that substances with appreciable aqueous solubility concentrate in the mucus at the proximal end of an airflow path across the nasal mucosa. This phenomenon is similar to the differential retention of substances in a gas–liquid chromatograph column and could produce spatial separation of substances across the olfactory epithelium (Mozell and Jagadowicz, 1973). For normal inspiration through the nostrils, the vestibule and anterior respiratory area innervated by the trigeminal and terminalis nerves and the area around the opening of the vomeronasal duct (in rodents) would be expected to accumulate the highest concentration of water-soluble substances. Both vomeronasal and trigeminal systems appear to respond well to water-soluble substances (Tucker, 1963a,b, 1971; Doty, 1975; Doty *et al.*, 1978).

For the trigeminal and terminalis systems, the free nerve endings observed in the nasal mucosa have not been seen to reach the surface of the epithelium (Graziadei and Gagne, 1973). Large molecules cannot penetrate effectively between cells because of the tight junctions that seal the surface of both olfactory and respiratory epithelia (Reese and Brightman, 1970; Kersjaschki and Horandner, 1976), but smaller molecules might. Any necessity for odor molecules to pass through cells to reach underlying nerve endings would be expected to show up as a requirement for greater lipid solubility for the molecule. This is not seen for nasal trigeminal stimulants but might be true for oral trigeminal stimulants (see Silver and Maruniak, 1982).

2. Nonvolatile Stimuli

For stimuli that dissolve in or are adsorbed by mucus, including water-soluble volatile stimuli and any nonvolatile stimuli that are introduced into the nose, there is an alternate mode of distribution to chemoreceptors via the circulation of the nasal mucus. In the hamster one can see a continuous stream of mucus passing down the ventral groove inside the nasal cavity in anesthetized animals (M. Meredith, unpublished observation). This stream passes over the entrance to the vomeronasal duct and may be responsible for the transport of nonvolatile materials to the duct from the nostril. Because it is quite possible that the circulation of mucus would continue for some time after death, this may explain the appearance of a nonvolatile fluorescent dye (rhodamine) in the vomeronasal lumen only a few minutes after its application to the nostril in the vole, even if the animal were dead (Wysocki, 1982). Wysocki *et al.* (1980) have also shown that rhodamine added to female guinea pig urine is transported, in male animals that have investigated the urine, not only to the vomeronasal lumen but also to the septal organ halfway up the nasal septum. They reported that no fluorescence could be detected over the olfactory epithelium farther up the nasal septum, but this may reflect a difference in holding capacity or a lack of sensitivity in the assay rather than the absence of transport to the olfactory area.

The flow of mucus, driven by cilia of the respiratory epithelium, appears in most species to be away from rather than toward the olfactory area, although the flow on the rodent nasal septum has not been reported (Lucas and Douglas, 1934; Bang, 1961). Nevertheless, the distribution of large molecules to the olfactory mucosa is certainly possible, as can be shown by the use of a horseradish peroxidase (HRP) tracer solution. The HRP can be taken up by olfactory receptor cells and transported through their axons to the olfactory bulb (Meredith *et al.*, 1980b). When a 10- to 25-μl drop of HRP is simply deposited in the nasal vestibule, this protein (MW approx. 40,000) apparently travels to all areas of the olfactory epithelium, because the HRP transported by olfactory axons can later be detected in all areas of the olfactory bulb. Whether this widespread distribution takes place by diffusion over the 24-hr survival period, by aerosol dispersion following rapid inspiration, or through the circulation of mucus is not known.

Some behaviorally important chemicals may prove to be nonvolatile. For example, mouse puberty acceleration pheromone (Vandenbergh *et al.*, 1975; Vandenbergh, 1980), hamster mounting pheromone (Singer *et al.*, 1980), and guinea pig sex identification substances (Beruter *et al.*, 1973) do not separate with the volatile fractions of their source materials. The induction of ovulation in persistent-estrous rats by male urine (Johns *et al.*, 1978) involves a chemical that has not been identified, but ovulation is prevented both by vomeronasal lesions and by prevention of contact with the urine. These results strongly suggest that a nonvolatile stimulus and a vomeronasal stimulus are necessary, but it is not yet established that these are the same. Wysocki *et al.* (1980) and Ladewig and Hart (1980) have demonstrated that nonvolatile dyes can reach the vomeronasal lumen, but there is as yet no direct evidence that the nonvolatile, biologically active materials discussed above do reach the lumen or that nonvolatile substances can stimulate vomeronasal receptors.

The lack of definite evidence is emphasized here only to make the point that the VNO should not be the only chemosensory system considered when nonvolatile stimuli are involved, nor should nonvolatile stimuli necessarily be expected when the vomeronasal system is implicated.

In some circumstances the loss of a behavior when contact is prevented may be open to an alternative explanation. In tests with animals having main olfactory system damage (e.g., Powers *et al.,* 1979), olfactory cues for the operation of the VNO pump might remain undetected so that volatile stimuli would not be delivered to vomeronasal receptors. The addition of extra cues (visual, tactile) associated with contact with the stimulus source could trigger the vomeronasal pump and allow the response to appear.

III. CHEMOSENSORY INPUT TO THE BRAIN

A. Neural Projections

The central projections of chemoreceptor systems are summarized schematically in Figs. 2 to 6. The diagrams are intended as a graphical representation of some of the possible chemoreceptor influences on various brain areas. Not all projections are shown (see legend). Each system has projections into limbic areas. The olfactory, gustatory, and trigeminal systems have thalamocortical projections as well. The nervus terminalis may influence thalamocortical activity via the septal–mediodorsal thalamus projection reported by Meibach and Siegel (1977) (in tissue not reacted to show LHRH). The vomeronasal system has no known neocortical representation except possibly via projections from the bed nucleus of stria terminalis to the midline thalamic nuclei (Swanson and Cowan, 1979) and thence to the medial orbital neocortex (Kretteck and Price, 1977a). What is known about the function of the different central projections is mainly derived from studies of behavioral deficits following the placement of lesions in various locations.

In chemosensory discrimination tasks thought to involve the olfactory system, rats could detect and discriminate odors after the lateral olfactory tracts were cut but not after combined cuts of the lateral olfactory tracts and the anterior limb of the anterior commissure (Slotnik and Berman, 1980). Cuts of the lateral olfactory tracts alone did eliminate mating in male hamsters, possibly because both olfactory and vomeronasal projections to the amygdala were cut (Macrides *et al.,* 1976). Lesions of the mediodorsal thalamus or olfactory cortex had little effect on detection or threshold but had a much greater effect on more sophisticated olfactory tasks in rats (Eichenbaum *et al.,* 1980). In hamsters, lesions of the thalamocortical olfactory projections appeared to interfere with odor preferences for conspecific

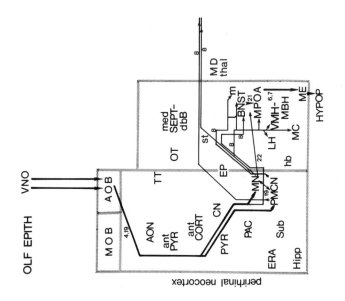

Fig. 3. Vomeronasal system.

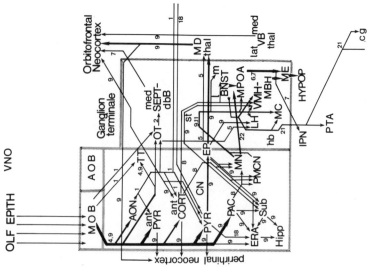

Fig. 2. Olfactory system. (See legend on p. 214.)

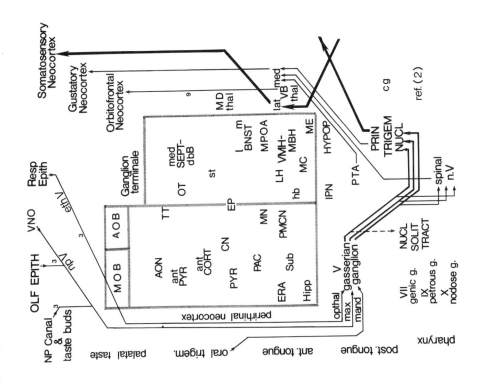

Fig. 5. Trigeminal system (right). (See legend on p. 214.)

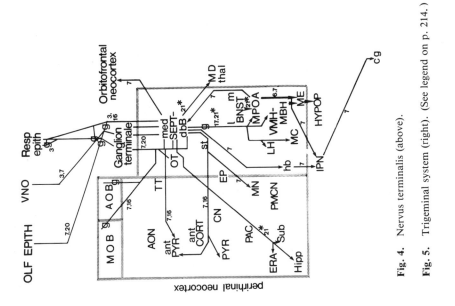

Fig. 4. Nervus terminalis (above).

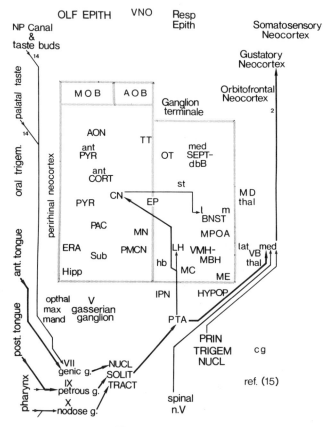

Fig. 6. Taste system.

Figs. 2–6. Schematic diagrams of the central connections of chemoreceptor systems. Fig. 2: main olfactory projections; Fig. 3: vomeronasal projections; Fig. 4: nervus terminalis and LHRH system (connections marked with an asterisk have not been shown to contain LHRH); Fig. 5: trigeminal projections; Fig. 6: gustatory projections. The diagrams represent one-half of the brain (midline to the right). The large left-hand block enclosed by shaded lines represents the paleocortex. The block to the right includes other limbic structures. Not all connections reported by the authors listed below are shown. For example, few centrifugal projections are shown, although many areas are reciprocally connected. Species differences among those species studied are generally minor, usually involving density rather than presence or absence of projections. Additional olfactory projections to neocortex via the ventrobasal thalamus and via the hypothalamus suggested by electrophysiological data and reviewed by Takagi (1982) are not included because the details of the pathway are not known. The separation of gustatory and somatosensory neocortex into two or more areas is not shown. Perirhinal neocortex includes all areas adjacent to the rhinal sulcus. In Fig. 2 all vomeronasal system projections to fourth-order targets are shown except those from BNST. BNST projections are not shown because it is not known which, if any, of these projections include axons from cells in the "third-order vomeronasal" part of BNST, which receives direct AOB projections. In the other females but had a minimal effect on mating (Sapolsky and Eichenbaum, 1980). Tanabe *et al.* (1975b) recorded odor responses in pyriform cortex, thalamus, and olfactory neocortex in monkeys and found increasing specificity of response to arbitrarily selected odorants at higher levels. Lesions in areas of frontal cortex that could be activated by electrical stimulation' of the olfactory bulb produced deficits in a simple behavioral odor discrimination task (Tanabe *et al.*, 1975a). A functional pathway via the hypothalamus was suggested because hypothalamic ablations eliminated the evoked responses produced in frontal cortex by olfactory bulb stimulation, but this possibility was not tested behaviorally. The pathways proposed on the basis of this type of experiment have been reviewed by Takagi (1982). These and other studies suggest that odor detection and simple discrimination do not require the thalamocortical projection and, if the behavioral test is sufficiently sensitive, may be demonstrable when remarkably little of the olfactory bulb output remains intact. The thalamocortical projections are apparently not required for mating behavior, at least in the rodents tested, suggesting that some quite complex species-typical behaviors involving odor identification can be accomplished at subcortical levels, possibly

---

figures, potentially important projections from a given nucleus are shown if that nucleus receives chemosensory input, even if the correspondence between the cells of origin of the efferent projection and the recipients of chemosensory input have not been definitely established as the same cells. Key to references: 1, Broadwell (1975a,b); 2, from Brodal (1981); 3, Bojsen-Moller (1975); 4, Davis *et al.* (1978); 5, Heimer (1972), Heimer *et al.* (1975); 6, Ibata *et al.* [*] (1979); 7, Jennes and Stumpf (1980); 8, Kevetter and Winans (1981a,b); 9, Kretteck and Price (1977a,b,c, 1978a,b); 10, Lehman (1982); 11, Leonard and Scott (1971); 12, Macrides *et al.* (1981); 13, Meibach and Siegel (1977); 14, Miller and Porcelli (1976); 15, Norgren (1977a,b); 16, Phillips *et al.* (1980); 17, Poulain and Carette (1978); 18, Price (1973); 19, Scalia and Winans (1975); 20, Schwanzel-Fukuda and Silverman (1980); 21, Swanson and Cohen (1979); 22, Winans (1982). Abbreviations: AOB, accessory olfactory bulb; AON, anterior olfactory nucleus; BNST (l, m): bed nucleus of stria terminalis (lateral, medial); cg, central gray (of midbrain); CN, central amygdaloid nucleus; ant CORT, anterior cortical amygdaloid nucleus; EP, endopyriform nucleus; ERA, entorhinal area; eth V, ethmoid branch of fifth cranial nerve; g., ganglion nervus terminalis; genic g., geniculate ganglion (VII); Hb, habenula; Hipp, hippocampus; HYPOP, hypophysis; IPN, interpeduncular nucleus; LH, lateral hypothalamus; MBH, medial basal hypothalamus (includes VMH); MC, mammilary complex; ME, median eminence; MD thal, mediodorsal thalamus; MN, medial amygdaloid nucleus; MOB, main olfactory bulb; MPOA, medial preoptic area; NP Canal, nasopalatine canal wall; npV, nasopalatine branch of fifth cranial nerve; nodose g., nodose ganglion (X); NUCL SOLIT TRACT, nucleus of solitary tract; OLF EPITH, olfactory epithelium; OT, olfactory tubercle; petrous g., petrous ganglion (IX); PRIN TRIGM N, principal trigeminal nucleus; PTA, pontine taste area; PMCN, posteromedial cortical nucleus; ant PYR, anterior pyriform cortex; PYR, pyriform cortex; RESP EPITH, respiratory epithelium; med SEPT–dbB, medial septal nucleus-diagonal band of Brocca; st, stria terminalis; Spinal V, Spinal trigeminal nucleus; Sub, subiculum; TT, taenia tecta; VB Thal, ventrobasal thalamus; VMH, ventromedial hypothalamus; VNO vomeronasal organ.* See also Hoffman and Gibbs (1982).

without involving cognitive processes. More abstract tasks involving odors may require the thalamocortical projections.

Lloyd-Thomas and Keverne (1982) have suggested that input through the vomeronasal system, whose principal projections are entirely subcortical, may actually be unavailable for cognitive processes but the evidence for this is sparse (see Section IV,B). Lesions in the central vomeronasal pathways may have dramatic effects on mating behavior but their effects on olfactory tasks involving arbitrary odors have not been studied.

Central vomeronasal projections include the medial amygdala and medial preoptic area, and lesions of both these areas produce serious deficits in mating behavior in male hamsters (Lehman *et al.,* 1981) and rats (Harris and Sachs, 1975; Ryan and Frankel, 1978). From experiments involving lesions of the amygdala, stria terminalis, and ventral amygdalofugal pathway, Winans (1982) and co-workers provided evidence that the medial amygdala lesions may interrupt a vomeronasal system projection passing via the ventral amygdalofugal pathway to the posterior bed nucleus of the stria terminalis adjacent to the medial preoptic area. The effects of these limbic lesions on discrimination of arbitrary odors was not reported, so the extent to which simple sensory deprivation is responsible for the behavioral deficits is not known.

The effects of lesions of the central projections of chemoreceptor systems are usually more difficult to interpret than those of peripheral lesions. Small lesions may affect more than one system because of convergence and will not eliminate all input from a system with multiple projections. The possibility that lesions prevent responses for reasons other than the removal of sensory input becomes more likely with central lesions, but a systematic assessment of this possibility, by measurement of sensory capacity after the induction of lesions that produce deficits in species specific behaviors, has not usually been attempted.

The more dramatic effect of lesions in the vomeronasal compared with the olfactory system in these few examples may result from differences in the tests used to assess deficits, it may indicate that the vomeronasal is a more specialized system functionally or that vomeronasal projections are more concentrated anatomically. The more dramatic effect of lesions aimed at vomeronasal targets may also be the consequence of the simultaneous removal of vomeronasal, olfactory and/or terminalis systems which converge on the lesioned area.

B. Social Stimulation and Release of Luteinizing Hormone

Bronson (1979; see also Chapter 7) has pointed out that luteinizing hormone (LH) release is a common initial hormonal response to social stimuli in both sexes. For example, LH is released within 30 min in prepubertal female mice exposed to male stimuli (Bronson and Maruniak, 1976). In male mice exposed to females, LH is released within 5 min and is followed by testosterone release (Coquelin and Bronson, 1980; Desjardins, 1981). In many cases the response to social stimuli with which the LH release is associated has been shown to be dependent on vomeronasal input (see Section IV), suggesting that the vomeronasal system may project centrally to LH-releasing systems in the ventral forebrain. (See also Beltramino and Talesnik, 1983.)

The recent finding that luteinizing hormone releasing hormone- (LHRH-) like activity has been localized by immunohistochemistry and radioimmunoassay to the olfactory bulb, accessory olfactory bulb, and to the interbulbar elements of the nervus terminalis suggests that this putative link between chemosensory input and LH release should be examined in more detail.

Neural control of LH release is mediated by the levels of LHRH liberated into the pituitary portal plasma from the terminals of cells in the basal hypothalamus (Silverman and Krey, 1978a,b) and medial preoptic area (MPOA) (Setalo et al., 1976). In females (and also in neonatally castrated males), a special neural mechanism develops for the production of the large surge in LH release necessary for ovulation (Gorski, 1971; Dyer et al., 1976; Raisman and Field, 1973), and this mechanism appears to be controlled from the MPOA (Koves and Halasz, 1970). The neonatal androgen level in intact males and neonatally androgenized females is thought to prevent the development of the LH-surge mechanism. Nevertheless, electrochemical stimulation (ECS) of the MPOA with an iron-depositing electrode, which results in LHRH release into the portal system (Eskay et al., 1976), produces LH release in both sexes so the lack of a surge mechanism does not preclude episodic release of LHRH (see also Desjardins, 1981). The MPOA and regions that connect to it are projection targets for the corticomedial amygdala (Leonard and Scott, 1971; Kevetter and Winans, 1981a,b; Winans, 1982), which in turn receives vomeronasal input from the accessory olfactory bulb (AOB) (Scalia and Winans, 1975; Davis et al., 1978). In females but not males, ECS in the corticomedial amygdala can also release LH (Velasco and Talesnik, 1969; Beltramino and Talesnik, 1978). This response and the somewhat weaker one produced by ECS in the AOB of females (Beltramino and Talesnik, 1979) appear to result from the activation of the ovulatory LH-surge mechanism because (a) the amount of LH released is similar to that preceding ovulation and much larger than that following social stimulation; (b) the response occurs only after a period of estrogen priming, as does the ovulatory surge. In related experiments in which the amygdala stimulation was used to produce ovulation in implanted ovaries, the ovulation could be elicited only in animals not exposed to neonatal androgen (Teresawa et al., 1969; Arai, 1971).

Stimulation of the corticomedial anygdala would be expected to activate vomeronasal projections, all of which must pass through this region. The failure to elicit statistically significant LH release in males (Velasco and Talesnik, 1969) may be related to the fact that peaks in LH release in response to social stimuli are smaller than the ovulatory surge and may have been missed in experiments investigating ovulation. However, failure of electrical stimulation of the vomeronasal pathway to release LH is not good evidence against the proposed vomeronasally elicited release, because the ECS is unlikely to mimic natural activity in the system. The mechanism of action of ECS is not known precisely but depends on the deposition of iron and may involve prolonged excitation, suppression, or poisoning of selected cell populations (Dyer and Burnett, 1976).

The notion that vomeronasal input may be concerned with LHRH and LH release in the male is supported by the fact that (*a*) sexual behavior of male rats is facilitated by LHRH injection (Moss *et al.*, 1975) and by MPOA stimulation (Malsbury, 1971), which also elicits LH release; and (*b*) male sexual behavior is reduced or eliminated by vomeronasal lesions in the mouse (Ingersoll, 1980) and hamster (Powers and Winans, 1975), by bulbectomy in the inexperienced rat (Larsson, 1975), and by MPOA lesions in the rat (Ryan and Frankel, 1978) and hamster (Bergondy *et al.*, 1982). Vomeronasal lesions can also prevent hormonal release in mice (Wysocki, 1982).

In the rat, MPOA lesions eliminated mating behavior but not LH release on exposure to females (Ryan and Frankel, 1978). The lesions appeared to have spared the ventrocaudal MPOA/anterior hypothalamus region (see Fig. 1 in Ryan and Frankel, 1978), where some LHRH cell bodies are located (Ibata *et al.*, 1979), but it is not known whether there is vomeronasal input to these cells or whether any such input would have survived the lesion. These experiments do suggest that LHRH release in response to social stimulation is not sufficient to elicit sexual behavior in the absence of an intact MPOA.

An even more direct pathway for chemical signals to elicit hormonal responses is suggested by the finding (Schwanzel-Fukuda and Silverman, 1980; Phillips *et al.*, 1980; Jennes and Stumpf, 1980) that the nervus terminalis contains immunoreactive LHRH and projects into a network of LHRH-containing cells and fibers in the anterior ventral forebrain. This network extends into the MPOA, although the precise connections of the supposed sensory cells are not known. The nervus terminalis fibers enter and/or leave the brain around the anterior cerebral artery and connect with the olfactory tubercle, diagonal band of Brocca, and medial septum (Phillips *et al.*, 1980; Schwanzel-Fukuda and Silverman, 1980) and with the caudal septum (Jennes and Stumpf, 1980). It is not clear how many, if any, of these fibers are the axons of LHRH cells in the peripheral ganglia and how many are the axons of LHRH cells in the basal forebrain. Nor is it clear how many are afferent (regardless of soma position) and how many are efferent. Schwanzel-Fukuda and Silverman (1980) concluded that most LHRH elements of the nervus terminalis are probably sensory and homologous with the bipolar cells observed by others in nonimmunoreacted tissue (Larsell, 1950; Pearson, 1941). Certainly there are neural connections between peripheral nervus terminalis fibers and the ganglion terminale and between the ganglion terminale and the olfactory tubercle, diagonal band of Brocca, and septum.

The possibility that the nasal LHRH system participates in LH release clearly needs further investigation, and such a conclusion would be premature. We do not yet know (*a*) if the nervus terminalis is, in fact, chemosensitive, (*b*) if any chemosensitive information is carried centrally, (*c*) if centrally directed chemosensory afferents reach the MPOA or other area concerned with LH release, or (*d*) if the mechanism by which LHRH mediates behavioral and physiological changes is, in fact, part of the same mechanism by which chemosensory input achieves the same result.

In fish, a system of LHRH containing cells and fibers extends from the forebrain to both the olfactory bulb (nervus terminalis) and optic tract (Münz *et al.,* 1982). Recent experiments by Demski *et al.* (1982) show that stimulation of either the olfactory or optic tract in males can produce sperm release, as can LHRH injections into the ventrical close to the central projection of the nervus terminalis. The caveats applicable to mammals, listed above, also apply to this system but it is clearly a promising preparation for the study of terminalis function.

In female rats the anterior septal LHRH-containing cells do not participate in the ovulatory LH surge (Silverman and Krey, 1978b), but that does not rule out their participation in the LH release elicited by chemical signals in either sex. LHRH-positive fibers derived from the network that connects to the nervus terminalis pass laterally through the ventral amygdaloid pathway to the corticomedial amygdala (Jennes and Stumpf, 1980; Phillips *et al.,* 1980). Experiments in the hamster showed that lesions in the medial but not in the basolateral amygdala eliminated male mating behavior (Lehman *et al.,* 1981; Lehman and Winans, 1982), but the effect on LH release was not reported. Macrides *et al.* (1976) found no changes in basal levels of testosterone after in animals with lateral olfactory tract lesions but did not look at acute changes in LH and testosterone levels in response to social stimuli. Lateral olfactory tract lesions might be used to distinguish between vomeronasal and terminalis contributions, because these systems project to common areas in the amygdala and MPOA via different routes. Lesions of the septal region specifically designed to interrupt the nervus terminalis projections have not been reported, but septal lesions are known to have many effects that are probably not attributable to sensory deafferentation (Paxinos, 1976; Donovick *et al.*, 1979). The results of central terminalis lesions might therefore be difficult to interpret.

The widespread occurrence of LHRH-containing cells and terminals and of neuronal responses to the iontophoresis of LHRH (Jennes and Stumpf, 1980; Samson *et al.*, 1980; Poulain and Carette, 1978; Moss, 1979) suggests that the peptide may simply serve as a neurotransmitter or neuromodulator (Hokfelt *et al.*, 1980) unconnected with LH release. If so, the nervus terminalis and LHRH systems associated with the main and accessory olfactory bulb may have no special significance for reproductive physiology or behavior. LHRH-positive projections outside the hypothalamus are commonly found in areas that do influence sexual behavior and may, as suggested by Moss (1979) and Pfaff (1980), coordinate physiological and behavioral responses to sexual stimuli. In this context the efferent components of the nervus terminalis to the olfactory epithelium and VNO (Larsell, 1950; Schwanzel-Fukuda and Silverman, 1980) and the LHRH connections to the olfactory bulb, AOB, and amygdala (Jennes and Stumpf, 1980) may serve to integrate or modulate nasal chemosensory input.

IV. EVIDENCE FOR VOMERONASAL INVOLVEMENT

In this section experiments are evaluated for evidence suggesting that particular sensory systems are involved in pheromonal responses. Most of these experiments involve lesions of one or more sensory systems. The various techniques used and the possible involvement of chemosensory systems other than those that were the target of the lesion are reviewed here. The evaluation in this section includes a speculative assessment of the implications of data that are suggestive even if not statistically significant. This is not a criticism of the original authors, who very properly restrict their interpretations to statistically significant results; the intention is to explore possible directions for future research. Five criteria are considered in this evaluation:

1. Has the vomeronasal contribution been definitely established?
2. Is a vomeronasal contribution necessary and/or sufficient?
3. In particular, does elimination of the sensory system produce at least the same reduction in performance as is produced by removal of the sensory cue?
4. Have contributions by other systems been (*a*) ruled out or (*b*) definitely shown to occur and are any such contributions necessary and/or sufficient?
5. Is there any evidence that nonvolatile rather than volatile chemicals were involved in the participation of the vomeronasal or other system?

Information on all these topics is not available from all the studies, many of which used experimental designs with redundant cues. For example, contact between individuals of opposite sex has been used even where chemical stimuli alone have been shown to be sufficient to communicate sexual information. Any residual response after lesions are made in one chemosensory system cannot necessarily be attributed to the surviving chemosensory systems in such tests because nonchemosensory information is also available.

Residual responses that are not statistically significantly different from control response in the absence of the stimulus are usually interpreted as proof that the lesioned sensory system is the only one involved in the response. The null hypothesis of the statistical test is set up in the reverse sense, however. Significant difference from control would indicate that there is some other contribution to the response, but a nonsignificant difference simply means that the null hypothesis cannot be rejected. Such results cannot be interpreted as definite evidence against alternative sensory input.

A. Ovulation in Light-Induced Persistent-Estrous Rats

Ovulation during the normal rat estrous cycle results from a release of LH, which is initiated by LHRH release (Eskay *et al.,* 1977; Sakar *et al.,* 1976) and is dependent on estrogen priming of the CNS release mechanism (Niell *et al.,* 1971; Ferin *et al.,* 1969). In rats exposed to constant light, the cyclic changes are arrested because the diurnal signal (Legan and Karsch, 1975; Freeman *et al.,* 1976) that normally controls the timing of the LH surge has been removed. A low level of circulating estrogen, sufficient to prime the LH-surge mechanism, is usually present in these animals. They apparently need only a trigger for the LH surge to elicit ovulation, and this can be supplied by male stimuli (Brown-Grant *et al.,* 1973). In the experiments of Johns *et al.* (1978) and Johns (1980) considered here, male exposure or male-soiled bedding reliably elicited ovulation in some percentage of constant-light, persistent-estrous females, as did clean bedding to which a sufficient quantity of male urine had been added. Vomeronasal function was impaired by lesions designed to occlude the vomeronasal entrance ducts. Groups with vomeronasal damage (VNX) showed significantly less ovulation than sham controls when exposed to male-soiled bedding, although some ovulations did occur. A comparison of the effects of vomeronasal damage and of cue removal can be made only by comparing across two experiments, but the control values for the two are essentially identical. The percentage of females that ovulated in the VNX group was lower than the percentage of intact females that ovulated after contact with clean bedding. Thus, the obstruction of the sensory system did produce at least as much diminution in performance as the removal of the sensory cue. In the limited circumstances of the experiment, then, the vomeronasal system (and/or any other system that the lesion affects) appears to be both necessary and sufficient. The lack of ovulation when contact with the stimulus was prevented in these experiments suggests that some relevant cues are not volatile odors but does not, by itself, necessarily implicate the vomeronasal system, because other potential chemoreceptors were not disabled.

B. Estrous Cyclicity and Puberty Acceleration in the Rat

Male stimuli can cause adult female rats housed in groups to accelerate their estrous cycles so that a greater proportion of the group is estrous at any given time (Chateau et al., 1973; Aron, 1979). If all animals were on 4-day cycles, 50% of them would be on their estrous or proestrous day at one time (2/4). If all were on 5-day cycles, the percentage would be 40% (2/5). Sanchez-Criado (1979,1982) showed that damage to the accessory olfactory bulb or the vomeronasal nerve results in a shift from 4- to 5-day cycles in many animals and therefore a decrease in the percentage of animals in proestrus or estrus.

Sanchez-Criado found in rats that the proportion of females in proestrus or estrus declined by 37% (from 47.2% to 29.7%) and 39% (from 49% to 30%) after lesions were placed in the accessory olfactory bulb or vomeronasal nerves, respectively, when compared with sham-lesioned animals. These changes in proportions are greater than the 20% change that would occur if all females switched from 4-day cycles to 5-day cycles. However, the observed changes are approximately equal to those that occur when females are isolated from male influence. According to figures given by Gallego and Sanchez-Criado (1979) isolation from male stimuli produces a 35% decrease in the proportion of females in proestrus or estrus for sham-operated animals and a 40% decrease for intact animals. Thus, the vomeronasal lesions alone appear to eliminate all the differences associated with the presence of males, suggesting that the vomeronasal system is both necessary and sufficient (in as far as its lesions do not affect other systems). Other systems, including the olfactory system, appeared to be incapable of maintaining the behavior, although no histological examination of the olfactory epithelium, to ensure its integrity and the absence of disease, were reported.

Female rats, like mice, also show earlier sexual maturation in the presence of males (Vandenbergh, 1976) or male odors (Sato et al., 1974). In an assay of accelerated puberty in female rats with vomeronasal nerve damage (Sanchez-Criado, 1979, 1982; Sanchez-Criado and Gallego, 1979), the times of vaginal opening and of first estrus for lesioned females in the presence of males were indistinguishable from those of intact females isolated from males. The advance in first estrus is only about one-third that produced in mice by exposure to male cues, but it is significant and does appear to depend on vomeronasal input.

No tests of the volatility or otherwise of the relevant stimuli for puberty acceleration or changes in estrous cycle length were made here.

C. Estrous Cyclicity in Group-Housed Mice

Mice housed in all-female groups show a prolongation of estrous cycle length, and many individuals become acyclic (Whitten, 1959). Individually housed females do not generally become acyclic but can be made so by the addition to their cages of the soiled bedding or urine of group-housed females (Whitten and Champlin, 1973). Reynolds and Keverne (1979) studied the vomeronasal contribution to this effect using cautery of the organ to block vomeronasal input. After vomeronasal damage the proportion of females in suppressed estrus fell from an average of 91% for all control groups to an average of 32% for all lesioned groups, a change relative to control animals of 65% (91 − 32/91 × 100 = 65%: 64% difference from sham-lesioned animals, which showed 88% suppression). This level of suppressed estrus was higher than that for females isolated from males, although the difference just escapes significance. Nevertheless, the possibility remains either that the VNO damage itself reduced estrous cycling or that another sensory system contributed to the detection of female grouping cues, even after vomeronasal damage. No additional tests were made to assess contributions from other systems. The nature of any chemical cues producing suppressed estrus cannot be deduced from these results.

Further experiments to investigate the hormonal basis of the suppression of estrus were also reported by Reynolds and Keverne (1979). Injections of bromocryptine (CB-154), a dopamine agonist, caused a 70% drop in the proportion of females in suppressed estrus 72 hr later. Following injections of the dopamine antagonist haloperidol into grouped females with VNO lesions, the proportion of females in suppressed estrus was high, similar to that for the unlesioned groups. Withdrawal of the haloperidol was followed by a drop in the proportion of the lesioned animals in suppressed estrus to a level similar to that in isolated animals. The dopamine systems influenced by these drugs maintain an inhibitory effect on prolactin secretion (Negro-Villar and Ojeda, 1981), so that these data are consistent with a role for prolactin in the suppression of estrus. Haloperidol has many actions other than an elevation of prolactin level, so that evidence from its use can be only supportive, at best, of other data on this point. However, CB-154 is fairly specific in its effects on pituitary hormone secretion, lowering prolactin level while having little effect on LH and follicle-stimulating hormone (FSH) levels (Advis *et al.,* 1981). It is not clear that the lowered prolactin level is the cause of the suppression of estrus, however. The authors point out that elevated prolactin levels have a feedback effect on dopamine turnover in the hypothalamus, and either drug may have its effect by altering dopamine systems unconnected with prolactin release. A useful test of the prolactin hypothesis would be the use of exogenous prolactin to replace that lost as a result of CB-154 treatment (Advis *et al.,* 1981). Any failure of normal levels of prolactin to protect against the effect of CB-154 could not be explained by the prolactin hypothesis.

In a testing *tour de force,* Ingersoll (1980) compared the effect of vomeronasal, olfactory, or combined lesions on the performance of SJ/LJ (congenitally blind) mice in seven different behavioral situations, including the regulation of the estrous cycle. Vomeronasal lesions were made by cautery of the entire vomeronasal organ on both sides, and olfactory damage was produced by intranasal infusion of 0.17 M $ZnSO_4$ (ZS). All lesions were verified by histology, although none were illustrated. Ingersoll observed that the performance of lesioned animals in Reynolds and Keverne's experiments could not be considered to be independent of that of other females in the group because these were also lesioned. He therefore repeated the experiment using 105 groups of 8 females, 1 female from each group being assigned as an experimental animal. There were thus 15 experimental animals, all of which showed suppression of estrus preoperatively, for each of seven treatments (olfactory, vomeronasal, or combined lesions, the three appropriate shams, and a no-treatment group). Confirming Reynolds and Keverne's results, 80% of the animals with vomeronasal lesions and 93% of animals with combined lesions returned to estrus within 72 hr and showed 4- to 5-day cycles for 20 days. In addition, only 20% of olfactory-lesioned animals showed estrous vaginal smears postoperatively, and all of these were suppressed again by the end of testing at 23 days after surgery. These results suggest that the female signal responsible for suppression of estrus (Champlin, 1971) is detected by the VNO and that the main olfactory system makes little or no contribution, at least in this laboratory situation. An alternative explanation is that the resumption of estrus in 20% of ZS-treated animals reflects a contribution from the olfactory or another system, and the later suppression of estrus in these animals reflects recovery from the effects of ZS treatment. All animals were tested for correct localization of food odor during the last 10 postoperative days, and no ZS-treated animals performed above chance. However, this kind of test, although well designed in itself, cannot provide definitive proof that an animal is unable to detect biologically significant odors (Alberts, 1974; Slotnik, 1979).

Vomeronasal lesions also produced 4- to 5-day estrous cycles in individually housed females whose cycles before the lesion were 7–9 days in length. Ingersoll suggested that these females may have been affected by their own odor but it is also possible that the vomeronasal lesion itself had some effect on estrous cycles.

Vandenbergh (1973) provided evidence that bulbectomy or ZS treatment can cause an increase in estrous cycle length in isolated female mice, from an average before the lesion of a little over 4 days to 6.5–7 days after the lesion. No histological analysis of ZS damage to the main and accessory olfactory system was reported but, regardless of one's assumptions, it is difficult to reconcile these findings and those of Ingersoll and of Reynolds and Keverne. Ingersoll found no effect of ZS treatment but a shortened estrous cycle length after vomeronasal lesions were made. Similarly, in Reynolds and Keverne's experiment the resumption of estrus after vomeronasal lesions were made also suggests a shortened estrous cycle. The situation is further complicated by a brief report from Barber and Raisman (1977), who found little effect of vomeronasal nerve lesions on estrous cycling in isolated female mice or on the synchronization of estrus by exposure to males. The latter results suggest that the vomeronasal system is not involved in the detection of male stimuli, but they might also be explained if lesioned vomeronasal nerves had time to regenerate before the animals were tested as has been suggested by Wysocki (1979). On the other hand, an estrous cycle length characteristic of females in the presence of males might be expected in this experiment after the introduction of males into a group of females with vomeronasal lesions. According to Ingersoll's results, lesioned females would already have 4-day estrous cycles characteristic of females housed with males. The brief description of Barber and Raisman's experiment does not suggest that this was the explanation for their results, but insufficient details are given.

Different strains of mice were used in these various experiments, and this may be the cause of some of the differences in results. Strains of mice have been reported to differ in the effects of lesions to the olfactory bulb and nasal mucosa (Vandenbergh, 1973; Schoots et al., 1978).

In contrast to the situation in mice, Sanchez-Criado found that vomeronasal system lesions in rats produce a lengthening of mean estrous cycle lengths to approximately equal those found for isolated females and significantly longer than the 4-day cycle in the presence of males. The lesions in rats were made by cautery of the vomeronasal nerves or of the accessory olfactory bulbs, whereas the vomeronasal lesions used in mice by Reynolds and Keverne and by Ingersoll involved cautery of the organ itself. The lesions in the two species would produce different types of ancillary damage, but it is difficult to imagine how the different behavioral results could be produced in this way. In both rats and mice, the introduction of males to isolated females causes a reduction in estrous cycle length, but Aron (1979) notes that rats differ from mice in the effect of grouping females. Grouped female rats showed shorter estrous cycles under most circumstances, whereas cycle length in mice is lengthened by grouping. Thus in both species vomeronasal lesions oppose the effects of female grouping.

D. Acceleration of Puberty in Female Mice

Wilson *et al.* (1980) and Kaneko *et al.* (1980) utilized a bioassay for puberty based on uterine growth in prepubescent mice exposed to male stimuli for 48 hr. Uterine growth is the first morphological sign of puberty, and it occurs earlier in females exposed to males (Vandenbergh *et al.*, 1975; Bronson and Maruniak, 1976). In the Kaneko *et al.* experiments, one olfactory bulb was removed to allow visual control of the destruction of all branches of the contralateral vomeronasal nerve. These procedures thus produced an animal with one functional olfactory bulb but no intact vomeronasal nerves. Although unilateral olfactory bulbectomy has only a minimal effect on an animal's performance on some odor-related tasks (Bennett, 1971; Devor and Murphy, 1973), it apparently does have an effect here. The uterine weight gain of unilaterally bulbectomized females is less than that of unoperated controls.

Bilateral bulbectomy in these experiments reduced uterine weight gain significantly compared with control animals that were isolated from males in an all-female room (Wilson *et al.*, 1980). Bilateral bulbectomy may therefore have effects on uterine weight gain in addition to any effects of the sensory deprivation. No isolated bulbectomized controls were reported, so interactions between male exposure and bulbectomy cannot be assessed. In view of these complications, the possibility that unilateral bulbectomy has effects in addition to unilateral sensory deprivation cannot be ignored. In spite of these considerations, it seems likely that the uterine weights of animals with both unilateral bulbectomy and vomeronasal nerve cut are in fact significantly lower than those of unilaterally bulbectomized females, although the authors do not make that particular calculation. If that were so, the authors' conclusion that vomeronasal input did have a significant effect on uterine growth in the presence of males, would be justified. No alternative procedures to reveal any other sensory inputs contributing to the performance were reported.

There appears to be some residual uterine growth even in animals with vomeronasal lesions in these experiments by Kaneko *et al.* (1980), but the more definitive experiments of Lomas and Keverne (1982) suggest that vomeronasal input can account for all of the effects of male stimuli. These authors used bedding soiled by strange males to produce accelerated estrus in prepubertal females. They recorded the day of vaginal opening and first estrus in addition to uterine weight gain and included control groups with sham lesions, a group isolated from male stimuli, and a group both isolated and lesioned. Groups of animals with bilateral cautery of the VNO reached first estrus later than isolated controls, suggesting that there may be some direct effect of the lesions on puberty. However, the lesioned animals exposed to male stimuli did not show first estrus until after the isolated lesioned group, so there is no residual performance to be accounted for by other than vomeronasal sensory input (and/or other systems affected by the lesion). Confirming the somewhat equivocal results of Kaneko *et al.* (1980), the uterine weight (corrected for body weight) in these experiments was less than 2% greater in lesioned animals exposed to male-soiled bedding for 48 hr than in unexposed lesioned animals. In unlesioned control animals similarly exposed, uterine weight was 44% greater than in unexposed controls.

In additional experiments the authors examined the effect of dopamine agonists and antagonists on puberty acceleration. These drugs were used in an attempt to examine the effects of modulation in prolactin secretion. Other reports, quoted by the authors, have come to contradictory conclusions about the effect of prolactin in accelerating or delaying puberty when dopaminergic drugs were used. Although these drugs affect prolactin secretion selectively compared with their effects on other pituitary hormones, they must also affect dopamine systems, which, although not directly concerned with gross levels of hormone release, may have more subtle effects. The interpretation of the role of prolactin is more convincing where prolactin levels and the effect of exogenous prolactin are measured, as, for example, in the Advis *et al.* (1981) demonstration of puberty delay following early CB-154 treatment in the rat.

In Lomas and Keverne's experiments on puberty acceleration, puberty did occur earlier when animals were injected on days 26 and 27 with bromocryptine to lower the prolactin level. Bromocryptine had no effect when injected on days 23–24, the days when exposure to male bedding accelerates puberty. The authors suggest that the female's ovaries are not sufficiently mature at that time for the effect of lowered prolactin level to be demonstrated. If this is the case, it is not obvious how a change in prolactin level could be the primary response that initiates puberty acceleration in females exposed to male stimuli.

No conclusion can be drawn about the volatility of the chemical stimuli involved in either of the experiments on puberty acceleration because contact with male stimuli was not restricted.

E. Pregnancy Block in Mice

One of the most dramatic effects of mouse urinary pheromones is the block of pregnancy that occurs in most strains when recently mated females are exposed to the urine of a strange male. This has been regarded as an artifact of the laboratory testing situation by Bronson (1979; Bronson and Coquelin, 1980), but it does allow the investigation of the sensory channels by which urinary components are detected, as well as the investigation of the urinary components themselves (see Chapter 6).

Bellringer *et al.* (1980) exposed females with bilateral vomeronasal cautery (VNX) to males of a different strain 48 hr after they were impregnated by a male of their own strain (impregnation determined by the presence of a vaginal plug). The VNX females returned to estrus less frequently (4/16 = 25%) than sham-operated females, impregnated and exposed to males in the same way (78%). Some VNX animals did return to estrus as judged by vaginal smear data, but the results suggest that vomeronasal input may be important in the discrimination of strain differences, a discrimination which must precede pregnancy block.

In experiments using male-soiled bedding rather than cohabitation with males as the stimulus for pregnancy block, 12 of 16 animals, including 4 that had shown estrous-type vaginal smears, were found to be carrying diapausing embryos. These embryos were found to be viable for culture *in vitro* and apparently could be made to implant *in vivo* by injecting gonadotropin. In as far as animals that had shown estrous smears could retain viable embryos, these results suggest that the extent of the pregnancy block produced by male bedding and thus the extent of the protection against pregnancy block by vomeronasal lesions may have been less than it appeared.

Experiments by Ingersoll (1980) support and extend the findings of Bellringer *et al.* (1980), providing independent evidence that vomeronasal lesions influence pregnancy block in impregnated females exposed to male stimuli. Eighty percent of animals with vomeronasal lesions and 87% of animals with combined vomeronasal and olfactory lesions failed to show pregnancy block when exposed to male-soiled bedding. Each had at least one fetus in the uterus 10 days after exposure to male-soiled bedding for 5 days. In sham-lesioned and control animals the proportions were reversed, with 80–86% of animals showing pregnancy block. No embryos were reported in females showing estrous-type vaginal smears.

In later experiments Lloyd-Thomas and Keverne (1982) also used male-soiled bedding to induce pregnancy block but classified as blocked only those females that both returned to estrus and had no implantation sites 6 days after impregnation. No diapausing embryos were reported. In these experiments none of the VNX females showed pregnancy block when exposed to alien male bedding, but 78–83% of control, sham-operated, or ZS-treated animals were blocked. The fact that ZS treatment did not reduce the incidence of pregnancy block suggests that the 20–25% pregnancy blockage found in VNX females in previous experiments may not have been produced by olfactory cues and may indeed have been spontaneous.

Animals with ZS lesions lost the ability to show a preference when presented with the bedding odors of intact and castrated males but, as also found by Ingersoll (1980), ZS-treated animals still showed pregnancy block. There was a difference of only 2% between ZS-treated and untreated animals in the percentage of pregnancies blocked, suggesting that olfactory detection of cues from the alien male was not important. Lloyd-Thomas and Keverne (1982) suggest that females distinguish between familiar and alien males by recognizing a cue produced by the familiar (stud) male. This suggestion is supported by the finding of Keverne and de la Riva (1982) that 6-hydroxydopamine lesions of the medial olfactory peduncle or posterior dorsal olfactory bulb eliminate the discrimination between stud and alien male: *Both* produce pregnancy block in lesioned females, and both must therefore produce cues that can elicit the block. Apparently, additional cues from the familiar male, which are detected by a system sensitive to the 6-hydroxydopamine lesions, result in inhibition of the pregnancy block response. 6-hydroxydopamine lesions by themselves did not result in pregnancy block. These results suggest that it is not the strange male that blocks pregnancy but rather the stud or familiar male that prevents the blockage.

Because ZS-treated females in the Lloyd-Thomas and Keverne study still showed pregnancy block in response to alien and not stud males, the distinction is presumably mediated by the vomeronasal system—If all pregnancy block effects are mediated by the vomeronasal system then this system must be capable of discriminating stimuli from different males. The validity of this conclusion rests, of course, on the efficacy of the ZS treatment in eliminating all nonvomeronasal chemoreception during the time of female exposure to male cues (on the second to fourth day after ZS treatment, or longer if the females were not inseminated on the first night with the stud). The olfactory capability of ZS-treated females reexposed to studs was apparently not tested postoperatively.

Keverne and de la Riva (1982) also found that females removed from their studs on the morning after impregnation and exposed for 48 hr to strange male bedding responded with pregnancy block when reexposed to their studs. Females placed with the same strange male whose bedding they had been exposed to immediately after removal from the stud did not show pregnancy block. These findings suggest that the animals are "imprinted" during this period on cues that can later initiate the process of pregnancy block protection.

No definite conclusions about the volatility or otherwise of the chemical cues can be drawn from these experiments except that intact females showed no preference for the odor of either male strain and could not be trained to discriminate them in 27 trials. Lloyd-Thomas and Keverne (1982) suggest that the failure to discriminate behaviorally even though a vomeronasally mediated physiological differentiation is possible indicates that vomeronasal input is not available to cognitive processes. Mice can be trained to discriminate between the odors of very closely related mice if enough trials are given (Yamazaki et al., 1980), although the sensory pathway is not known.

In additional experiments by Bellringer et al. (1980) mated females injected with bromocriptine (CB 154) to lower prolactin levels tended to return to estrus (64%). This is not unexpected because prolactin is thought to be essential for the survival of the corpus luteum in the initial stages of pregnancy in rodents (Smith, 1980). It has been shown (a) that exogenous gonadotropin [pregnant mare serum gonadotropin (PMSG) but not LH or FSH] produces pregnancy block in mice by preventing implantation, perhaps by the leuteolytic properties of the gonadotropin (Hoppe and Whitten, 1972), and (b) that exogenous prolactin or lactation (elevated prolactin level) can protect against pregnancy block (Parks and Bruce, 1961). These findings suggest that either elevated gonadotropin levels or lowered prolactin levels are responsible for pregnancy block. The results of Bellringer et al. are consistent with the lowered prolactin level hypothesis, but Chapman et al. (1970) were unable to show a significant reduction in prolactin level following female exposure to alien males. The development of a method for frequent blood sampling in mice (Coquelin and Bronson, 1980, 1981) should make it possible to address the question of hormonal mediation of pheromone responses more directly.

F. Testosterone Response to Females in Male Mice

When males are exposed to females following a period of isolation or housing in all-male groups, they show a rise in serum testosterone levels (Macrides et al., 1975). Wysocki and Katz (Wysocki, 1982) showed that surgical removal of both vomeronasal organs (VNX) prevents this rise in serum testosterone level. Basal testosterone levels in isolated males or those housed in all-male groups are reported to be adequate to maintain sexual behavior (Davidson, 1977). It has been suggested (Macrides et al., 1975) that the testosterone peak may be unnecessary for copulation but may facilitate the production of male characteristic behaviors and signals, including pheromones. These signals in turn would elicit hormonal changes in the female and induce receptivity. Studies of young and aged mice in which LH and testosterone levels were sampled at frequent intervals suggest that periodic testosterone peaks, whether spontaneous or induced, are preceded and probably elicited by a sharp peak in LH levels but that basal levels of both hormones are low (Desjardins, 1981; Coquelin and Bronson, 1980). These studies suggest that successful copulation is associated with the frequency of spontaneous testosterone peaks in stimulated males. In rats, the correlation between episodic LH release and testosterone levels is not so well established (Desjardins, 1981) but there is some evidence that transitory increases in testosterone level may facilitate copulatory behavior (Malmnas, 1977). It thus seems possible that the testosterone peak produced by exposure to females may assist in ensuring copulatory success as well as providing signals that synchronize male and female readiness to mate.

Wysocki and Katz did not measure LH levels, but they did show that testosterone and dihydrotestosterone (DHT) levels did not rise in VNX, sexually experienced males after exposure to a female. Levels in intact males did rise on exposure to a female. Basal levels of both testosterone and DHT in VNX mice isolated from females were slightly but not significantly lower than in isolated intact animals. After exposure to females, testosterone and DHT levels in VNX animals were very slightly higher, although still below the unstimulated level for intact animals. The differences are so small that there is no reason to suspect any contribution from other sensory systems in this test. This finding is actually somewhat surprising because, in rats at least, it is possible to condition LH and testosterone peaks in experienced animals to arbitrary volatile odor cues (Graham and Desjardins, 1980) and such cues would be expected to be detectable by the main olfactory system. (See Section VI for further discussion.)

G. Male Sexual Behavior in Hamsters and Mice

The first report of vomeronasal involvement in sexual behavior was that of Powers and Winans (1975), who found that 40% of males with intracranial vomeronasal nerve cuts (VNX) showed severe deficits in sexual behavior. In contrast, no deficits were found in males treated with intranasal zinc sulfate (ZS) by a procedure previously shown to eliminate performance on an olfactory task (Powers and Winans, 1973). The vomeronasal system thus appeared to be both necessary and sufficient for normal sexual behavior in at least some individuals. The main olfactory system appeared not to be necessary for any individual, although it was sufficient for some. One or the other system appeared to be necessary for all individuals, because ZS treatment eliminated all mating behavior in males that continued to mate after their vomeronasal nerves were cut.

A replication of these experiments (Meredith *et al.,* 1980a; Meredith, 1980; R.J. O'Connell, M. Meredith, and D.M. Marques, unpublished) using the same lesion techniques confirmed that ZS treatment had no significant effects on mating behavior in laboratory tests, implying that the vomeronasal input is sufficient to maintain sexual behavior (or that some other system damaged by vomeronasal nerve cuts but not by ZS treatment was involved). In these experiments vomeronasal nerve cuts alone were not effective in producing deficits in mating behavior when males were tested with naturally cycling, behaviorally receptive females. Subsequent ZS treatment eliminated mating behavior with cycling females in all vomeronasal nerve cut animals, as in the Powers and Winans experiments. Murphy (1980) also failed to find deficits in tests of the mounting behavior of VNX males with intact females. Naturally cycling receptive females may provide more cues (chemical or otherwise) to the male than do hormone-primed ovariectomized animals so that the removal of vomeronasal input is less critical, especially in sexually experienced animals. This view has indirect support from experiments in which there was a severe restriction on the female cues available to the test male. Anesthetized male hamsters scented with hamster vaginal fluid provide sufficient cues that intact males will mount and attempt intromission (Macrides *et al.,* 1977; Meredith *et al.,* 1980a). In such tests mounting and thrusting was significantly reduced in animals with vomeronasal nerve lesions alone. These results imply that both vomeronasal and olfactory systems can contribute to the induction of mating behavior in sexually experienced male hamsters.

Zinc sulfate treatment in hamsters eliminates most of the main olfactory receptors, but some always survive, usually in the ventral and lateral regions (Winans and Powers, 1977; Meredith *et al.,* 1980b). Any remaining olfactory input is insufficient to maintain mating behavior, as demonstrated by the loss of behavior in animals with combined vomeronasal nerve cuts and ZS treatment. The main olfactory bulb damage produced by vomeronasal nerve cuts is in the same region as that maximally affected by ZS treatment and should not affect any residual olfactory capability (Meredith *et al.,* 1980b).

It is possible that other systems are compromised by lesions intended to damage vomeronasal or olfactory systems. This possibility can be examined more closely here than in most cases because two types of vomeronasal system lesions were used. Nasopalatine nerve lesions (Meredith *et al.,* 1980a) were designed to prevent stimulus access to vomeronasal receptors, but they also damage the nasopalatine trigeminal and autonomic projections. They do not damage the main olfactory system. On the other hand, the Powers and Winans vomeronasal nerve lesions do damage the medial olfactory bulb but not the nasopalatine projection. When combined with ZS treatment (which has no effect by itself) both of these lesions produce significant deficits in mating behavior. These deficits cannot, therefore, be attributed solely to the ancillary damage done by either lesion. It is possible, although anatomically unlikely, that the ventral septum cautery used to lesion the nasopalatine nerves also damages the septal organ. Intracranial vomeronasal nerve cuts might also damage septal organ projections so that both types of lesion could have damaged the same two systems. However, if septal damage rather than vomeronasal damage were the important result of lesions aimed at the vomeronasal system, the ineffectiveness of ZS treatment would have to be explained. The septal organ would have to survive ZS treatment to account for the results according to this hypothesis, and that is unlikely.

As mentioned in Section II,B, there is evidence that nonvolatile chemicals in hamster vaginal fluid (HVF) can elicit mounting behavior. Attraction of males to the odor of HVF is dependent on the olfactory system and can be drastically reduced by olfactory lesions when contact is prevented, suggesting that volatile substances are involved. The attraction to HVF smeared on the anogenital area of anesthetized males persists after the induction of olfactory lesions, suggesting attraction mediated by the vomeronasal system (Powers *et al.,* 1979; Meredith, 1980). Powers *et al.* (1979, 1981) suggest that the vomeronasal system can detect the attractants only when contact with the stimulus is possible, but there is an alternative explanation: that in anosmic (ZS-treated) animals, vomeronasal pumping is initiated only when the stimulus animal is encountered, and only then are stimuli delivered to receptors. Whether the vomeronasally mediated attraction is to dimethyl disulfide, a volatile sex attractant in hamster vaginal fluid (Singer *et al.,* 1980), or to other volatile or nonvolatile components is not known. Electrophysiological experiments show that dimethyl disulfide and other volatile stimuli can stimulate the vomeronasal system if delivered to the receptors (Meredith and O'Connell, 1979; Tucker, 1963a,b, 1971), and we have some preliminary evidence that volatiles from hamster vaginal fluid can elicit mounting as well as attraction, although at a reduced rate and via unknown sensory pathways (Meredith, 1982).

In mice, male copulatory behavior was examined by Ingersoll (1980) and shown to be unaffected by ZS treatment. Ejaculation was eliminated by either vomeronasal or combined vomeronasal and olfactory lesions, and animals with combined lesions also failed to mount. Mounting in animals with vomeronasal lesions alone was severely depressed (by 71%) but not eliminated, suggesting that olfactory input may have some facilitatory influence on this behavior. Anogenital sniffing was severely reduced after the vomeronasal system was lesioned but only slightly reduced after the olfactory system was lesioned. Ingersoll suggests that this result reflects a reduction of interest in the genital area of females rather than a reduction in sniffing per se. In comparison with investigations of hamster behavior, these results suggest a greater dependence on vomeronasal input in the mouse.

Both mice (Wysocki et al., 1982) and guinea pigs (Beauchamp et al., 1982) showed less discrimination between male and female chemosensory cues when deprived of their vomeronasal organs, suggesting that vomeronasal lesions might impair precopulatory behavior. When tested in small cages, male guinea pigs lacking vomeronasal organs or with bilateral bulbectomy did not show significant deficits in mating behavior but in a more natural situation mating by bulbectomized guinea pigs was impaired (Beauchamp et al., 1982).

H. Maternal Behavior in Rats and Hamsters

Virgin female rodents tend to avoid or to kill newborn pups placed into their cages, but they eventually show various aspects of normal maternal behavior if continuously exposed to pups. The initial aversion is thought to be due to an aversion to the odor of pups, because the latency for virgin females to become maternal can be reduced by lesions of chemoreceptor pathways (Fleming and Rosenblatt, 1974a,b). Fleming et al. (1979) showed that vomeronasal nerve cuts alone were effective in reducing the latency for virgin female rats to retrieve pups and assume a nursing posture over them. The reduction in latency after damage to the main olfactory bulbs was not statistically significant. This difference cannot be interpreted as a demonstration that the vomeronasal and not the olfactory system is involved in detecting pup odors. The combination of vomeronasal nerve cuts and main olfactory bulb damage was significantly more effective than either vomeronasal nerve cuts alone or main bulb damage alone in reducing the latency to become maternal, indicating contributions from both systems. The olfactory bulb damage was produced by inserting a surgical blade into the lateral side of the anterior third of the bulb, a procedure that would probably disconnect no more than 25% of the olfactory input to the brain (the output axons of less than half of the anterior third of the bulb plus those receptor axons terminating posterior to the cut that do not reach the lateral bulb from below). This type of lesion should do no damage to other systems but is not a good test of the importance of main olfactory input. More extensive main olfactory bulb damage might well have had significant effects by itself. In ovariectomized, hysterectomized, hormone-treated, virgin female rats, Mayer and Rosenblatt (1980) also showed a significant decrease in latency following a form of ZS treatment claimed to damage both olfactory and vomeronasal systems. No histological verification was given.

In hamsters, virgin females given experience with pups fall reliably into two groups: those that carry pups and those that kill them. Marques (1979) found that vomeronasal nerve cuts converted 7 of 12 (68%) animals shown preoperatively to be killers into carriers and that subsequent olfactory damage by ZS treatment converted to carriers 4 of the 5 remaining killers. Zinc sulfate lesions converted 29% of killers, and combined lesions converted all but 1 killer in each group. Thus, in hamsters as in rats, both olfactory and vomeronasal systems appear to contribute to the behavior of virgin females to pups. The contributions of other systems are not known.

It has not been definitely established that the effects investigated by Marques or those investigated by Fleming and Rosenblatt or Mayer and Rosenblatt are due to the prevention of chemosensory input. Radical olfactory bulbectomy, which is known to have nonsensory effects on behavior (Cain, 1974a,b; Cain and Paxinos, 1974; Alberts, 1974), affects virgin female behavior with pups more than peripheral deafferentation does (Fleming and Rosenblatt, 1974a,b; Marques, 1979). This finding does not demonstrate, however, that peripheral deafferentation has no nonsensory effects.

I. Other Behaviors

There are four other series of experiments in which the contribution of particular chemosensory systems to intraspecific communication have been investigated. The situations tested are simply listed here because published results are sparse. Ingersoll (1980) concluded that aggressive interactions and dominance in male mice depend on both the vomeronasal and olfactory systems. In three other cases there was some evidence that vomeronasal input was not involved in the behavior. These are (a) the preference among male hamsters for conspecific females as partners in mating behavior (Murphy, 1980), (b) the reinitiation of copulatory behavior in sexually satiated male hamsters presented with a new female (R.E. Johnston, personal communication, 1981), and (c) nipple finding and suckling in neonatal rat pups (Singh et al., 1977). In the last case bulbectomy and ZS treatment produced similar deficits in suckling (Singh et al., 1976, 1977), and there is some evidence that a small region of the olfactory bulb, near but not within the AOB, may be important in this behavior (Teicher et al., 1980).

Note additional evidence for vomeronasal influence on LH release in female rats exposed to male odors (Beltramino and Talesnik, 1983).

V. METHODS FOR THE DEMONSTRATION OF CHEMOSENSORY PATHWAYS

Four basic methods provide some evidence that a particular chemosensory pathway is involved:

1. Prevention of stimulus access: The behavioral or physiological response should disappear when the causative stimulus is no longer detected.
2. Lesions of the receptors or the neural pathway to the brain: The response disappears when information transfer to the brain is blocked.
3. Demonstration that all active stimuli reach or activate only one particular sensory system and not other systems.
4. Selective stimulation of the neural pathway electrically or chemically in an attempt to produce the response in the absence of the pheromone.

A. Prevention of Access

Access to the main olfactory mucosa or septal organ might be blocked by occluding the clefts between turbinates or by laying the occluding material over the septal organ. Damage to underlying nerves and distribution of the occluding material to other systems would be difficult to avoid, however. The method of unilateral bulbectomy and contralateral nostril occlusion used by Devor and Murphy (1973) probably does not completely block access in most rodents (including the hamster) because there is communication between the two sides of the nose through the septal window. Neither of these methods is selective for the olfactory system alone because trigeminal and terminalis endings are also present in the olfactory area. Access of stimuli to the vomeronasal epithelium has been blocked by cautery of the duct (Johns, 1980). Serial sections of decalcified tissue would be necessary to determine the extent of damage, as with all intracranial lesions, but even with this evidence it would be difficult to be sure that no pathway to intact receptors had been established through the friable necrotic tissue by forceful action of the vomeronasal pump. Occlusion of the nasopalatine canal in species in which the organ opens into it does have some behavioral effect (McGrath *et al.,* 1981; Verberne, 1976), but the degree and longevity of the blockage have to be carefully monitored. Blockage of stimulus access to the trigeminal and terminalis systems would be difficult to achieve selectively because of the widespread distribution of their endings. Tracer studies might be useful to show blockage of access in each of these systems but are not conclusive for reasons given below.

B. Lesions

Olfactory bulbectomy is no longer used to demonstrate olfactory input because it also damages other chemoreceptor systems and it may have behavioral effects in addition to those caused by the removal of sensory input

(Cain, 1974a,b; Alberts, 1974; Meisel *et al.*, 1982). Some of the results of bulbectomy once thought to be nonsensory effects are probably not (Murphy, 1976) but enough remain to make the method unattractive except for an initial screening procedure. Although bulbectomy is nonselective, it still does not remove all chemoreceptor input from the nose. The nasopalatine and posterior nasal branches of the trigeminal system would be unaffected, although the ethmoidal trigeminal branch which passes rostro-laterally over the olfactory bulb would be damaged. A better method for eliminating all nasal chemoreception might be nasal infusion with local anesthetics (Doty and Anisko, 1973), especially if there is some evidence for blockage of trigeminal receptors such as the failure to respond to ether (Banks *et al.*, 1963). Lesions of the olfactory nerves (Larsson, 1971) are as nonselective as bulbectomy but, in addition, are difficult to make complete (Graziadei and Monti-Graziadei, 1980).

The only nonsurgical olfactory lesion shown to spare vomeronasal input is the intranasal infusion of ZS (Alberts and Galef, 1971; Alberts, 1974). There appears to be no regeneration in areas where the receptor epithelium is sloughed off from the lamina propria after infusion with 0.17 M ZnSO$_4$ (Winans and Powers, 1977; Harding *et al.*, 1978), but not all receptors are destroyed and there is usually some regeneration. Behavioral recovery is reported to be fairly rapid in the hamster (Powers and Winans, 1973) and less so in the mouse (Harding *et al.*, 1978). Recovery may vary with species, or it may depend on the stringency of the method used to assess olfactory performance (Slotnik and Guttman, 1977). The degree of protection of the vomeronasal receptors during ZS treatment may depend on the method used. Ether anesthesia (Winans and Powers, 1977; Meredith *et al.*, 1980a,b) may protect the vomeronasal epithelium by increasing secretions in and around the vomeronasal duct. The use of atropine or other drugs to increase access to the olfactory area may result in vomeronasal damage (e.g., Mayer and Rosenblatt, 1980), but this possibility has not been systematically investigated. Zinc sulfate treatment almost certainly damages the exposed septal organ receptors and, where the epithelium is sloughed from the lamina propria, the terminals of the trigeminal and terminalis fibers must be damaged. These terminals probably regenerate, however, possibly with different time courses from that of the recovery of olfactory receptors, and might be responsible for short-term behavioral recovery in some circumstances.

The incomplete and nonselective nature of damage and the variable results obtained by different workers make ZS treatment less than satisfactory for the selective elimination of olfactory input. At present, there is no better alternative, although an immunological method might be devised (Goldberg *et al.*, 1979).

In the vomeronasal system there are four possible lesion sites:

1. The organ itself can be cauterized (Reynolds and Keverne, 1979; Vaccarezza *et al.,* 1979; Ingersoll, 1980) or removed entirely (Wysocki, 1982). Ancillary damage would include the trigeminal nerves to the nasopalatine canal, ventral septum, and ventral swell body (Bojsen-Moller and Fahrenkrug, 1971) as well as both trigeminal and terminalis nerves to the VNO. Extensive lesions with intranasal electrodes or traction on the septal mucosa during removal of the organ might also damage the septal organ.

2. Intracranial section of the vomeronasal nerve by cutting the nerves where they pass between the main bulbs has been used extensively (Powers and Winans, 1975; Winans and Powers, 1977; Marques, 1979; Meredith *et al.,* 1980a). It damages the medial side of the main bulb (Winans and Powers, 1977), generally deafferenting the glomeruli posterior to the line of the cut, and probably damages the nervus terminalis network between the bulbs. Some terminalis fibers might pass below the level of the cut and enter olfactory and vomeronasal nerve bundles (Bojsen-Moller, 1975; Schwanzel-Fukuda and Silverman, 1980), but LHRH-positive fibers entering the vomeronasal nerves at the AOB (Jennes and Stumpf, 1980) must be cut. Damage to terminalis fibers cannot be directly assessed using simple histology, but histology is essential to determine the extent of the lesion. In cases in which the AOB glomeruli degenerate completely, it can be assumed that all vomeronasal input has been cut off (Winans and Powers, 1977), but at 1 to 2 weeks survival complete degeneration does not always occur, even when no intact fibers can be demonstrated by HRP transport from the mucosa (Meredith *et al.,* 1980a,b). At longer survival times regeneration may occur (Barber and Raisman, 1978). The method of unilateral bulbectomy (UOBX) followed by contralateral vomeronasal nerve section under direct vision (Kaneko *et al.,* 1980) has the advantage of minimizing damage to the intact bulb. Terminalis damage is probable, however, and the UOBX itself represents a 50% reduction in olfactory input.

3. It should be possible to cut or cauterize the vomeronasal nerves in most species where they pass across the nasal septum anterior to the olfactory area (e.g., Verberne, 1981). Restricted lesions should avoid damage to the dorsal (ethmoidal) and ventral (nasopalatine) trigeminal nerve trunks, but damage to the septal organ would have to be assessed in each case. Selective lesions of septal organ nerves might also be possible except in the guinea pig, where the septal organ and vomeronasal nerves appear to run together. A comparison of lesions rostral and caudal to the septal organ in the guinea pig might reveal septal organ influence.

4. Sanchez-Criado (1982) found similar deficits in reproductive functions

in female rats with AOB lesions or intracranial vomeronasal nerve cuts. Accessory olfactory bulb lesions may not damage the main olfactory bulb (MOB), but in rodents they do damage the axons of posteromedial main bulb output cells where these pass through the AOB granule cell layer (Johnson *et al.,* 1982). Lesions of centrally projecting neurons such as MOB or AOB output cells may lead to transsynaptic degeneration of the central target neurons (Heimer and Kalil, 1978), which could produce additional behavioral deficits.

No method is ideal for selectively eliminating vomeronasal input, but the successive use of different techniques, as discussed above for nasopalatine nerve lesions, could make more definitive interpretations possible.

Trigeminal and taste systems can be eliminated by cutting or disabling the relevant nerves extracranially (Allen, 1928; Stone *et al.,* 1968), without damage to most other systems. Trigeminal lesions may have adverse effects on behavior, not because of the removal of chemosensory input but because of the elimination of tactile responses from the snout. More peripheral trigeminal lesions avoiding the external nasal nerves to the snout could be used, but these lesions may damage autonomic fibers to the nasal cavity and vomeronasal pump. Selective terminalis lesions would be practically impossible to produce because of the proximity of the terminalis nerves to other nerves. It might be possible to isolate the system from the CNS by lesions of its central connections between the main bulbs. Ancillary damage to medial olfactory projections might be controlled for by separate lesions, or a selective immunological blockade using anti-LHRH antibody might be possible if the sensory pathway does in fact use LHRH. It is conceivable that some of the effects of lesions aimed at other systems may occur through damage to the nervus terminalis. All intranasal and intracranial lesions aimed at other systems could damage some component of the nervus terminalis, even if only the part passing to the VNO itself.

C. Exclusive Stimulation

The demonstration that one system is activated by a stimulus and another is not requires that all induced activity be detected. Neither single-unit nor multiunit electrophysiology can ensure this. 2-Deoxyglucose autoradiography (Kennedy *et al.,* 1975) allows all parts of the brain to be examined, but not all activated elements can be shown to take up 2-deoxyglucose (e.g., interneurons and motor neurons involved in spinal reflexes; Proshansky *et al.,* 1980). Neither electrophysiology nor 2-deoxyglucose methods can show whether the activity recorded is produced by a pheromone or by behaviorally irrelevant components of unpurified stimulus substances, and neither method can indicate whether the activity recorded contributes to the response or is ignored by the animal.

The use of tracer materials to demonstrate the effective stimulation of one set of receptors and not another depends on the sensitivity of the detection system used by the experimenter compared with that used by the animal. Errors in both directions are possible. The animal may respond to concentrations not detectable by the experimenter and sensory systems reached by detectable levels of tracer may not be sensitive enough to respond to the stimulus. Postmortem detectability of the tracer must be a matter of degree depending on the concentration achieved. Detection may also be related to differential retention rather than exclusive stimulation. Moreover, tracers that are physicochemically different from actual stimulus substances may not be distributed to receptors in the same way. Finally, all experiments using inert tracers are subject to artifactual migration of tracer due to blood pressure and secretion changes at death or on freezing, however rapidly this can be brought about. Tracers such as HRP and labeled amino acids, which can be detected after slow uptake into living cells (Barber and Raisman, 1977; Meredith *et al.*, 1980b), are not subject to this problem but also cannot be used to investigate short-term stimulus movements.

D. Artificial Stimulation

Because electrical stimulation can never mimic the natural pattern of neural activity in more than one neuron (Ranck, 1975), the production of a normal behavioral or physiological response by electrical or electrochemical stimulation of a sensory pathway is unlikely, unless the system is geared to respond to quantity rather than quality of neural input. The olfactory system seems an unlikely candidate for this type of organization because the many molecules to which it responds are probably discriminated on the basis of neural patterns of activity (Moulton, 1976; Mackay-Sim and Kubie, 1982). The vomeronasal system may be a more promising candidate for reasons given in the next section, but this possibility has not been evaluated experimentally. As discussed above the release of LH in response to electrochemical stimulation in the vomeronasal pathway is apparently a more complicated situation than a simple mimicry of the sensory input that produces LH release during social stimulation.

In summary, it would appear that the use of carefully controlled lesions is the method of choice for revealing a contribution from a particular sensory system to a behavioral response.

VI. THE VOMERONASAL SYSTEM AS A PHEROMONE DETECTOR

The vomeronasal system was originally regarded merely as a secondary olfactory system. In some circumstances it does appear to work in conjunction with the olfactory system but it is not unreasonable to ask, first, why the vomeronasal epithelium should be necessary at all, if the olfactory system is a universal molecular analyzer, and, second, why in mammals it should be sequestered in a separate chamber needing a pump mechanism for access. Three possible explanations are the following:

1. The vomeronasal receptors might be especially sensitive to some chemical signal but more vulnerable to damage than the olfactory receptors and therefore not exposed continuously.
2. Detection of some chemicals might require a different glandular secretion over the receptor surface, and this could be supplied in the separate vomeronasal lumen.
3. Afferent information entering the brain over the vomeronasal pathway might be so potent in eliciting behavioral or physiological responses in naive animals that inadvertent stimulation would have to be avoided, presuming inappropriate responses to have some evolutionary disadvantage.

The first two suggestions are not immediately susceptible to experimental test. The last hypothesis is suggested in part by the privileged pathway from the vomeronasal system to the ventromedial forebrain. This privileged pathway and the sequestered receptors could have evolved as a two-stage system, making reproduction more reliable. Inexperienced animals, especially those of solitary or colonizing species, would benefit from a system that would reliably elicit the appropriate behavioral or physiological response on their first encounter with the appropriate environmental cues. A detector system with such a potent influence would tend to elicit responses out of context unless, like insect pheromone detectors, its receptors were very specific. In mammals neither the olfactory nor the vomeronasal system has been shown to be remarkably specific (although the vomeronasal system has not been tested extensively). However, the vomeronasal pump might confer some additional specificity if operated only when the spectrum of environmental signals, both chemical and nonchemical, met some moderately specific criteria for example, the presence of another animal resembling the parent. The vomeronasal system could then make the final discrimination and initiate the response on the basis of pheromonal cues. The initial screening by the olfactory and other sensory systems would prevent some false positive responses, and the final discrimination would prevent others, without either stage of the two-stage process being extremely specific.

If this hypothesis is correct, one might expect inexperienced animals to be more dependent on their vomeronasal systems than experienced animals. Animals having previous experience with particular situations involving chemical cues could learn the finer distinctions of the behavioral situation and would no longer need to rely on preprogrammed vomeronasal cues to initiate appropriate behavior.

Of 15 situations reviewed above in which vomeronasal damage produces significant deficits in performance, 8 involve animals inexperienced with the stimuli used. These are (a) ovulation in persistent-estrous rats (Johns et al., 1978), (b) acceleration of puberty in female mice (Kaneko et al., 1980; Lomas and Keverne, 1982), (c) pregnancy block in mice (Bellringer et al., 1980; Ingersoll, 1980; Lloyd-Thomas and Keverne, 1982), (d) suppression of estrus in mice (Reynolds and Keverne, 1979; Ingersoll, 1980), (e) suppression of estrus in rats (Sanchez-Criado, 1982), (f) acceleration of puberty in rats (Sanchez-Criado, 1982), (g) ultrasonic calling in male mice exposed to females (Wysocki et al., 1982), and (h) maternal behavior in virgin female rats (Fleming et al., 1979).

In the first seven of these eight situations the response decreases by 85 to 100% after vomeronasal damage, suggesting that responses that are preprogrammed and can appear in inexperienced animals are dependent almost exclusively on vomeronasal input. In six situations in which experienced animals were tested, there was 25% or more residual behavior after vomeronasal damage in all but one case and 50% or more in all but two.

Unfortunately, most of the responses shown to depend on vomeronasal input have not been examined in both experienced and inexperienced animals. Some of the experiments may necessarily involve inexperienced animals; for example, there is no opportunity to observe the effects of chemical cues on puberty acceleration more than once in the same animal. In other cases experienced and inexperienced animals could have been used, but in only one case was that comparison actually made. Wysocki et al. (1982) showed that ultrasonic calling by the male in response to female urine appeared only after males had had sexual experience with females. This calling behavior could be maintained in experienced mice by nonvomeronasal chemoreceptive input, even after vomeronasal damage. That is, experienced but not inexperienced males still gave ultrasonic calls to female urine after vomeronasal damage (although they gave significantly fewer). This result suggests that conditioned olfactory cues, probably detected by the main olfactory system, had been associated with the unconditioned cues present in urine. The fact that inexperienced VNX mice did not make the association, giving no ultrasonic calls even after extensive social interaction with receptive females, is consistent with the notion (Wysocki *et al.,* 1982) that the unconditioned cues in urine can be detected only by the vomeronasal system. These VNX mice did not mate, however, so may have been lacking some reinforcement for making the association.

Graham and Desjardins (1980) demonstrated that the LH peak and consequent testosterone peak produced in males by exposure to females could be conditioned in rats to an irrelevant olfactory cue. By analogy, experienced male mice would be expected to show the female-induced peak in testosterone levels even after vomeronasal damage, but they do not (Wysocki, 1982). This is especially surprising because experienced VNX males can detect female cues and respond with ultrasounds (Wysocki *et al.,* 1982). Two possible explanations come to mind: (*a*) that LH release is more difficult to condition and the number of pairings was insufficient to condition the more difficult conditioned response and (*b*) that conditioned stimuli are detected by the vomeronasal system as well as the olfactory system but that LH release can be conditioned only via the vomeronasal input, whereas ultrasound production can be conditioned to the simultaneous olfactory input from the same or a different stimulus. Vomeronasal damage would thus prevent the activation of the LH-release system, which had been conditioned to respond to a new stimulus. It would be interesting to know if conditioning in mice, established by the method of Graham and Desjardins, would survive vomeronasal damage. The results of ZS lesions that damage the main olfactory but not the vomeronasal receptors might also be instructive.

In other situations where only inexperienced animals have been tested it will be interesting to ascertain whether experienced animals are as dependent on the vomeronasal organ or whether other sensory inputs can take over.

With the exception of Wysocki's experiments on testosterone levels, experienced animals given vomeronasal lesions did not reduce their performance to the level expected in the absence of relevant sensory cues. The most notable example among those reviewed above is the mating behavior of male hamsters. Severe deficits in mounting and intromission with females were recorded in only 40% of VNX males in one experiment (Powers and Winans, 1975) and in only one animal (approx. 14%) in another experiment (Meredith, 1980; Meredith *et al.,* 1980a). The animals used by both sets of authors in these experiments were deliberately selected to be reasonably vigorous maters, in order to eliminate false negative results from animals that would not mate reliably regardless of the presence or absence of lesions. There was therefore an opportunity for input from nonvomeronasal chemoreceptors to be conditionally associated with the (unknown) unconditioned stimulus. The ability of the olfactory input to maintain the behavior may therefore be secondary. It should be noted, however, that Macrides *et al.* (1977) could not demonstrate induced mounting with the sexual attractant dimethyl disulfide despite its known detectability and significance to males and its presence in the same source (hamster vaginal fluid) as chemical cues for mounting (Singer *et al.,* 1976). Macrides' animals had some sexual experience but had not made the association. A more consistent dependence on vomeronasal input for the initial mating performance compared with the vomeronasal dependence in sexually experienced animals might still be demonstrated if a reasonable number of inexperienced VNX males were tested. Macrides *et al.* (1977) did show somewhat less mounting by inexperienced intact animals in response to anesthetized male hamsters scented with vaginal fluid, compared with mounting by the same males after sexual experience. In the rat, sexual behavior in isolated, inexperienced animals is practically eliminated by bulbectomy, whereas bulbectomy after sexual experience has very little effect (Larsson, 1975), suggesting that in this species an unconditional chemosensory signal could be associated with nonchemosensory cues. Whether the important input in naive animals is olfactory or vomeronasal or carried by some other system is not known.

There are other examples of chemosensory responses by experienced animals where both vomeronasal and olfactory systems are implicated, but whether the olfactory input is conditioned in these cases is unknown. The fact that inexperienced animals depended almost exclusively on vomeronasal input in seven of the eight cases, whereas experienced animals used both olfactory and vomeronasal input in five of six cases, may be simply a chance result of the choices of experimental design and the types of response studied. It is consistent, however, with the hypothesis that the genetically determined or early imprinted ability to respond to chemical cues depends on input through the vomeronasal system but that this dependence is obscured once the animal gains experience, by its ability to associate other (conditioned) cues with the original unconditioned response.

If one considers the variety of functions reported for the vomeronasal system in reptiles, one might expect that additional examples of vomeronasal influence would be found in mammals (Burghardt, 1980). The examination of a greater number of response types in greater depth could be a useful test of the hypothesis connecting "preprogrammed" responses and a dependence on vomeronasal input.

VII. CONCLUSION

The vomeronasal system appears to be involved, in mammals, in species-typical responses to chemosensory signals. It is suggested that the system may be especially important in eliciting appropriate responses in inexperienced animals and that experienced animals may be conditioned through experience to respond to the input from other chemosensory or nonchemosensory systems. Lesion experiments are the most easily interpreted of experiments designed to show which chemosensory system is involved in a particular behavior. Because some lesions cannot be made complete and because most lesions damage more than one system, the contribution to species-typical behavioral responses by chemosensory input through other than the olfactory and vomeronasal systems has not been ruled out, although it has not yet been clearly demonstrated either.

ACKNOWLEDGMENTS

Parts of my own work described here were supported by NIH grant NS14453 to R. J. O'Connell and by NIH fellowship NS05849. The notion of vomeronasal organ importance in inexperienced animals emerged during discussions with D. M. Marques and R. J. O'Connell, in Dr. O'Connell's laboratory, and with C. J. Wysocki of the Monell Chemical Senses Center. I thank Dr. D. Ingersoll of Fordham University for permission to quote from his thesis research and Drs. M. E. Freeman, D. Ingersoll, A. Mackay-Sim, D. M. Marques, S. S. Winans, and C. J. Wysocki for comments on all or part of earlier versions of the manuscript.

REFERENCES

Adams, D. R., and MacFarland, L. Z. (1971). *Comp. Biochem. Physiol.* **40A**, 971–974.
Advis, J. P., Smith-White, S., and Ojeda, S. R. (1981) *Endocrinology* **109**, 1321–1330.
Alberts, J. R. (1974). *Physiol. Behav.* **12**, 657–670.
Alberts, J. R., and Galef, B. G., Jr. (1971). *Physiol. Behav.* **6**, 619–621.
Allen, W. F. (1928). *Am. J. Physiol.* **87**, 319–325.
Arai, Y. (1971). *Endocrinol. Jpn.* **18**, 211–214.
Aron, C. (1979). *Physiol. Rev.* **59**, 229–284.
Atema, J. (1971). *Brain, Behav. Evol.* **4**, 273–294.
Bailey, K. (1978). *Behaviour* **65**, 309–319.
Bang, B. G. (1961). *J. Morphol.* **109**, 57–71.
Banks, E. M., Bishop, R., and Norton, H. W. (1963). *Proc. Int. Congr. Zool., 16th, 1963* Vol. 2, p. 25 (from Alberts, 1974).
Barber, P. C., and Raisman, G. (1974). *Brain Res.* **81**, 21–30.
Barber, P. C., and Raisman, G. (1977). *Abstr., Int. Congr. Physiol. Sci., 27th, 1977* p. 51.
Barber, P. C., and Raisman, G. (1978). *Brain Res.* **147**, 297–314.
Beauchamp, G., Doty, R. L., Moulton, D. G., and Mugford, R. A. (1976). *In* "Mammalian Olfaction Reproductive Processes and Behavior" (R. L. Doty, ed.), pp. 144–160. Academic Press, New York.
Beauchamp, G. K., Martin, I. G., Wysocki, C. J. and Wellington, J. L. (1982). *Physiol. Behav.* **29**, 329–336.
Beidler, L. M. (1977). *In* "Chemical Signals in Vertebrates" (D. Müller-Schwarze and M. M. Mozell, eds.), pp. 483–488. Plenum, New York.
Bellringer, J. F., Pratt, H. P. M., and Keverne, E. B. (1980). *J. Reprod. Fertil.* **59**, 223–228.

Beltramino, C., and Talesnik, S. (1978). *Brain Res.* **144,** 95–107.

Beltramino, C., and Talesnik, S. (1979). *Neuroendocrinology* **28,** 320–328.

Beltramino, C., and Talesnik, S. (1983). *Neuroendocrinology* **36,** 53–58.

Bennett, M. H. (1971). *Physiol. Behav.* **7,** 597–599.

Berüter, J., Beauchamp, G. K., and Muetterties, E. L. (1973). *Biochem. Biophys. Res. Commun.,* **53,** 264–271.

Bergondy, M. L., Winans, S. S., and Powers, J. B. (1982) *Neurosci Abstr.* **8,** 972.

Blier, Z. (1930). *Am. J. Physiol.* **93,** 398–406.

Boelens, H. (1976). *In* "Structure-Activity Relationships in Chemoreception" (G. Benz, ed.), pp. 197–210. IRL, London.

Bojsen-Moller, F. (1964). *Anat. Rec.* **150,** 11–24.

Bojsen-Moller, F. (1975). *J. Comp. Neurol.* **159,** 245–256.

Bojsen-Moller, F., and Fahrenkrug, J. (1971). *J. Anat.* **110,** 25–37.

Bossert, W. H., and Wilson, E. O. 1963. *J. Theor. Biol.* **5,** 443–469.

Broadwell, R. D. (1975a). *J. Comp. Neurol.* **163,** 329–346.

Broadwell, R. D. (1975b). *J. Comp. Neurol.* **164,** 389–410.

Brodal, A. (1981). "Neurological Anatomy," 3rd ed. Oxford Univ. Press, London and New York.

Bronson, F. H. (1979). *Q. Rev. Biol.* **54,** 265–299.

Bronson, F. H., and Coquelin, A. (1980). *In* "Chemical Signals in Vertebrates and Aquatic Invertebrates" (D. Müller-Schwarze and R. M. Silverstein, eds.), pp. 243–266. Plenum, New York.

Bronson, F. H., and Maruniak, J. A. (1976). *Endocrinology* **98,** 1101–1108.

Brookover, C. (1910). *J. Comp. Neurol.* **20,** 49–118.

Brown-Grant, K., Davidson, J. M., and Greig, F. (1973). *J. Endocrinol.* **57,** 7–22.

Burghardt, G. M. (1980). *In* "Chemical Signals in Vertebrates and Aquatic Invertebrates" (D. Müller-Schwarze and R. M. Silverstein, eds.), pp. 275–302. Plenum, New York.

Cain, D. P. (1974a). *J. Comp. Physiol. Psychol.* **80,** 213–220.

Cain, D. P. (1974b). *Psychol. Bull.* **81,** 654–671.

Cain, D. P., and Paxinos, G. (1974). *J. Comp. Physiol. Psychol.* **86,** 202–212.

Cain, W. S., and Murphy, C. L. (1980). *Nature (London)* **284,** 255–257.

Caprio, J. (1982). *In* "Chemoreception in Fishes" (T. J. Hara, ed.), pp. 109–134. Elsevier, Amsterdam.

Champlin, A. K. (1971). *J. Reprod. Fertil.* **27,** 233–241.

Chapman, V. M., Desjardins, C., and Whitten, W. C. (1970). *J. Reprod. Fertil.* **21,** 333–337.

Chateau, D., Roos, J., and Aron, C. (1973). *C. R. Hebd. Seances Acad. Sci., Ser. D* **276,** 2823–2826.

Coquelin, A., and Bronson, F. H. (1980). *Endocrinology* **100,** 1224–1229.

Coquelin, A., and Bronson, F. H. (1981). *Endocrinology* **109,** 1605–1610.

Davidson, J. M. (1977). *Int. Rev. Physiol.* **13,** 225–254.

Davis, B. J., Macrides, F., Youngs, W. M., Schneider, S. P., and Rosene, D. L. (1978). *Brain Res. Bull.* **3,** 59–72.

Demski, L. S., Dulka, J. G., and Northcutt, R. G. (1982) *Neurosci. Abstr.* **8,** 611.

Desjardins, C. (1981). *Biol. Reprod.* **24,** 1–19.

Devor, M., and Murphy, M. R. (1973). *Behav. Biol.* **9,** 31–42.

Donovick, P. J., Burright, R. G., and Bengelloun, W. A. (1979). *Neurosci. Biobehav. Rev.* **3,** 83–96.

Doty, R. L. (1975). *Physiol. Behav.* **14,** 855–859.

Doty, R. L., and Anisko, J. J. (1973). *Physiol. Behav.* **10,** 395–397.

Doty, R. L., Brugger, W. E., Jurs, P. C., Orndorff, M. A., Snyder, P. J., and Lowry, L. D. (1978). *Physiol. Behav.* **20,** 175–185.

Doving, K. B. (1966). *J. Neurophysiol.* **29**, 675–683.

Dravnieks, A. (1975). *In* "Methods in Olfactory Research" (D. G. Moulton, A. Turk, and J. W. Johnston, Jr., eds.), pp. 1–62. Academic Press, New York.

Dyer, R. G., and Burnett, F. (1976). *J. Endocrinol.* **69**, 247–254.

Dyer, R. G., MacLeod, N. K., and Ellendorf, F. (1976). *Proc. R. Soc. London, B Ser.* **193**, 421–440.

Eichenbaum, H., Shedlack, K. J., and Eckman, K. W. (1980). *Brain Behav. Evol.* **17**, 255–275.

Eccles, R. (1982). *Physiol. Behav.* **28**, 1011–1015.

Eccles, R., and Lee, R. L. (1980). *Acta Oto-Laryngol.* **91**, 127–134.

Eccles, R., and Wilson, H. (1973). *J. Physiol. (London)* **230**, 213–223.

Eskay, R. L., Mical, R. S., and Porter, J. C. (1977). *Endocrinology* **100**, 263–270.

Estes, R. D. (1972). *Mammalia* **36**, 315–341.

Ferin, M., Tempone, A., Zimmering, P., and Van DeWiele, R. L. (1969). *Endocrinology* **85**, 1070–1078.

Fleming, A. S., Vaccarino, F., Tambosso, L., and Chee, P. (1979). *Science* **203**, 372–373.

Fleming, A. S., and Rosenblatt, J. S. (1974a). *J. Comp. Physiol. Psychol.* **86**, 221–232.

Fleming, A. S., and Rosenblatt, J. S. (1974b). *J. Comp. Physiol. Psychol.* **86**, 233–246.

Freeman, M. C., Dupke, K. C., and Croteau, C. M. (1976). *Endocrinology* **99**, 223–229.

Gallego, A., and Sanchez-Criado, J. E. (1979). *Acta Endocrinol. (Copenhagen), Suppl.* **225**, 256.

Garcia, J., and Rusiniak, K. W. (1980). *In* "Chemical Signals in Vertebrates and Aquatic Invertebrates" (D. Müller-Schwarze and R. M. Silverstein, eds.), pp. 141–156. Plenum, New York.

Gesteland, R. C. (1978). *In* "Handbook of Perception" (E. C. Carterette and P. Friedman, eds.), Vol. 6A, pp. 259–276. Academic Press, New York.

Getchell, T. V., Heck, G. L., DeSimone, J. A., and Price, S. (1980). *Biophys. J.* **29**, 397–411.

Goldberg, S. J., Turpin, J., and Price, S. (1979). *Chem. Senses Flavour* **4**, 207–214.

Gorski, R. A. (1971). *Front. Neuroendocrinol.* **2**, 237–290.

Graham, J. M., and Desjardins, C. (1980). *Science* **210**, 1039–1041.

Graziadei, P. P. C. (1977). *In* "Chemical Signals in Vertebrates" (D. Müller-Schwarze and M. M. Mozell, eds.), pp. 435–454. Plenum, New York.

Graziadei, P. P. C., and Gagne, H. T. (1973). *Z. Zellforsch. Mikrosk. Anat.* **138**, 315–326.

Graziadei, P. P. C., and Monti-Graziadei, G. A. (1980). *J. Neurocytol.* **9**, 145–162.

Guillot, M. (1967). *Recherches* **16**, 173–198.

Harding, J. W., Getchell, T. V., and Margolis, F. L. (1978). *Brain Res.* **140**, 271–285.

Harris, V., and Sachs, B. D. (1975). *Brain Res.* **86**, 514–518.

Heimer, L. (1972). *Brain Behav. Evol.* **6**, 484–523.

Heimer, L., and Kalil, R. (1978). *J. Comp. Neurol.* **178**, 559–610.

Heimer, L., DeOlmos, J., Hardy, H., and Rosards, M. J. (1975). *Neursci. Abstr.* **1**, 680.

Hoffman, G. E. and Gibbs, E. F. (1982). *Neuroscience* **7**, 1979–1993.

Hokfelt, T., Johannsson, O., Ljungdahl, A., Lundberg, J. M., and Schultzberg, M. (1980). *Nature (London)* **284**, 515–521.

Holley, A., and Doving, K. B., (1977). *Proc. Int. Symp. Olfaction Taste, 6th, 1977,* pp. 113–124.

Hoppe, P. C., and Whitten, W. K. (1972). *Biol. Reprod.* **7**, 254–259.

Hornung, D. E., and Mozell, M. M. (1977a). *J. Gen. Physiol.* **69**, 343–361.

Hornung, D. E., and Mozell, M. M. (1977b). *Brain Res.* **128**, 158–163.

Ibata, Y., Watanabe, K., Kinoshita, H. Kubo, S., Sano, Y., Sin, S., Hashimura, E., and Imagawa, K., (1979). *Cell Tissue Res.* **198**, 381–395.

Ingersoll, D. (1980). Ph.D. Thesis, Department of Psychology, City University of New York, New York.

Jacobs, V. L., Sis, R. F., Chenoweth, P. J., Klemm, W. R., Sherry, C. J., and Copock, C. E. (1980). *Theriogenology* **13**, 353–356.

Jacobs, V. L., Sis, R. F., Chenoweth, P. J., Klemm, W. R., and Sherry, C. J. (1981). *Acta Anat.* **110**, 48–58.

Jellinek, J. S. (1964). *Ann. N.Y. Acad. Sci.* **116**, 725–734.

Jennes, L., and Stumpf, W. E. (1980). *Cell Tissue Res.* **209**, 239–256.

Johns, M. A. (1980). *In* "Chemical Signals in Vertebrates and Aquatic Invertebrates" (D. Müller-Schwarze and R. M. Silverstein, eds.), pp. 341–364. Plenum, New York.

Johns, M. A., Feder, H. H., Komisaruk, B. R., and Mayer, A. D. (1978). *Nature (London)* **272**, 97–120.

Johnson, J. I., Switzer, R. C., III, and Kirsch, J. A. W. (1982). *Brain Behav. Evol.* **20**, 97–117.

Johnston, R. E. (1977). *In* "Chemical Signals in Vertebrates" (D. Müller-Schwarze and M. M. Mozell, eds.), pp. 225–250. Plenum, New York.

Johnston, R. E., Zahorik, D. M., Immler, K., and Zakon, H. (1978). *J. Comp. Physiol. Psychol.* **92**, 85–93.

Kaneko, N., Debski, E. A., Wilson, M. C., and Whitten, W. K. (1980). *Biol. Reprod.* **22**, 873–878.

Kennedy, C., DesRosiers, M. H., Jehle, J. W., Reivich, M., Sharpe, F., and Sokoloff, L. (1975). *Science* **187**, 850–853.

Kersjaschki, I. D., and Horandner, H. (1976). *J. Ultrastruct. Res.* **54**, 420–444.

Keverne, E. B., and de la Riva, C., (1982). *Nature (London)* **296**, 148–150.

Kevetter, G. A., and Winans, S. S. (1981a). *J. Comp. Neurol.* **197**, 80–98.

Kevetter, G. A., and Winans, S. S. (1981b). *J. Comp. Neurol.* **197**, 99–111.

Knappe, H. V. (1964). *Zool. Garten, Leipzig* [N. S.] **28**, 188–193.

Koves, K., and Halasz, B. (1970). *Neuroendocrinology* **6**, 180–193.

Kretteck, J. E., and Price, J. L. (1977a). *J. Comp. Neurol.* **171**, 157–192.

Kretteck, J. E., and Price, J. L. (1977b). *J. Comp. Neurol.* **172**, 687–722.

Kretteck, J. E., and Price, J. L. (1977c). *J. Comp. Neurol.* **172**, 723–752.

Kretteck, J. E., and Price, J. L. (1978a). *J. Comp. Neurol.* **178**, 225–254.

Kretteck, J. E., and Price, J. L. (1978b). *J. Comp. Neurol.* **178**, 255– 280.

Ladewig, J., and Hart, B. L. (1980). *Physiol. Behav.* **24**, 1007–1071.

Ladewig, J., Price, E. O., and Hart, B. J. (1980). *Behav. Neural. Biol.* **30**, 312–322.

Laffort, P., and Dravnieks, A. (1974). *J. Theor. Biol.* **38**, 335–345.

Larsell, O. (1950). *Ann. Otol., Rhinol., Laryngol.* **59**, 414–438.

Larsson, K. (1971). *Brain Behav. Evol.* **4**, 463–471.

Larsson, K. (1975). *Physiol. Behav.* **14**, 195–199.

Legan, S. J., and Karsch, F. J. (1975). *Endocrinology* **96**, 57.

Lehman, M. N. (1982). Ph.D. Thesis, University of Michigan, Ann Arbor.

Lehman, M. N., and Winans, S. S. (1982). *Brain Res.* **240**, 27–41.

Lehman, M. N., Winans, S. S., and Powers, J. B. (1981). *Science* **210**, 557–559.

Leonard, C. M., and Scott, J. W. (1971). *J. Comp. Neurol.* **141**, 313–330.

Lloyd-Thomas, A., and Keverne, E. B. (1982). *Neuroscience* **7**, 907–912.

Lomas, D. E., and Keverne, E. B. (1982). *J. Reprod. Fertil.* **66**, 101–107.

Lucas, A. M., and Douglas, L. C. (1934). *Arch. Otolaryngol.* **20**, 518–541.

McClintock, M. K. (1978). *Horm. Behav.* **10**, 264–276.

McCotter, R. (1912). *Anat. Rec.* **6**, 299–318.

McGrath, T. J., Jacobs, V. L., Sis, R. F., and Klemm, W. R. (1981). *Zentralb. Veterinaer med., Reihe C* (in press).

Mackay-Sim, A., and Kubie, J. L. (1982). *Chem. Senses* **6**, 249–258.

Mackay-Sim, A., Shaman, P., and Moulton, D. G. (1982). *J. Neurophysiol.* **48**, 584–596.

Macrides, F. (1976). *In* "Mammalian Olfaction, Reproductive Processes, and Behavior" (R. L. Doty, ed.), pp. 29–66. Academic Press, New York.

Macrides, F., Bartke, A., and Dalterio, S. (1975). *Science* **189**, 1104–1106.

Macrides, F., Firl, A. C., Schneider, S. P., Bartke, A., and Stein, D. G. (1976). *Brain Res.* **109**, 97–109.

Macrides, F., Johnson, P. A., and Schneider, S. P. (1977). *Behav. Biol.* **20**, 377–386.

Macrides, F., Davis, B. J., Youngs, W. M., Nadi, S., and Margolis, F. L. (1981). *J. Comp. Neurol.* **203**, 495–514.

Malcolmson, K. G. (1959). *J. Laryngol. Otol.* **73**, 73–98.

Malmnäs, C. O. (1977). *J. Reprod. Fertil.* **51**, 351–354.

Malsbury, C. W. (1971). *Physiol. Behav.* **7**, 797–805.

Marques, D. M. (1979). *Behav. Neural Biol.* **26**, 298–329.

Marshall, D. A., and Moulton, D. G. (1977). *Proc. Int. Symp. Olfaction Taste, 6th, 1976,* p. 197.

Masera, R. (1943). *Arch. Ital. Anat. Embryol.* **48**, 157–212.

Mayer, A. D., and Rosenblatt, J. (1980). *J. Comp. Physiol. Psychol.* **94**, 1040–1059.

Meibach, R. C., and Siegel, A. (1977). *Brain Res.* **119**, 1–20.

Meisel, R. L., Lumia, A. R., and Sachs, B. D. (1982). *Exp. Neurol.* **77**, 612–624.

Meredith, M. (1980). *In* "Chemical Signals in Vertebrates and Aquatic Invertebrates" (D. Müller-Schwarze and R. M. Silverstein, eds.), pp. 303–326. Plenum, New York.

Meredith, M. (1982). *In* "Olfaction and Endocrine Regulation" (W. Breipohl, ed.), pp. 223–236. IRL, London.

Meredith, M., and Marques, D. M. (1981). *Abstr. Assoc. Chemorecept. Sci Meeting 1981,* p. 18.

Meredith, M., and O'Connell, R. J. (1979). *J. Physiol. (London)* **286**, 301–316.

Meredith, M., Marques, D. M., O'Connell, R. J., and Stern, F. L. (1980a). *Science* **207**, 1224–1226.

Meredith, M., Marques, D. M., Stern, F. L., O'Connell, R. J., and Davis, B. J. (1980b). *Abstr. Assoc. Chemorecept. Sci Meeting 1980,* p. 27.

Miller, I. J. (1982). *Chemical Senses* **7**, 99–108.

Miller, I. J., and Porcelli, L. J. (1976). *Anat. Rec.* **184**, 480.

Moss, R. L. (1979). *Annu. Rev. Physiol.* **41**, 617–31.

Moss, R. L., Dudley, C. A., Foreman, M. M., and McCann, S. M. (1975). *In* "Hypothalamic Hormones" (M. Motta, P. G. Crosignani, and L. Martini, eds.), pp. 269–278. Academic Press, New York.

Moulton, D. G. (1976). *Physiol. Rev.* **56**, 578–593.

Moulton, D. G. (1978). *In* "Handbook of Behavioral Neurobiology: Sensory Integration" (R. B. Masterton, ed.), Vol. 1, pp. 91–118. Plenum, New York.

Moulton, D. G., and Beidler, L. M. (1967). *Physiol. Rev.* **47**, 1–52.

Mozell, M. M., and Jagadowicz, M. (1973). *Science* **181**, 1247–1249.

Murphy, M. R. (1976) *In* "Mammalian Olfaction Reproductive Processes and Behavior" (R. L. Doty, ed.), pp. 96–118. Academic Press, New York.

Murphy, M. R. (1980). *Behav. Neural Biol.* **30**, 323–340.

Münz, H., Claas, B., Stumpf, W. E., and Jennes, L. (1982). *Cell Tiss. Res.* **222**, 313–323.

Negro-Villar, A., and Ojeda, S. R. (1981). *Int. Rev. Physiol.* **24**, 47–155.

Negus, V. (1958). "Comparative Anatomy of the Nose and Paranasal Sinuses." Livingston, Edinburgh.

Niell, J. D., Freeman, M. C., and Tilson, S. A. (1971). *Endocrinology* **89**, 1453–1468.

Norgren, R. (1977a). *In* Chemical Signals in Vertebrates" (D. Müller-Schwarze and M. M. Mozell, eds.), pp. 515–530. Plenum, New York.

Norgren, R. (1977b). *Proc. Int. Symp. Olfaction Taste, 6th, 1976* pp. 225–232.

Pager, J. (1974). *Physiol. Behav.* **13,** 523–526.

Panhuber, H. (1982). *Physiol. Behav* **28,** 149–155.

Parks, A. S., and Bruce, H. M. (1961). *Science* **134,** 1049–1054.

Paxinos, G. (1976). *Physiol. Behav.* **17,** 81–88.

Pearson, A. A. (1941). *J. Comp. Neurol.* **75,** 39–66.

Pfaff, D. W. (1980). "Estrogens and Brain Function." Springer-Verlag, Berlin and New York.

Pfaff, D. W., and Gregory, E. (1971). *J. Neurophysiol.* **34,** 208–216.

Phillips, H. S., Hostetter, G., Kerdelhue, B., and Kozlowski, G. P. (1980). *Brain Res.* **193,** 574–579.

Poulain, P., and Carette, B. (1978). *Brain Res.* **137,** 154–157.

Powers, J. B., and Winans, S. S. (1973). *Physiol. Behav.* **10,** 361–368.

Powers, J. B., and Winans, S. S. (1975). *Science* **187,** 961–963.

Powers, J. B., Fields R. B., and Winans, S. S. (1979) *Physiol Behav.* **22,** 77–84.

Powers, J. B., Bergondy, M., and Bopeley, L. (1981). *Neurosci. Abstr.* **7,** 663.

Price, J. L. (1973). *J. Comp. Neurol.* **150,** 87–108.

Proshansky, E., Kauer, J. S., Stewart, W. B., and Egger, M. D. (1980). *J. Comp. Neurol.* **194,** 505–517.

Raisman, G., and Field, P. M. (1973). *Brain Res.* **54,** 1–29.

Ranck, J. B. (1975). *Brain Res.* **98,** 417–440.

Reese, R. S., and Brightman, V. (1970). *In* "Taste and Smell in Vertebrates" (G. E. W. Wolstenholme and J. Knight, eds.), pp. 115–142. Churchill, London.

Regnier, F. E., and Goodwin, M. (1977). *In* "Chemical Signals in Vertebrates" (D. Müller-Schwarze and M. M. Mozell, eds.), pp. 115–134. Plenum, New York.

Reynolds, J., and Keverne, E. B. (1979). *J. Reprod. Fertil.* **57,** 31–35.

Ryan, E. L., and Frankel, A. I. (1978). *Biol. Reprod.* **19,** 971–983.

Sakar, D. K., Chiappa, S. A., Fink, G., and Sherwood, N. M. (1976). *Nature (London)* **264,** 461–463.

Samson, W. K., McCann, S. M., Chud, L., Dudley, C. A., and Moss, R. L. (1980). *Neuroendocrinology* **31,** 66–72.

Sanchez-Criado, J. E. (1979). *Rev. Esp. Fisiol.* **35,** 137–142.

Sanchez-Criado, J. E. (1982). *In* "Olfaction and Endocrine Regulation" (W. Breipohl, ed.), 1982 pp. 209–221. IRL, London.

Sanchez-Criado, J. R., and Gallego, A. (1979). *Acta Endocrinol. (Copenhagen), Suppl.* **225,** 255.

Sapolsky, R. M., and Eichenbaum, H. (1980). *Brain Behav. Evol.* **17,** 276–290.

Sato, N., Haller, E. W., Powell, R. D., and Henkin, R. I. (1974). *J. Reprod. Fertil.* **36,** 301–309.

Scalia, F., and Winans, S. S. (1970). *Science* **170,** 330–332.

Scalia, F., and Winans, S. S. (1975). *J. Comp. Neural.* **161,** 31–56.

Schoots, A. F. M., Crusio, W. E., and Van Abeelen, J. H. F. (1978). *Physiol. Behav.* **21,** 779–784.

Schwanzel-Fukuda, M., and Silverman, A. J. (1980). *J. Comp. Neurol.* **191,** 213–225.

Setalo, G., Vigh, S., Schally, A. V., Arimura, A., and Flerko, B. (1976). *Brain Res.* **103,** 597–602.

Shepherd, G. M. (1972). *Physiol. Rev.* **52,** 864–917.

Shepherd, G. M. (1974). "The Synaptic Organization of the Brain." Oxford Univ. Press, London and New York.

Silver, W. L., and Maruniak, J. A. (1982). *Chem. Senses* **6,** 295–305.

Silver, W. L., and Moulton, D. G. (1982). *Physiol. Behav.* **28,** 927–931.

Silverman, A. J., and Krey, L. C. (1978a). *Brain Res.* **157,** 233–246.

Silverman, A. J., and Krey, L. C. (1978b). *Brain Res.* **157**, 255–267.

Singer, A. G., Agosta, W. C., O'Conell, R. J., Pfaffman, C., Bowen, D. V., and Field, F. H. (1976). *Science* **191**, 948–950.

Singer, A. G., Macrides, F., and Agosta, W. C. (1980). *In* "Chemical Signals in Vertebrates and Aquatic Invertebrates" (D. Müller-Schwarze and R. M. Silverstein, eds.), pp. 365–375. Plenum, New York.

Singh, P. J., Tucker, A. M., and Hofer, M. A. (1976). *Physiol. Behav.* **17**, 373–382.

Singh, P. J., Menaker, S., and Hofer, M. A. (1977). *Neurosci. Abstr.* **3**, 83.

Skeen, L. C. (1977). *Brain Res.* **124**, 147–153.

Slotnik, B. M. (1979). *Science* **203**, 1139–1140.

Slotnik, B. M., and Berman, E. J. (1980). *Brain Res. Bull.* **5**, 141–145.

Slotnik, B. M., and Guttman, L. A. (1977). *J. Comp. Physiol.* **91**, 942–950.

Smith, M. S. (1980). *Int. Rev. Physiol.* **22**, 207–276.

Stewart, W. B., Kauer, J. S., and Shepherd, G. M. (1979). *J. Comp. Neurol.* **185**, 715–734.

Stone, H., Williams, B., and Carregal, E. J. A. (1968). *Exp. Neurol.* **21**, 11–19.

Swanson, L. W., and Cowan, W. M. (1979). *J. Comp. Neurol.* **186**, 621–656.

Takagi, S. F. (1982). *Chem. Senses* **6**, 329–334.

Tanabe, T., Yarita, H., Iino, M., Ooshima, Y., and Takagi, S. F. (1975a). *J. Neurophysiol.* **38**, 1269–1283.

Tanabe, T., Iino, M. and Takagi, S. F. (1975b). *J. Neurophysiol.* **38**, 1284–1296.

Teicher, M. H., Stewart, W. B., Kauer, J. S., and Shepherd, G. M. (1980). *Brain Res.* **194**, 530–535.

Teresawa, E., Kawakami, M., and Sawyer, C. H. (1969). *Proc. Soc. Exp. Biol. Med.* **132**, 497–501.

Todd, J. H., Atema, J., and Bardach, J. E. (1967). *Science* **158**, 672–673.

Tucker, D. (1963a). *In* "Olfaction and Taste" (Y. Zotterman, ed.), pp. 45–69. Pergamon, Oxford.

Tucker, D. (1963b). *J. Gen. Physiol.* **46**, 453–489.

Tucker, D. (1971). *In* "Handbook of Sensory Physiology" (L. M. Beidler, ed.), Vol. 4, Part 1, pp. 151–181. Springer-Verlag, Berlin and New York.

Vaccarezza, O. L., Requero, M., Berra, M., and Tramezzani, J. H. (1979). *Acta Physiol. Latinoam.* **29**, 95–99.

Van Buskirk, R. L., and Erickson, R. P. (1977). *Brain Res.* **135**, 287–305.

Vandenbergh, J. G. (1973). *Physiol. Behav.* **10**, 257–261.

Vandenbergh, J. G. (1976). *J. Reprod. Fertil.* **46**, 451–453.

Vandenbergh, J. G. (1980). *In* "Chemical Signals in Vertebrates and Aquatic Invertebrates" (D. Müller-Schwarze and R. M. Silverstein, eds.), pp. 229–242. Plenum, New York.

Vandenbergh, J. G., Whitsett, J. M., and Lombardi, J. R. (1975). *J. Reprod. Fertil.* **43**, 515–523.

Velasco, M. E., and Talesnik, S. (1969). *Endocrinology* **84**, 132–139.

Verberne, G. (1976). *Z. Tierpsychol.* **42**, 113–128.

Verberne, G., Ruardy, L., and Nijenhuis, E. D. (1981). *Vakbl. Biol.* **4**, 74–79.

Whitten, W. K. (1959). *J. Endocrinol.* **18**, 102–104.

Whitten, W. K. (1963). *Asia Oceania Congr. Endocrinol., 2nd, 1963* Sydney Australia 11 A.04 (quoted by Kaneko *et al.,* 1980).

Whitten, W. K., and Champlin, A. K. (1973). *In* "Handbook of Physiology" (R. O. Greep, ed.), Sect. 7, Vol. II, pp. 109–123. Am. Physiol. Soc., Washington, D.C.

Wilson, E. O., and Bossert, W. H. (1963). *Recent Prog. Horm. Res.* **19**, 673–711.

Wilson, M. C., Beamer, W. G., and Whitten, W. K. (1980). *Biol. Reprod.* **22**, 864–872.

Winans, S. S. (1982). *In* "Olfaction and Endocrine Regulation" (W. Breipohl, ed.), pp. 23–34. IRL, London.

Winans, S. S., and Powers, J. B. (1977). *Brain Res.* **126,** 325–344.

Wysocki, C. J. (1979). *Neurosci. Biobehav. Rev.* **3,** 301–341.

Wysocki, C. J. (1982). *In* "Olfaction and Endocrine Regulation" (W. Breipohl, ed.), pp. 195–208. IRL, London.

Wysocki, C. J., Wellington, J. L., and Beauchamp, G. K. (1980). *Science* **207,** 781–783.

Wysocki, C. J., Nyby, J., Whitney, G., Beauchamp, G. K., and Katz, Y. (1982). *Physiol. Behav.* **29,** 315–327.

Yamazaki, K., Yamaguchi, M., Boyse, E. A., and Thomas, L. (1980). *In* "Chemical Signals in Vertebrates and Aquatic Invertebrates" (D. Müller-Schwarze and R. M. Silverstein, eds.), pp. 267–274, Plenum, New York.

9

Pheromones and Reproduction in Domestic Animals

M. K. Izard

Department of Zoology
North Carolina State University
Raleigh, North Carolina

I. INTRODUCTION

Animals communicate information concerning reproduction to conspecifics in order to coordinate reproductive activities. Chemical communication with pheromones is one means of transmitting such information.

The term "pheromone" was proposed by Karlson and Butenandt (1959) to designate substances that are secreted externally by an animal and cause a specific reaction in a receiving individual of the same species; the reaction involves either the release of a specific behavior or a physiological change in the recipient's endocrine or reproductive system. These pheromones are thought to exert their effects either orally or through olfaction (Karlson and Butenandt, 1959; Karlson and Luscher, 1959). The concept of pheromonal

253

PHEROMONES AND REPRODUCTION IN MAMMALS
Copyright © 1983 by Academic Press, Inc.
All rights of reproduction in any form reserved.
ISBN 0-12-710780-0

communication presented by Karlson and Butenandt (1959) was originally applied to insects because the field of mammalian chemical communication was relatively new at that time.

Wilson and Bossert (1963) provided a useful classification of pheromones, again based on pheromonal communication in insects, which employed Karlson and Butenandt's original distinction between two end points: either an immediate behavioral response or a change in the endocrine or reproductive system of the recipient. Releasing pheromones were defined as pheromones that cause an immediate but reversible change in behavior, invoking a classical stimulus–response paradigm mediated by the central nervous system. Priming pheromones were defined as pheromones that initiate a chain of physiological events, either through inhibition or stimulation, in which endocrine, reproductive, and possibly other systems could be altered.

As it became increasingly clear that pheromonal communication played an important role in mammalian behavior and reproductive processes, it also became clear that Wilson and Bossert's concept of releasing pheromones could not appropriately be used with respect to mammalian behavioral responses to pheromones. The rigidity of response implied by the term "releasing pheromone" did not necessarily occur in mammals with their more flexible behavior patterns (Bronson, 1968). In place of "releasing pheromone," Bronson (1968) suggested that the term "signalling pheromone" be used to denote mammalian pheromones that evoke a behavioral response, because a signal implies only the transfer of information and not the nature of the response. In mammals, signalling and priming pheromones are thought to act through olfaction to stimulate responses in recipient animals.

Due to the flexibility of mammalian behavior and its dependence on a number of factors, including hormonal status, learning, and experience, a behavioral response to a mammalian olfactory signal may be less obvious or less well defined than an insect's behavioral response to a pheromone. In addition, a behavioral or physiological response in a particular context may be dependent not only on olfactory cues, but on tactile, visual, or auditory cues or a combination thereof. Beauchamp *et al.* (1976) suggested that the uncritical use of the term "pheromone" gives rise to misconceptions in the interpretation of mammalian behavioral research. Since the challenge of Beauchamp *et al.* (1976) concerning the applicability of the pheromone concept to mammals, a number of authors have been reluctant to use the term "pheromone" and prefer to substitute other phrases to denote mammalian olfactory communication.

While recognizing the problems inherent in applying to mammals a concept originally applied to insects and appreciating the concerns of Beauchamp *et al.* (1976), I continue to use the term "signalling pheromone" to denote an olfactory cue that transfers specific information and consequently elicits a specific behavior and "priming pheromone" to denote an olfactory cue that elicits a measurable physiological response.

Both signalling and priming pheromones have been shown to play important roles in the communication of information pertaining to reproduction in rodents (see Bronson, 1971; Vandenbergh, 1975; Milligan, 1980; and chapters in this volume). Until recently, however, research designed to investigate the involvement of pheromones in the reproduction of domestic animals was limited. Nonetheless, judging by the number of journal articles on the subject that have appeared in the past 5 years, interest in pheromonal communication in the reproduction of domestic animals is increasing. This surge of interest has a practical basis, because the success of livestock operations is to a large extent dependent on efficient reproduction. Pheromones have an unrealized potential for improving reproductive efficiency in livestock operations.

In this chapter I discuss signalling and priming pheromones as they relate to reproduction in domestic farm animals, particularly cattle, swine, sheep, and goats. The evidence implicating signalling and priming pheromones in communication between conspecifics is reviewed. In addition, I will discuss instances in which pheromones are being used, or have the potential for being used, to improve reproduction in livestock operations.

II. SIGNALLING PHEROMONES

A. Signalling Pheromones Produced by Females

Olfactory cues that transmit specific information and result in specific and immediate behavioral responses in the male appear to be produced in the urine or vaginal secretions of females of many species. These odors are present at estrus or proestrus, but not at any other time. The male, through investigation of the female's urine and anogenital region, can use these olfactory cues to determine the stage of the female's estrous cycle. These signalling pheromones may have more than one behavioral function, in that they can serve as attractants and/or inducers of sexual activity.

Males of a number of ungulates routinely investigate the anogenital region or urine of females (Grau, 1976). Among the domestic ungulates, such investigatory behavior is seen in horses (Waring *et al.,* 1975), sheep (Banks, 1964; Lindsay, 1965), goats (Shank, 1972; Ladewig *et al.,* 1980), and domestic cattle (Hafez and Bouissou, 1975). The components of anogenital investigation include sniffing, licking, and nuzzling of the anogenital region. These behaviors often elicit urination from the female under investigation. The male then puts his nose and mouth directly in the stream of urine or sniffs and licks the urine-soaked substrate. A behavior known as flehmen frequently follows, with the male showing the typical flehmen posture of raised head with open mouth and curled upper lip.

Flehmen is found in many ungulate species, the pig being a notable exception (Estes, 1972), and can be seen in both males and females in response to several odors (Estes, 1972; Grau, 1976). It is most commonly shown by the male after contact with female urine or the anogenital region. It is thought to be related to the functioning of the vomeronasal organ (VNO), a bilateral blind sac, which in cattle, sheep, and goats opens into the incisive duct (also called the nasopalatine canal) (Estes, 1972). The VNO has been implicated as a specialized chemoreceptor involved in the detection of estrus and in the release, control, and coordination of sexual activity (Estes, 1972; see also Chapter 8). It is thought to contain receptors for low-volatile pheromones in urine and vaginal secretions (Johns, 1980; Wysocki, 1979).

Several studies of domestic animals suggest a relationship among flehmen, the VNO, and signalling pheromones produced by the female. Ladewig and Hart (1980) followed the path of a tracer dye (sodium fluorescein) from the oral cavity into the VNO during flehmen in male goats. After introduction of the dye into the oral cavity, the goats were presented with urine samples to induce flehmen behavior. The maxilla were removed, frozen, and sectioned after the goats were injected with an anesthetic overdose. Only in subjects performing flehmen was the dye seen in the posterior two-thirds of the VNO, where the sensory epithelium is located (Ladewig and Hart, 1980). Ladewig and Hart (1980) concluded from these results that if the dye represented behaviorally significant olfactory cues taken into the mouth by the goats during investigation of urine, only the subjects displaying flehmen would have detected the cues. Therefore, flehmen appears to function in the transport of nonvolatile olfactory signals from the oral cavity to the sensory epithelium of the VNO.

In other experiments Ladewig et al. (1980) found that flehmen in male goats occurred more frequently in response to urine from diestrous as opposed to estrous does. Ladewig et al. (1980) concluded that the goats had already distinguished between the estrous and nonestrous samples by regular olfactory perception prior to flehmen and that flehmen and the VNO were used to confirm or refine information already received. For example, the detection of proestrus may require the more refined chemoreception afforded by the VNO.

During mating tests with restrained stimulus animals, flehmen in test subjects was most often seen after mounting or copulation, suggesting that another function of VNO stimulation through olfactory stimuli may be to maintain and stimulate sexual activity (Ladewig *et al.*, 1980). Olfactory bulbectomy eliminated flehmen behavior, although occlusion of the nasopalatine canal at the oral opening did not reduce the frequency of flehmen in the goats (Ladewig *et al.*, 1980). It was suggested that flehmen behavior after occlusion of the nasopalatine canal may have represented the continuation of a species-specific behavior pattern in the absence of sensory input. An alternative explanation proposed by Ladewig *et al.* (1980) is that chemical stimuli may have dissolved in the nasal cavity and entered the VNO through the unblocked end of the nasopalatine canal.

The former explanation is more likely to be correct, because in bulls the number of flehmen responses is not reduced even if the nasopalatine canal is completely plugged so that the nasal as well as the oral opening is occluded (McGrath, 1981). The work of McGrath (1981) and Jacobs *et al.* (1980) has shown that a bull may identify and direct his attention to receptive cows on the basis of information contained in reproductive tract fluids. McGrath (1981) collected data on flehmen responses in bulls before and after occlusion of the nasopalatine canal. Although the number of flehmen responses did not change, the duration of individual acts of flehmen increased after occlusion. These results were independent of the estrous status of stimulus cows. Far fewer services were performed on both receptive and non-receptive cows if the nasopalatine canal was plugged. More services were performed on estrous cows than nonestrous cows both before and after plugging of the nasopalatine canal, indicating that detection of estrous status was unimpaired by blocking the access of substances to the VNO and must therefore be possible by using the main olfactory system. The tongue compression strokes described by Jacobs *et al.* (1980) decreased in number but not duration after plugging of the nasopalatine canal (McGrath, 1981). Jacobs *et al.* (1980) have suggested that pressure applied to the palate during a tongue compression stroke may cause intermittent suction in the VNO, permitting the entrance of substances from the oral or nasal cavity.

There has been controversy concerning the role of olfaction in the detection of estrus in the bovine. In 1946 Hart *et al.* reported that urine and vaginal mucus of estrous cows, when rubbed on the vaginal membranes of nonestrous cows, attracted and stimulated bulls through olfaction. Almquist and Hale (1956), noting that bulls being ejaculated for semen responded to teasers of either sex equally, concluded that sex-related odors were associated with sexual excitation at best secondarily. Hale (1966) went on to demonstrate that blinded bulls had a reduced probability of identifying sexual situations and initiating sexual responses when restrained teasers were presented. He concluded that vision played an important role in the immediate and direct control of certain aspects of sexual behavior, whereas olfactory stimuli had not been demonstrated to play such a role.

Donavan (1967) showed that feces of estrous cows were attractive to bulls and ruled out the possibility of any other secretions or excretions having attractive properties.

The inconsistencies seen in these early studies of olfaction in the bovine probably stem from the fact that the bull can use a combination of factors associated with the female to determine if she is receptive, including visual, tactile, auditory, and olfactory stimuli. In addition, bulls that are routinely used for the collection of semen for artificial insemination (AI) often become conditioned to the collection procedure and will mount teaser animals of either sex (Hale, 1966).

Recent work indicates that odors probably play a significant role in signalling the reproductive state of cows. Paleologou (1977) demonstrated that a volatile odor in the cervicovaginal mucus of estrous cows is a source of sexual attraction for bulls. When placed in glass dishes and presented to a bull, cervicovaginal mucus elicited sniffing. No interest was shown in mucus from metestrous or diestrous cows. When cervicovaginal mucus from estrous cows was applied to a dummy, bulls mounted the dummy but did not mount a dummy smeared with mucus from metestrous and diestrous cows. Urine from estrous cows also stimulated sexual activity in bulls when applied to nonestrous cows (Sambraus and Waring, 1975).

Vaginal secretions have been shown to have pheromonal properties in many species (Adams, 1980; see also Chapters 1 and 3). The production of vaginal pheromones in primates appears to depend on interactions between vaginal bacteria and the vaginal secretions controlled by ovarian hormones (Keverne, 1974). The concentrations of volatile fatty acids in vaginal secretions of cows are elevated on the day before estrus and fall sharply thereafter (Hradecký, 1978). These changes in the concentrations of volatile fatty acids show signs of being secondary manifestations of hormonal changes in the cow mediated by the vaginal microflora. Changes in concentrations of volatile fatty acids may be the basis for the bull's determination of estrous status in cows.

It may be possible to use olfactory cues emitted by estrous cows as the basis for a system for detecting estrus. In the dairy industry, cows are routinely bred by AI. Detection of estrus and correct timing of AI in relationship to estrus are necessary to obtain satisfactory conception rates. However, a basic problem facing producers is the failure to detect estrus. In most dairy operations, the detection of estrus is only about 50% effective (Williamson *et al.,* 1972; Esslemont, 1974). This problem has become more serious as herd sizes have increased and man-hours per cow have decreased (Hodgson, 1973; Esslemont, 1974). Difficulties in detecting estrus have also hindered the use of AI in the beef industry, thereby limiting the rapid selection and genetic progress that has occurred as a result of the use of AI in the dairy industry.

One approach to this problem may be to use the olfactory abilities of other species to detect estrus in cows. Both dogs and rats can be trained to discriminate between urine samples from estrous and diestrous cows by olfactory means (Kiddy *et al.,* 1978; Ladewig and Hart, 1981). Dogs are also able to detect estrus-related odors in vaginal secretions and milk (Kiddy *et al.,* 1978, 1980; Kiddy and Mitchell, 1981). The results of these studies using rats and dogs indicate that there are changes in the concentration of a detectable odor or odors that are correlated with changes in the behavioral and presumably hormonal status of the cow. At present, it is uncertain whether dogs and rats use the same olfactory cues that would be used by a bull to determine when a cow is approaching estrus or is in estrus.

As determined by trained dogs, estrus-related odors begin to appear slowly during the 3 days before estrus and reach a peak in intensity on the day of estrus (Kiddy and Mitchell, 1981). However, rats cannot discriminate between urine samples collected on the day of estrus and those collected 1 day before estrus, although they can discriminate between samples collected 2 days before estrus and those collected on the day of estrus (Ladewig and Hart, 1981).

The work of these researchers has important implications, because in the future it may be possible to develop practical methods of using dogs or rats to detect estrus for herdsmen in both the beef and dairy industries. It is also possible that the response of dogs or rats could be used as a bioassay for the odors related to estrus. This would permit the identification of the compounds involved and might lead to the development of biochemical approaches to the detection of estrus.

Studies with sheep have shown that the means by which rams detect ewes in estrus probably involves olfactory cues. Flehmen in rams is most frequently seen when they are investigating proestrous ewes (Tompkins and Bryant, 1974). Kelley (1937) found that rams could detect estrus by an odor found in vaginal secretions. He was able to confuse rams by rubbing vaginal secretions of estrous ewes onto the vulva of nonestrous ewes. However, Banks *et al.* (1963) found no decrement in the ability of rams to select estrous ewes when anosmia was induced by intranasal zylocaine. Anosmia induced by olfactory bulb removal gave different results. Lindsay (1965) found that, whereas normal rams could discriminate between estrous and nonestrous ewes and preferentially approached estrous ewes, bulbectomized rams approached both categories of ewes at random. They subsequently determined which ewes were in heat by attempting to mount. Successful copulation occurred if ewes did not move away. The incidence of the precopulatory behaviors of sniffing and licking the vulva was decreased in these bulbectomized rams.

Fletcher and Lindsay (1968) tested the ability of intact, deaf, anosmic (after bilateral olfactory ablation), and blindfolded rams to mate with tethered and free estrous ewes. Both blindfolded and anosmic rams showed a reduced level of sexual activity. This could be attributed to an impaired ability to seek out the tethered estrous ewes. Although the ability of the anosmic rams to discriminate between estrous and nonestrous ewes was impaired, there was no effect on actual copulation with untethered ewes.

It has been remarked that boars do not appear to discriminate between estrous and diestrous sows. In fact, both are actively pursued (Signoret, 1970). In a T maze, boars are only slightly more attracted by estrous sows than by nonestrous sows (Signoret, 1970). However, olfactory cues can probably play a role in enhancing copulatory behavior in the boar. Placing mucus from the vulva of an estrous sow on a dummy will sometimes induce a reluctant boar to mount (Booth, 1980a).

Improving libido in males having semen collected for AI might be one means by which signalling pheromones that stimulate sexual activity could be practically applied. These pheromones might also be useful in facilitating the training of young males to mount dummies, which are often used in semen collection procedures.

Undoubtedly, a female presents a combination of olfactory, visual, tactile, and auditory cues, all of which a male has at his disposal to use in determining whether the female is in estrus or will soon be in estrus. The preceding discussion suggests, however, that signalling pheromones alone can suffice for discriminating between estrous and nonestrous females. Furthermore, it appears that signalling pheromones can stimulate and promote copulatory behavior in males.

B. Signalling Pheromones Produced by Males

What about females? Can olfactory stimuli from males play a role in attracting and stimulating sexual behavior in females? Although very little work has been done on the attraction of females by males, it does appear that males emit a sex attractant which estrous females can detect and respond to.

Estrous sows, given a choice in a T maze between intact boars and castrated males, will spend more time in the proximity of the intact boar (Signoret, 1972). The hormonal state of the sow is important, since anestrous sows divide their time equally between intact males and castrated males. An examination of the sensory stimuli used by estrous sows to discriminate between intact and castrated males made it possible to eliminate auditory and visual cues from the boar as relevant factors involved in discrimination. After removal of the olfactory bulbs, estrous sows were unable to discriminate between a male and a female on the basis of sight and hearing alone (Signoret, 1974). These observations suggest that boars emit an odor, or signalling pheromone, that attracts estrous sows.

A testosterone-treated sow attracts an estrous sow as effectively as a boar (Signoret, 1972), suggesting that the sex attractant emitted by males is androgen dependent. Signoret (1976) suggested that odoriferous steroids secreted by boars may be sex attractants, but this possibility has not been confirmed.

Rams also appear to attract estrous ewes. An estrous ewe will seek out a ram over a long distance (Inkster, 1957; Lindsay and Robinson, 1961; Hulet *et al.*, 1962). In one study rams were tethered so that mating depended on the ewes' ability to seek out the rams. At the end of a 52-day breeding period, 66% of ewes were bred by a tethered ram, compared with an 84% breeding rate if rams were free (Inkster, 1957). Similar results were seen by Lindsay and Robinson (1961). Fletcher and Lindsay (1968) showed that bulbectomized ewes had a decreased ability to compete for the attention of tethered rams, resulting in a decrease in the number of bulbectomized ewes that actually mated when compared to controls. These observations suggest that rams emit an odor, or signalling pheromone, that attracts estrous females. No compounds that are responsible for attraction of the female have yet been identified.

The chemical composition of a signalling pheromone produced by boars that stimulates sexual activity in sows has been identified. This signalling pheromone elicits the immobilization response in estrous sows, a behavior shown by most estrous sows when confronted with a mature boar (Signoret, 1970). During the immobilization response or standing reaction, a receptive sow stands immobile, with arched back and cocked ears, allowing the boar to mount and copulate. This stance can also be elicited by a human using the back pressure test (Altmann, 1941). An estrous sow will stand immobile when a human sits astride her, and she will actively resist forward pressure (Signoret, 1976). This reaction can be used as an aid in the detection of estrus. However, only 50% of estrous sows show the immobilization response in the absence of a boar. Olfactory, auditory, and visual stimuli from a boar can increase the response of estrous sows to the back pressure test (Signoret and du Mesnil du Buisson, 1961). Olfactory stimuli in particular appear to be the most important, accounting for a 60% increase in positive responses in sows previously negative to the back pressure test in the absence of a boar (Signoret and du Mesnil du Buisson, 1961), although auditory cues are almost as effective.

Warmed preputial fluid from boars was found to be as effective as whole male odor (Signoret, 1970) in eliciting the immobilization response. Preputial fluid consists of urine and secretions of the male reproductive tract that collect in the preputial diverticulum of boars (Booth, 1980a). Patterson (1966, 1968) identified some of the volatile compounds in boar preputial fluid, including several phenols, aliphatic acids, and aromatic acids. None of these compounds alone elicited the immobilization response in estrous sows. Patterson (1968) also found trace amounts of 5α-androst-16 en-3-one (5α-androstenone) in the preputial fluid. 5α-androstenone and its alcohol, 3α-hydroxy-5α-androst-16-ene (3α-androstenol) are members of a major group of testicular steroids in the boar, which include the compounds responsible for boar taint (Booth, 1980a). Although 5α-androstenone and 3α-androstenol originate in the testis, *in vitro* and *in vivo* studies have demonstrated that androgens are not their precursors (Gower, 1972; Booth, 1980b). Both of these compounds accumulate in high concentrations in the submaxillary salivary glands of boars (Patterson, 1968; Booth, 1975) and are also found in the saliva, fat, and sweat glands (Stinson and Patterson, 1972).

Perry *et al.* (1980) presented evidence that the submaxillary salivary gland of the boar and its secretions are essential for normal estrous behavior in gilts. The effect of boars with and without submaxillary salivary glands on the estrous behavior of gilts was examined. Gilts exposed to a boar without submaxillary salivary glands did not show estrous behavior as early and did not show as great a peak of estrous behavior as gilts exposed to boars with intact salivary glands. These observations suggest that substances released from the submaxillary salivary glands play a positive role in synchronizing and promoting reproductive behavior. These substances are probably the 19-carbon androgen steroids that accumulate in the submaxillary salivary gland.

Melrose *et al.* (1971) demonstrated that aerosol preparations containing 5α-androstenone or 3α-androstenol could be used to induce the immobilization response in estrous sows not responsive to the back pressure test in the absence of a boar. The advantages of such a preparation when used for the detection of estrus in pigs before AI was realized, and an aerosol preparation containing 5α-androstenone is now marketed commercially as Boar Mate (Antec. A. H. International, Ltd.). It is the only mammalian pheromone to be synthesized and sold as a means of improving reproductive efficiency in livestock operations.

Melrose *et al.* (1971) also demonstrated that a mixture of preputial fluid and urine could induce the immobilization response in estrous sows previously negative to the back pressure test. From a practical standpoint, the use of the synthetic signalling pheromone is preferable, because aerosol preparations eliminate the possibility of disease transmission.

In the study of Melrose *et al.* (1971), estrous sows reacted equally well to 5α-androstenone and 3α-androstenol. The alcohol may be the active compound, because the ketone is readily metabolized *in vitro* by sow epithelial tissue to androstenol with a 75% yield (Gennings *et al.*, 1977). On the other hand, high-affinity binding receptors for both 5α-androstenol and 3α-androstenone have been isolated from the olfactory but not the respiratory mucosa of sows (Gennings *et al.*, 1977). In addition, unit activity of neurons in the mitral cell layer of the porcine olfactory bulb is altered by olfactory presentation of 5α-androstenone (MaCleod *et al.*, 1979). This work may lead to insight into how external steroids influence the brain.

For domestic animals, in most cases the chemical characteristics of signalling pheromones and the metabolic pathways by which they are produced are unclear. Little is known about the way in which the production of signalling pheromones is influenced by hormonal status. In some cases, the site of production of signalling pheromones is unknown. More information is needed in these areas in order to facilitate the practical use of signalling pheromones in improving the reproduction of domestic animals.

III. PRIMING PHEROMONES

Chemical stimuli that have physiological effects, the priming pheromones, have been shown to be involved in the reproduction of mammals, especially rodents. In domestic mammals, priming pheromones from the male have an influence on the induction of puberty, the termination of seasonal anestrus, and the shortening of postpartum anestrus. Each of these effects involves the termination of an anestrous state in the female by chemical signals from the male. Recently, priming pheromones from females have been shown to affect ovarian activity in other females. Table I summarizes the reproductive phenomena that are known to be affected by priming pheromones and the probable sources of these pheromones.

A. Priming Pheromones and Puberty

In a number of rodents the presence of a male has been shown to hasten the onset of puberty in females (Vandenbergh, 1969; see also Chapter 4). In mice, an androgen-dependent priming pheromone in the urine of adult males is responsible for this effect (Colby and Vandenbergh, 1971; Lombardi *et al.*, 1976). If young female mice with advanced onset of puberty are mated, they adjust physiologically to pregnancy and retain the accelerated growth seen in nonpregnant females of the same age (Eisen and Leatherwood, 1976). Among domestic animals the effect of the male on

TABLE I

Sources of Priming Pheromones in Domestic Animals

Function	Species	Source	References
Acceleration of puberty	Pig	Submaxillary salivary gland?	Kirkwood and Hughes (1980), Kirkwood *et al.* (1981)
	Cow	Bull urine	Izard (1981), Izard and Vandenbergh (1982a)
Termination of seasonal anestrus and synchroniza-tion of estrus	Sheep	Wool and wax, possibly urine	Knight and Lynch (1980)
	Goat	Urine? Mohair?	Shelton and Morrow (1965), Shelton (1980)
Shortening of postpartum anestrus	Pig	5α-Androstenone from sub-maxillary salivary gland	Hillyer (1976)
Synchronization of estrus	Cow	Cervical mucus	Izard (1981), Izard and Vandenbergh (1982b)

puberty in young females has been examined in both the pig and the cow. For both of these species evidence has accumulated showing that puberty in the female can be affected by priming pheromones from the male.

Many factors influence the age at puberty in gilts, including transport, type of housing, breed, season of year during sexual maturation, and social environment (Bourn *et al.*, 1974; Mavrogenis and Robison, 1976; Christenson, 1981). Perhaps the most effective of these factors is the social environment, in particular the presence of a boar. The presence of a boar can accelerate puberty in gilts by about 1 month (Brooks and Cole, 1970). Furthermore, if boars are introduced to gilts at about 190 days of age (the approximate mean age of puberty), a marked synchrony in attainment of the pubertal estrus occurs (Brooks and Cole, 1970).

The age of the gilt at exposure to the boar has an influence on the interval from first boar contact to puberty, as well as on the degree of synchronization of the pubertal estrus (Hughes and Cole, 1976; Kirkwood and Hughes, 1979). Kirkwood and Hughes (1979) exposed nine groups of gilts to 30 min of daily boar contact beginning at different ages and measured factors associated with puberty. Optimization of the age at puberty, the interval from the onset of boar introduction to puberty, and the degree of synchronization of pubertal estrus occurred when the boar was introduced between 160 and 170 days of age. Gilts reached puberty the earliest (166 days of age) when boar exposure began at 139 days of age. When boar exposure began at earlier ages (125 or 132 days of age), the age at puberty was increased, as was the interval from first contact with the boar to puberty. If boars are introduced to gilts at very young ages (90–120 days of age), a delayed and variable response to the boar's presence is seen (Brooks and

Cole, 1969). Presumably, at very young ages, when gilts are physiologically incapable of responding to the stimulus of the boar, conditioning or habituation to his presence occurs, so that later responses to the boar are attenuated (Brooks and Cole, 1969).

Although the sensory cues involved in the boar's effect on puberty were thought to be olfactory cues (Signoret, 1970, 1976), it was not until recently that studies were conducted to examine directly the role of olfaction in the induction of puberty in gilts. Kirkwood and Hughes (1980) attempted to advance puberty in gilts using 5α-androstenone, the signalling pheromone produced by the boar which, as mentioned above, is marketed commercially as an aerosol spray (Boar Mate) to aid in the detection of estrus. At 165 days of age, gilts were allocated to one of four treatment groups, as described in Table II. To expose the gilts to 5α-androstenone, a 10-sec burst of the commercially marketed aerosol spray was applied daily to food on the pen floor. In addition, each gilt was sprayed for 2 sec on the nostrils. Unfortunately, the results of this study were inconclusive because boar-exposed gilts were not significantly younger at puberty than the other groups, as they should have been. This was probably a consequence of using young boars (Kirkwood and Hughes, 1980, 1981). However, the gilts treated with the pheromone spray did not appear to reach puberty much earlier than control gilts.

In a small trial with only four animals in each of three treatment groups, the effectiveness of the signalling pheromone spray in inducing puberty was compared with the effectiveness of daily introduction into a pen previously occupied by a boar. By the age of 235 days, four gilts going to the boar pen were pubertal, two gilts receiving pheromone spray were pubertal, and no control gilts were pubertal (Kirkwood and Hughes, 1980). Although the results of such a small trial are by no means conclusive, it appeared that exposing the gilts to a pen previously occupied by a boar and presumably

TABLE II

Influence of Pen Change and Pheromone Exposure on Puberty Attainment in the Gilt[a]

Treatment	No. of gilts	Mean age at puberty (days)[b]
30 min of daily contact with a boar	10	203.6 ± 6.9
30 min of pen change daily	10	210.7 ± 2.4
30 min of pen change and daily exposure to 5α-androstenone	10	219.5 ± 5.3
Control	10	226.0 ± 8.3

[a] Data drawn from Kirkwood and Hughes (1980).
[b] Mean value ± SE.

permeated with his odor was effective in inducing early puberty. Apparently, priming pheromones remaining in the boar's pen after his removal were sufficient to induce early puberty. The evidence presented by Kirkwood and Hughes (1980) suggests that 5α-androstenone, a known signalling pheromone, is unlikely to have priming effects on puberty.

In another experiment designed to assess the role of olfaction in the boar's effect on puberty in gilts, Kirkwood et al. (1981) removed the olfactory bulbs of 6- to 7-week-old gilts. Beginning at 160 days of age, they were exposed to vasectomized boars for 30 min daily until puberty was reached. Bulbectomized gilts reached puberty at about the same age as gilts that received no boar exposure, whereas sham-operated and unoperated gilts that received boar exposure reached puberty more than 3 weeks earlier (Table III). The results of Kirkwood et al. (1981) demonstrate that olfaction plays a major role in the induction of puberty by the boar and again suggest that a priming pheromone is responsible for the boar's effect.

In a related study Kirkwood and Hughes (1981) found that very young boars (6.5 months of age) are ineffective in advancing puberty in gilts, whereas boars 11 months of age or older are capable of decreasing gilt age at puberty. This inability of young boars to advance puberty in gilts has been attributed to a lack of production of the priming pheromone or to a decreased ability to produce the pheromone as compared with older boars (Kirkwood and Hughes, 1981). This supposed lack of pheromones in young boars does not appear to be due to decreased levels of circulating testosterone, because serum testosterone levels in the young boars used by Kirkwood and Hughes were higher than those of the older boars.

There are age differences in the ability of boars to produce the gonadal 19-carbon steroids 5α-androstenone and 3α-androstenol (Booth, 1975), as well as age differences in the morphological and biochemical development of the submaxillary salivary gland (Booth et al., 1973), from which sig-

TABLE III

Influence of Olfactory Bulbectomy on Puberty Attainment in the Gilt [a]

Treatment	No. of gilts	Mean age at puberty (days) [b]
Bulbectomized, boar-exposed	9	229.9 ± 14.6
Sham-operated, boar-exposed	9	204.0 ± 2.5
Unoperated, boar-exposed	9	207.6 ± 8.5
Control, not exposed to boar	9	234.4 ± 7.8

[a] Data drawn from Kirkwood et al. (1981).
[b] Mean value ± SE.

nalling pheromones are released (Patterson, 1968). Both maturation of the submaxillary salivary gland and increases in the production of the 19-carbon steroids begin to occur at approximately 6 months of age (Booth, 1975; Booth *et al.,* 1973).

If Kirkwood and Hughes (1980) and Kirkwood *et al.* (1981) are correct in their suggestion that the submaxillary salivary gland is the probable source of priming pheromones as well as signalling pheromones, a lack of mature salivary glands may have prevented the young boars used by Kirkwood and Hughes (1981) from affecting gilt age at puberty.

The effect of the boar on age at puberty in gilts can be seen in traditional nonconfinement systems of swine production (Brooks and Cole, 1970) and in total confinement systems (Thompson and Savage, 1978). There has been a trend in recent years to use the total confinement system for intensified swine production. Gilts reared in confinement are capable of reproducing, but first estrus is delayed as a result of physiological stresses imposed by their environment (Thompson and Savage, 1978), so that only 40–80% of gilts show regular estrous cycles at breeding age (Christenson, 1981). The average age at first estrus for gilts reared in confinement (235 days) can be reduced to an average age of 225 days by boar exposure (Thompson and Savage, 1978). Apparently, the boar's presence provides enough stimulation to overcome some of the adverse effects of confinement on puberty (Thompson and Savage, 1978). Because the success of the total confinement system depends on reproductive efficiency, the effect of the boar can be used to lower the age at first farrowing, thereby increasing lifetime production.

At comparable ages, gilts reaching early puberty through boar contact have higher ovulation rates than controls and have experienced more estrous cycles (Paterson and Lindsay, 1980). They therefore have a higher reproductive potential. The advantages conferred by early mating on long-term productivity are discussed by Brooks and Smith (1980).

Although hormone treatments have been used to induce puberty in gilts, the degree of success of such treatments in inducing a pubertal ovulation is variable, and cyclic activity often does not persist (Hughes and Cole, 1978; Paterson and Lindsay, 1981). Furthermore, these treatments are costly and involve extra time and labor. The effect of the boar and presumably priming pheromones emitted by the boar can be used advantageously to improve reproductive efficiency in swine operations, both confinement and nonconfinement.

Many factors influence the age of puberty in heifers. In beef heifers, these factors include age and breed of dam, breed of sire and sires within breed (Laster *et al.,* 1976), heterosis (Wiltbank *et al.,* 1966), environmental temperature (Dale *et al.,* 1958), weight as affected by nutrition (Crichton *et al.,* 1959; Short and Bellows, 1971), and growth rates before and after weaning (Clanton *et al.,* 1964; Wiltbank, 1967). Until recently, the possibility that priming pheromones are an additional factor influencing the age of puberty in heifers had not been examined.

An experiment has been completed which was designed to test the hypothesis that a priming pheromone present in bull urine affects the age at puberty in heifers. This study was an attempt to extend basic research on pheromones and puberty acceleration in mice (see Chapter 4) to the cow, an economically important species. Although there was no existing experimental evidence that bulls produce priming pheromones that advance the age of puberty in heifers, conversations with local producers revealed the belief that young heifers housed near a bull grew faster than heifers isolated from a bull.

In this experiment 15 prepubertal crossbred beef heifers (approximately 10 months of age) were sprayed once per week in the nose and mouth with 3 ml of Angus bull urine. Nineteen control heifers were sprayed with water [for details of the experimental procedure see Izard (1981) and Izard and Vandenbergh (1982a)]. After 7 weeks of treatment with either bull urine or water, the heifers were palpated via the rectum and classified as either pubertal or prepubertal on the basis of palpable evidence of ovarian activity. Significantly more of the heifers sprayed with bull urine (67%) had reached puberty after the treatment period than had the heifers that were sprayed with water (32%) (Table IV). Therefore, it appears that bulls do excrete a urinary priming pheromone, similar to the urinary priming pheromone of male mice (Colby and Vandenbergh, 1974), that can hasten the onset of puberty in heifers.

Heifers of low body weight did not respond to spraying with bull urine, presumably because of immaturity. Gonzalez-Padilla *et al.* (1975b) showed that body weight can affect the response to hormones injected to induce estrus in prepubertal heifers. A body-weight-dependent response of female mice to the puberty-accelerating pheromone produced by male mice has also been demonstrated (Eisen, 1975).

Soon after the heifers in the preceding experiment were palpated to determine if they had reached puberty, they were put with bulls for a 90-day breeding period, and their subsequent calving dates were recorded. Exposure to bull urine had an effect on the mean day of calving, so that bull urine-treated heifers calved earlier than water-treated heifers (Table IV). Furthermore, the time of calvings was such that urine-treated heifers that reached puberty had a shorter calving season than water-treated heifers.

The finding that a pheromone in bull urine affects both the percentage of heifers reaching puberty and the subsequent calving date of those heifers

TABLE IV

Effects of Bull Urine on Puberty Attainment and Calving Date in Beef Heifers[a]

Treatment	No. of heifers	Percentage reaching puberty in 7 weeks	No. of heifers calving	Mean day of calving
Bull urine	15	67	13	34.4
Water	19	32	15	46.8

[a] Data drawn from Izard and Vandenbergh (1982a).

has implications for the management of reproduction in beef cattle. A large proportion of beef heifers do not reach puberty before or near the beginning of their first breeding season (Wiltbank *et al.,* 1969; Arije and Wiltbank, 1971). Although hormone treatments have been used to induce puberty in heifers (Gonzalez-Padilla *et al.,* 1975a,b; Short *et al.,* 1975; Berardinelli, 1976), these treatments are expensive and involve too much labor to be of use to the average producer. Perhaps a priming pheromone in the urine of bulls could be used to induce earlier puberty in heifers just as pheromonal cues from the boar have been used to accelerate puberty in gilts. It would not be surprising if this effect also occurred in dairy cattle.

Heifers that calve early in the calving season continue to calve early throughout their lifetime (Lesmeister *et al.,* 1973), alleviating the problems of a prolonged calving season (Wiltbank, 1970). A reduction in the length of the calving season leads to more effective management of labor at calving and more effective management of the calf crop at weaning. Therefore, priming pheromones in bull urine have additional potential applications for concentrating the calving season in beef heifers, because heifers exposed to bull urine have a shorter calving season (Izard and Vandenbergh, 1982a).

There is limited anecdotal evidence that the ram may have an effect on the attainment of puberty in ewe lambs, but there is no experimental evidence to substantiate the existence of this so-called ram effect (Dýrmundsson, 1981). In a study by Dýrmundsson and Lees (1972) the sudden introduction of a ram to ewe lambs resulted in a synchronized first estrus but did not influence the age at first estrus. If, in fact, the ram does accelerate puberty in ewe lambs through a priming pheromone, sheep would be ideal animals in which to investigate hormonal responses to priming pheromones. They are more convenient experimental animals than cows, and there is an extensive literature base on peripubertal hormone levels in sheep (see Foster and Ryan, 1979, for references).

B. Priming Pheromones and Termination
   of Seasonal Anestrus

In several mammalian species the male is believed to play a role in the termination of seasonal anestrus and the subsequent initiation of estrus or ovulation. Among domestic animals the role of the male in the termination of seasonal anestrus has been demonstrated in sheep and goats. As a group of ewes approaches the transition between seasonal anestrus and the onset of the breeding season, the introduction of a ram to the group stimulates reproductive function so that estrus occurs 15–20 days after the ram is introduced (Underwood *et al.*, 1944; Thompson and Schinckel, 1952; Edgar and Bilkey, 1963). Because the ewes react as a group to the stimulation of the ram, the result is synchrony of estrus in the ewes (Underwood and Shier, 1941; Underwood *et al.*, 1944).

A similar effect has been observed in goats. The introduction of a buck to a group of does just before the start of the breeding season results in initiation of synchronized estrus 5–10 days after the onset of exposure to the buck (Shelton, 1960; Shelton and Morrow, 1965; Ott *et al.*, 1980). For either the buck or the ram to exhibit these priming effects he must be a novel stimulus, because ewes and does exposed continuously to males do not show induction or synchronization of estrus.

On the basis of observations of corpora lutea at slaughter, Schinckel (1954a) concluded that ewes are induced to ovulate within 6 days of the introduction of a ram. This ovulation is unaccompanied by estrus (a silent ovulation) due to the lack of a waning corpus luteum but is followed approximately 17–18 days later (the length of a normal estrous cycle) by estrus and ovulation. More recent evidence, based on laparoscopic examination of ewes exposed to rams, suggests that 50% of ewes ovulate as early as 41 hr after the onset of ram exposure (Oldham *et al.*, 1979). About half of seasonally anovular ewes that ovulate in response to the ram's stimulation develop a corpus luteum with a normal life span and show estrus and ovulation about 18 days after ram introduction. The other half show premature regression of the corpus luteum followed by a second ovulation unaccompanied by estrus and formation of a second corpus luteum with a normal life span (Oldham and Martin, 1979). These ewes contribute to a second peak of estrous activity that has been observed approximately 24 days after ram introduction (Schinckel, 1954b; Lyle and Hunter, 1967; Fairnie, 1976).

Short cycles such as those seen in sheep have also been reported in goats after male stimulation (Ott *et al.*, 1980). However, goats differ from sheep in that both ovulation and estrus occur within 10 days of the introduction of a buck (Shelton, 1980).

Physical or visual contact is not necessary for the ram to induce estrus in ewes (Watson and Radford, 1960), suggesting that chemical cues may be involved. Furthermore, anosmic ewes fail to respond to the introduction of the ram (Morgan *et al.,* 1972). Male goats have a characteristic strong seasonal odor (Shelton, 1960). A "buck jar" containing the odor of the buck can be used as an aid in the detection of estrus in does (Smith, 1978). These observations have led to the suggestion that olfactory stimuli produced by the ram and the buck are responsible for the induction and synchronization of estrus in ewes and does in a manner similar to the synchronization of estrus in mice (Whitten, 1958). Experiments using both sheep and goats have been conducted to determine if pheromones produced in secretions of the male can initiate estrus as effectively as the presence of the male.

Knight and Lynch (1980) tested the capacity of ram urine or a combination of wax, collected from around the eyes and from the flanks of rams, and shorn wool to induce ovulation in ewes early in the breeding season. In these experiments the proportion of ewes ovulating after 3 days of treatment was measured by laparoscopy. In one experiment ewes were sprayed with ram urine or water six times daily for 3 days. Another group of ewes had contact with two rams. The proportion of ewes ovulating in the group of ewes sprayed with urine was intermediate between those sprayed with water and those exposed to rams (Table V). In a second experiment one group of ewes had wax rubbed on their nostrils and wool held over their muzzles for 1 min the first day. On the second day of treatment the same wool was again held over their muzzles, then left scattered around the pen for the rest of the treatment period. A second group of ewes was isolated from rams, and a third group had contact with four rams. Treatment with wax and wool was equally as effective as contact with rams in inducing

TABLE V

Effect of Ram Secretions on Percentage of Ewes Ovulating [a]

Treatment	No. of ewes	Percentage ovulating after 3 days
Ram contact	14	43
Ram urine	18	22
Water	17	0
Ram contact	26	50
Wax and wool	29	48
Isolated from ram	30	7

[a] Data drawn from Knight and Lynch (1980).

ovulation (Table V). The results of these studies indicate that pheromones in the wool and/or wax of rams are sufficient to stimulate ewes to ovulate early in the breeding season. The results also suggest that, although there may be some pheromonal activity in ram urine, it does not appear to be a major source of the stimulus pheromones.

Attempts to determine if priming pheromones emitted by the buck are responsible for the induction and synchronization of estrus in does have not given such unequivocal results. In a study designed to determine the effect of various degrees of male stimulation on the initiation of estrus in Angora does, Shelton and Morrow (1965) were unable to show an effect of buck odor alone. Exposure to male odor was accomplished by housing the treatment group in an area previously occupied by several bucks. Additional olfactory stimulation was provided by a sack of mohair shorn from rutting bucks, which was hung near the does' feed trough. This treatment group showed only a slight increase over controls in the percentage of does ovulating in that time (Table VI). However, Shelton and Morrow (1965) noted that in their opinion it was not possible to retain strong buck odor in an area throughout the 14- to 17-day experimental period without the presence of the buck.

In further experiments that examined the role of factors associated with the buck in the initiation of estrus in Angora does, Shelton (1980) exposed does to buck odor by housing them in an area previously occupied by rutting bucks. In addition, urine from rutting bucks was collected daily and placed in containers in the does' pen. According to Shelton (1980), only moderate success in concentrating buck odor was attained. However, there was a significant increase over controls in the percentage of does that ovulated after 9 to 12 days of treatment, although this increase was less than that seen in does that were in contact with bucks (Table VI).

TABLE VI

Effect of Buck Odors on Percentage of Does Ovulating

Treatment	No. of does	Percentage ovulating
Buck contact	42	90
Buck odor (vacated pen and shorn mohair)	38	26
No buck contact	36	19
Data drawn from Shelton and Morrow (1965)		
Buck contact	66	69
Buck odor (vacated pen and urine)	70	22
No buck contact	66	12
Data drawn from Shelton (1980)		

There appeared to be a positive relationship between a number of additional factors associated with the buck to which the does were exposed and the number of does that ovulated, leading Shelton (1980) to conclude that the initiation of estrus was due to a combination of several exteroceptive factors associated with the buck, including tactile, auditory, visual, and olfactory stimuli. However, it does appear that a priming pheromone in the urine of bucks can increase the number of does ovulating within a target period. This observation supports a hypothesis advanced by Coblentz (1976) concerning the function of scent-urination in ungulates. Most male ungulates, including goats, impregnate their pelage with urine during the breeding season, a behavior termed scent-urination by Coblentz (1976). On the basis of behavioral observations, Coblentz (1976) proposed that one function of scent-urination may be to hasten and synchronize the onset of estrus in females.

The problems encountered in the preceding experiments in concentrating the odor of the buck suggest that direct application of a test substance to a female in such a way that olfactory stimulation is ensured may be a more appropriate method of treatment. The role of priming pheromones in the induction of estrus in goats deserves more attention.

Although it has been clearly established that the introduction of a ram to ewes early in the breeding season causes ovulation within 3 days of initial contact with the ram (Knight *et al.,* 1978; Oldham *et al.,* 1979) and that pheromones in the wool or the wax of rams are responsible for this effect (Knight and Lynch, 1980), the mechanism by which the pheromones induce ovulation is still unknown. However, there is some evidence that stimulation of luteinizing hormone (LH) release is involved. Chesworth and Tait (1974) showed that increases in plasma LH concentrations of anestrous ewes in the middle of the nonbreeding season occur within 10 hr of the introduction of the ram. These increases are small (2–3 ng/ml) compared with the 80–200 ng/ml surges of LH that precede ovulation in ewes during the breeding season (Goding *et al.,* 1969). In ewes at the onset of the breeding season, ovulation was preceded by LH peaks that began at a mean of 35 hr after the introduction of the ram (Knight *et al.,* 1978). These ewes did not show the peak of estradiol 17B that normally precedes the release of LH in the estrous cycles of ewes unstimulated by rams (Goding *et al.,* 1969). As pointed out by Knight *et al.* (1978) the ram may stimulate release of LH independently of the positive feedback effect of estrogen on the hypothalamus. Such an input, through olfaction, would suggest the involvement of the VNO, which has neural connections with the hypothalamus (Scalia and Winans, 1975) and is thought to be a mediator of effects of priming pheromones that influence ovarian function (Johns, 1980; see also Chapter 8).

The role of the ram in synchronizing estrus in ewes can be used in a practical way to improve reproduction. Artificial insemination can be used to a greater extent if the timing of estrus is predictable. This procedure could sharply increase opportunities for genetic improvement. If breeding, either by AI or natural mating, is concentrated within a short period of time, then lambing will occur within a short time period, making management of labor more effective. In addition, lambs will be of comparable age and weight and can be marketed in a uniform group. In breeds such as the Romney the effect of ram introduction can be used to offset the slow onset of seasonal breeding activity in the ewes (Knight and Lynch, 1980).

The effect of the ram alone on the induction and synchronization of estrus or the effect of the ram in conjunction with hormone treatments can be used to improve reproductive efficiency in breeding flocks. Treatment with progesterone or synthetic progestagens for 2 weeks suppresses estrus in ewes. Withdrawal of hormone treatment is usually followed promptly by estrus and ovulation. In ewes injected daily for 2 weeks with progesterone, the introduction of a ram following the cessation of progesterone injections resulted in a reduction in the variance of the interval to onset of estrus (Lamond, 1964). In addition, more ewes showed estrus when the ram was introduced after progesterone injections than those in groups having the ram with them continuously. However, this effect was evident only at the beginning and end of the breeding season. Hormone treatments involve a great deal of labor if ewes must be injected daily for 2 weeks.

The use of intravaginal sponges permeated with a synthetic progestagen eliminates the need for daily injections. The presence of a vasectomized teaser ram during 2 weeks of treatment with a progestagen-impregnated intravaginal sponge increased the synchronization of lambing over that of ewes without ram contact (Hunter et al., 1971). Unfortunately, fertility is usually low at the first estrus after progesterone or progestagen treatment. While fertility is normal at subsequent ovulations, the synchronizing effect may be lost or diminished by the second estrus. Such hormone treatments must be improved before they can be routinely used by producers.

The influence of the buck on the induction and synchronization of estrus in does may be of less use in the management of reproduction of goats, because young goats are rarely marketed for meat, at least in the United States. However, if increased opportunities to use AI result from increased synchronization of breeding, producers of goat's milk can expect to see the same benefits and improvements in their herds as were seen in dairy cattle when the use of AI became routine. Furthermore, as pointed out by Ott et al. (1980), male stimulation in the late anestrous period would be important for breeding programs that require does to be bred as early as possible in the breeding season.

There is limited evidence that the boar may play a role in the induction of estrus in anestrous sows. Šipilov (1965) reported that the presence of a boar can stimulate a large proportion of anestrous, nonlactating sows to come into estrus. To my knowledge, no further work has been done on this aspect of the boar's influence. It would be interesting to determine if priming pheromones play a role in this effect.

C. Priming Pheromones and the Postpartum Interval

In addition to induction of early puberty and induction of estrus at the termination of seasonal anestrus, males can also have effects on the timing of postpartum estrus in females.

To ensure efficient reproduction in the swine, beef cattle, and dairy cattle industries, producers must rebreed sows and cows as soon after parturition and uterine involution as possible. For swine early rebreeding helps producers get a maximum number of farrowings per year from their sows. Early rebreeding in the beef and dairy industries is important to ensure yearly calving intervals.

Sows go through a period of postpartum anestrus, the cause of which is thought to be inhibition of the synthesis of LH and the release of follicle-stimulating hormone (FSH) via the suckling stimulus (Crighton and Lamming, 1969; Peters et al., 1969). Several researchers have been successful in reliably inducing estrus in lactating sows by grouping sows with their litters in the presence of a boar (Šipilov, 1965; Rowlinson et al., 1975; Petherick et al., 1977). In fact, the introduction of the boar to a group of sows and their litters is an essential management practice in systems of production that rely on rebreeding at lactational estrus for efficient operation. Rowlinson et al. (1975), working in a commercial unit, grouped Landrace sows and their litters at 3 weeks postpartum and introduced a boar the next day. Lactational estrus was shown by all 180 sows in the experiment. The interval from grouping to lactational estrus was 11.15 ± 0.28 days, with a conception rate of 84.9%. These sows had a mean farrowing interval of 153 days, with a potential yearly performance of 2.35 litters per sow.

Other workers have not been as successful in inducing lactational estrus with the boar (Guthrie et al., 1978; Petchey and English, 1980). However, Petchey and English (1980) were able to decrease the interval from weaning to first estrus and conception by introducing the boar to the sow and her litter before weaning. In this study boar presence during lactation reduced the interval between weaning and first breeding. A few sows were bred during lactation, and there was a reduction in the proportion of sows that took longer than 10 days to exhibit estrus after weaning. Petchey and English

(1980) hypothesized that the presence of the boar increases levels of pituitary FSH in lactation and that these higher FSH levels at weaning provoke a more rapid onset of estrus and ovulation.

Hillyer (1976) tested the possibility that a signalling pheromone (5α-androstenone) produced by the boar could shorten the interval between weaning and breeding. Sows at a commercial unit were weaned after a 35-day suckling period and allocated to one of two treatment groups or a control group. Sows were sprayed either once or twice on the nose with the commercially available 5α-androstenone (Boar Mate). There was a significant reduction in the average number of days from weaning to successful breeding in both treatment groups when compared to controls (Table VII).

It is noteworthy that an identified signalling pheromone can also act as a priming pheromone. Pheromones having dual signalling and priming effects have been identified in insects. For example, 9-oxodecenoic acid, a pheromone produced by the queen honeybee, inhibits queen rearing and suppresses oogenesis in workers, two priming functions. In addition, 9-oxodecenoic acid attracts drones during the nuptial flight, a releasing function (Butler, 1964). To my knowledge, Hillyer's study (1976) is the first demonstration of dual priming and signalling functions of a mammalian pheromone.

Although it is possible to use hormone therapy to induce postpartum estrus in sows (Cole and Hughes, 1946; Allen et al., 1957), inconsistent results and the commercial unacceptability of frequent hormone injections have prevented the incorporation of hormone therapy into commercial management practices. According to Rowlinson et al. (1975), systems that result in stimulation of endogenous hormone release are more acceptable. It appears that the effect of the boar, through priming pheromones, is to stimulate postpartum reproductive function. The success of this practice

TABLE VII

Effect of 5α-Androstenone on Days from Weaning to Successful Breeding in Swine [a]

Treatment	No. of sows	Mean days from weaning to conception
Pheromone spray on day 2 after weaning	34	10.3
Pheromone spray on day 2 and day 4 after weaning	71	9.0
Control	92	27.2

[a] Data drawn from Hillyer (1976).

has led to its incorporation into the management routines of commercial swine operations.

The length of postpartum anestrus and its effects on reproductive efficiency in cattle have led to a great deal of research on factors influencing calving-to-estrus intervals (see Carter *et al.,* 1980, for references), postpartum changes in hormone levels (see Britt *et al.,* 1981), and means of counteracting postpartum decline in ovarian activity (see Inskeep and Lishman, 1979; Britt *et al.,* 1981).

There is some evidence that the presence of a bull may influence postpartum ovarian activity, but these studies have been virtually ignored. Petropavlovskiĭ and Rykova (1958) exposed newly calved cows to a vasectomized bull for 3 to 4 hr twice daily. These cows conceived from fertile matings earlier than control cows that were isolated from stimuli from bulls. Nersesjan (1959) introduced vasectomized bulls to a group of postpartum cows. The number of cows that took less than 60 days to conceive after insemination was greater in the group that had bull contact than in a group of cows without bull contact. In addition, more of the cows with bull contact conceived from insemination at their first postpartum estrus. If a vasectomized bull is introduced to a breeding herd 30 days before the start of the breeding season, postpartum ovarian activity is increased. A group of cows teased in this manner all mated within 21 days of the start of the breeding season, whereas 52 days were required for the completion of breeding in unteased controls (Skinner and Bonsma, 1964). Teased cows would therefore calve earlier. A similar effect was seen by Izard and Vandenbergh (1982a), although treatment with bull urine was the only form of teasing that experimental heifers received. Heifers that were exposed to bull urine before the breeding season calved earlier in the calving season than control heifers.

It has been suggested that the decline in ovarian activity after calving is due to ovarian insensitivity to gonadotropins or to a deficiency in gonadotropin levels (Radford *et al.,* 1978). If the presence of the bull increases gonadotropin levels, the effects seen by Petropavlovskiĭ and Rykova (1958), Nersesjan (1959), and Skinner and Bonsma (1964) might be accounted for. Postpartum hormone levels are well known (see Britt *et al.,* 1981, for references), and hormonal changes due to the bull or odors associated with the bull could be easily measured. It would be of interest to investigate this area to determine if pheromonal effects are involved.

D. Priming Pheromones and Female–Female Interactions

Previous portions of this discussion on priming pheromones in domestic animals have dealt with male influences on ovarian function in the female.

Female ovarian function can also be influenced by cues originating from other females. For example, the age at puberty in young female mice is increased by priming pheromones produced by grouped females (Vandenbergh, 1973; Drickamer, 1974; see also Chapter 4). Synchrony of estrus or ovulation within a group of females is seen in several species (McClintock, 1981; see also Chapter 5). In rats synchrony of estrus is generated by airborne chemical cues or priming pheromones (McClintock, 1978, 1981).

In at least one species of domestic animal, the cow, there is evidence that female–female interactions affect ovarian function and that these interactions are mediated by priming pheromones. Cows whose estrous cycles are synchronized through the use of synthetic progestagens or prostaglandin $F_{2\alpha}$ ($PGF_{2\alpha}$) appear to enhance cycling in herd mates so that untreated cows in the same herd tend to show estrus along with or slightly after the treated cows (Weston and Ulberg, 1976; Zimbelman et al., 1977). The possible role of pheromones in this phenomenon was suggested by Weston and Ulberg (1976).

Two studies have been completed that were designed to determine if priming pheromones produced by estrous cows are responsible for influencing the timing of estrus in other cows (Izard, 1978, 1981; Izard and Vandenbergh, 1982b). This objective was carried out by first pretreating dairy heifers with $PGF_{2\alpha}$. In dairy and beef cows, $PGF_{2\alpha}$ is used to synchronize estrus in order to expedite the detection of estrus and the use of AI. If given to cows during the luteal phase of the estrous cycle, $PGF_{2\alpha}$ causes regression of the corpus luteum and the subsequent onset of the follicular phase of the cycle (Lauderdale, 1972). However, the timing of the onset of estrus is variable (Nancarrow et al., 1974). In the following experiments, synchrony was generated externally by the use of $PGF_{2\alpha}$, and then secretions from estrous cows were tested for their capacity to reduce the variance in the onset of estrus in the synchronized heifers.

Urine contains sexually stimulating odors in many species (Shorey, 1976). Bovine cervical mucus undergoes a number of hormonally induced changes associated with the estrous cycle (Hammond, 1927; Alliston et al., 1958; Foulkes et al., 1981). In order to maximize the changes of detecting pheromonal activity in the first experiment, a combination of urine and cervical mucus was tested for its capacity to influence the timing of estrus. Once daily for 3 days after $PGF_{2\alpha}$ injection, heifers received oronasal treatment with a mixture of urine and cervical mucus collected from estrous cows. The heifers were observed for estrous behavior and bred 12 hr after the onset of estrus. When compared to heifers that received oronasal treatment with water, there was a significant reduction in the variance of the onset of estrus, so that estrus following $PGF_{2\alpha}$ injection was more synchronized (Izard, 1978; Izard and Vandenbergh, 1982b). A subsequent study using a similar experimental protocol showed that oronasal treatment with cervical mucus alone could increase the sychronization of estrus after $PGF_{2\alpha}$ injection (Izard, 1981; Izard and Vandenbergh, 1982b). These results indicate that cervical mucus from estrous cows contains a priming pheromone that affects ovarian function in heifers (Fig. 1). This principle of pheromonal communication has been used in state-owned institutional herds in North

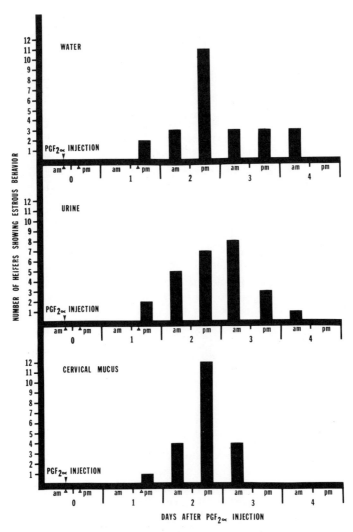

Fig. 1. Timing of the onset of estrus after $PGF_{2\alpha}$ injection. Heifers were exposed to water, urine from estrous cows, or cervical mucus from estrous cows at times denoted by arrows.

Carolina in conjunction with $PGF_{2\alpha}$ to set up a rhythm breeding program (L. C. Ulberg, personal communication).

Unfortunately, the conception rate in heifers treated with cervical mucus was only 25%, as compared with 64% in water-treated heifers and 58% in urine-treated heifers. This finding is surprising because cervical mucus in combination with urine did not depress conception rates (Izard and Vandenbergh, 1982b). Further investigation is needed to explore the cause of the lower conception rate in cervical-mucus-treated heifers.

If the decreased conception rate proves to be an aberrant result or the problem can be solved, an improvement in the synchronization of estrus following $PGF_{2\alpha}$ injections by a priming pheromone can improve cattle breeding programs. Such treatment will have a positive effect whether AI occurs after estrus detection or is used at a set time after $PGF_{2\alpha}$ injection. In the latter situation, breeding at a set time after $PGF_{2\alpha}$ injection eliminates the need for the detection of estrus. However, the degree of synchrony presently obtainable with $PGF_{2\alpha}$ usually yields fairly low conception rates if set-time AI is used. An increase in the degree of synchrony, as was seen in the cervical mucus group, should improve conception rates with set-time AI. If cows are artificially inseminated in relation to estrus, estrus must be detected. As shown by Hurnik *et al.* (1975), estrous behavior intensifies as the number of animals in estrus at the same time increases. Therefore, an increase in synchrony should increase estrous behavior, and consequently the detection of estrus should be improved.

Information is not yet available on the hormonal responses to the priming pheromones of domestic animals. In some cases these hormonal responses may prove to be analogous to the responses seen in mice and discussed in Chapter 7. The basic studies on the physiological responses to priming pheromones that have been conducted in mice can serve as a foundation on which to base future investigations in domestic animals.

IV. CONCLUSIONS

Signalling and priming pheromones induce sharp shifts in behavior or physiology in insects (Butler, 1964). In contrast, the effects of signalling and priming pheromones in domestic animals appear to take the form of minor adjustments to ongoing reproductive processes and behavior. The pheromonal stimuli may act synergistically with visual, auditory, or tactile cues to increase the magnitude of their effects.

The pheromonal mechanisms present in domestic animals are likely to have evolved as adaptive mechanisms ensuring reproductive success for the wild stocks. Modern husbandry practices—isolation of the sexes, crowding, artificial insemination, etc.—may prevent these mechanisms from functioning. By discovering and blending such mechanisms with modern husbandry practices, improvements in reproductive efficiency are possible.

Further work is needed not only to identify additional contexts in which priming and signalling pheromones have effects on the reproductive physiology and behavior of domestic animals, but to develop efficient practical means of incorporating presently known pheromonal effects into the management of reproduction of domestic animals. The identification, characterization, and synthesis of pheromonal compounds would facilitate their application to livestock management.

Research in the next decade may produce major advances in our knowledge of pheromones and the role they play in the reproduction of domestic animals. In the words of A. V. Nalbandov, "Of many unsolved problems I find myself greatly attracted to the role pheromones play in reproductive sexuality especially in domestic animals. If I were starting out in the field, I would certainly want to concentrate my efforts in this area" (Nalbandov, 1978; reprinted by permission from pp. 8 and 9.)

REFERENCES

Adams, M. G. (1980). *Symp. Zool. Soc. London* **45**, 57–86.

Allen, A. D., Lasley, J. F., and Uren, A. W. (1957). *J. Anim. Sci.* **16**, 1097–1098 (abstr.).

Alliston, C. W., Patterson, T. B., and Ulberg, L. C. (1958). *J. Anim. Sci.* **17**, 322–325.

Almquist, J. O., and Hale, E. B. (1956). *Proc.—Int. Congr. Anim. Reprod. Artif. Insemin., 3rd, 1956* Vol. 3, pp. 84–85.

Altmann, M. (1941). *J. Comp. Psychol.* **31**, 473–479.

Arije, G. F., and Wiltbank, J. N. (1971). *J. Anim. Sci.* **33**, 401–406.

Banks, E. M. (1964). *Behaviour* **23**, 249–279.

Banks, E. M., Bishop, R., and Norton, H. W. (1963). *Proc. Int. Congr. Zool., 16th, 1963* Vol. 2, p. 25.

Beauchamp, G. K., Doty, R. L., Moulton, D. G., and Mugford, R. A. (1976). *In* "Mammalian Olfaction, Reproductive Processes, and Behaviour" (R. L. Doty, ed.), pp. 143–160. Academic Press, New York.

Berardinelli, J. G. (1976). M.S. Thesis, West Virginia University, Morgantown.

Booth, W. D. (1975). *J. Reprod. Fertil.* **42**, 459–472.

Booth, W. D. (1980a). *Symp. Zool. Soc. London* **45**, 287–311.

Booth, W. D. (1980b). *J. Reprod. Fertil.* **59**, 155–156.

Booth, W. D., Hay, M. F., and Dott, H. M. (1973). *J. Reprod. Fertil.* **33**, 163–166.

Bourn, P., Carlson, R., Lantz, B., and Zimmerman, D. R. (1974). *J. Anim. Sci.* **39**, 987 (abstr.).

Britt, J. H., Cox, N. M., and Stevenson, J. S. (1981). *J. Dairy Sci.* **64**, 1378–1402.

Bronson, F. H. (1968). *In* "Perspectives in Reproduction and Sexual Behavior" (M. Diamond, ed.), pp. 341–361. Indiana Univ. Press, Bloomington.

Bronson, F. H. (1971). *Biol. Reprod.* **4**, 344–357.

Brooks, P. H., and Cole, D. J. A. (1969). *Proc. Easter Sch. Agric. Sci. (Univ. Nottingham),* 74–77.

Brooks, P. H., and Cole, D. J. A. (1970). *J. Reprod. Fertil.* **23**, 435–440.

Brooks, P. H., and Smith, D. A. (1980). *Livest. Prod. Sci.* **7**, 67–78.

Butler, C. G. (1964). *Symp. R. Entomol. Soc. London* **2**, 66–67.

Carter, M. L., Dierschke, D. J., Rutledge, J. J., and Hauser, E. R. (1980). *J. Anim. Sci.* **51**, 903–910.

Chesworth, J. M., and Tait, A. (1974). *Anim. Prod.* **19**, 107–110.

Chrichton, J. A., Aitken, J. N., and Boyne, A. W. (1959). *Anim. Prod.* **1**, 145–162.

Christenson, R. K. (1981). *J. Anim. Sci.* **52**, 821–830.

Clanton, D. C., Zimmerman, D. R., and Albin, R. C. (1964). *J. Anim. Sci.* **23**, 870 (abstr.).

Coblentz, B. (1976). *Am. Nat.* **110**, 549–557.

Colby, D. R., and Vandenbergh, J. G. (1974). *Biol. Reprod.* **11**, 268–279.

Cole, H. H., and Hughes, E. H. (1946). *J. Anim. Sci.* **5**, 25–29.

Crighton, D. B., and Lamming, G. E. (1969). *J. Endocrinol.* **43**, 507–509.

Dale, H. E., Ragsdale, A. C., and Cheng, C. S. (1958). *Fed. Proc., Fed. Am. Soc. Exp. Biol.* **17**, 31 (abstr.).

Donavan, C. A. (1967). *VM/SAC, Vet. Med. Small Anim. Clin.* **62**, 1047–1051.

Drickamer, L. C. (1974). *Dev. Psychobiol.* **7**, 257–265.

Dýrmundsson, O. R. (1981). *Livest. Prod. Sci.* **8**, 55–65.

Dýrmundsson, O. R., and Lees, J. L. (1972). *J. Agric. Sci.* **79**, 39–45.

Edgar, D. G., and Bilkey, D. A. (1963). *Proc. N. Z. Soc. Anim. Prod.* **23**, 79–87.

Eisen, E. J. (1975). *J. Anim. Sci.* **40**, 816–825.

Eisen, E. J., and Leatherwood, J. M. (1976). *J. Anim. Sci.* **42**, 52–62.

Esslemont, R. J. (1974). *Q. Rev. ADAS* **12**, 175–184.

Estes, R. D. (1972). *Mammalia* **36**, 315–341.

Fairnie, I. J. (1976). *In* "Proceedings of the International Sheep Breeding Congress" (G. T. Tomes, D. E. Robertson, and R. J. Lightfoot, eds.), pp. 500-508. W.A.I.T. Press, Perth.

Fletcher, I. C. and Lindsay, D. R. (1968). *Anim. Behav.* **16**, 410–414.

Foster, D. L., and Ryan, K. D. (1979). *Endocrinology* **105**, 896–904.

Foulkes, J. A., Hartley, P. E., and Stewart, D. L. (1981). *Res. Vet. Sci.* **30**, 14–17.

Gennings, J. N., Gower, D. B., and Bannister, L. H. (1977). *Biochim. Biophys. Acta* **496**, 547–556.

Goding, J. R., Catt, K. J., Brown, J. M., Kaltenbach, C. C., Cumming, I. A., and Mole, B. J. (1969). *Endocrinology* **85**, 133–142.

Gonzalez-Padilla, E., Wiltbank, J. N., and Niswender, G. D. (1975a). *J. Anim. Sci.* **40**, 1091–1104.

Gonzalez-Padilla, E., Niswender, G. D., and Wiltbank, J. N. (1975b). *J. Anim. Sci.* **40**, 1105–1109.

Gower, D. B. (1972). *J. Steroid Biochem.* **3**, 45–103.

Grau, G. A. (1976). *In* "Mammalian Olfaction, Reproductive Processes, and Behaviour" (R. L. Doty, ed.), pp. 219–241. Academic Press, New York.

Guthrie, H. D., Pursel, V. G., and Frobish, L. T. (1978). *J. Anim. Sci.* **47**, 1145–1151.

Hafez, E. S. E., and Bouissou, M. F. (1975). *In* "The Behaviour of Domestic Animals" (E. S. E. Hafez, ed.), pp. 203–245. Baillière, London.

Hale, E. B. (1966). *J. Anim. Sci.* **25**, Suppl., 36–44.

Hammond, J. (1927). "The Physiology of Reproduction in the Cow." Cambridge Univ. Press, London/New York.

Hart, G. H., Mead, S. W., and Regan, W. M. (1946). *Endocrinology* **39**, 221–223.

Hillyer, G. M. (1976). *Vet. Rec.* **98**, 93–94.

Hodgson, R. E. (1973). *J. Dairy Sci.* **56**, 614–620.

Hradecký, P. (1978). *Vet. Morfol. Fysiol.* **31**, 1–21.

Hughes, P. E., and Cole, D. J. A. (1976). *Anim. Prod.* **23**, 89–94.

Hughes, P. E., and Cole, D. J. A. (1978). *Anim. Prod.* **27**, 11–20.
Hulet, C. V., Blackwell, R. L., Ercanbrack, S. K., Price, D. A., and Wilson, E. O. (1962). *J. Anim. Sci.* **21**, 870–874.
Hunter, G. L., Belonje, P. C., and Van Niekerk, C. H. (1971). *Agroanimalia* **3**, 133–140.
Hurnik, J. F., King, G. J., and Robertson, H. A. (1975). *Appl. Anim. Ethol.* **2**, 55–68.
Inkster, I. J. (1957). *N.Z. Sheep Farm. Annu.* pp. 163–169.
Inskeep, E. K., and Lishman, A. W. (1979). *Beltsville Symp. Agric. Res.* **3**, 277–289.
Izard, M. K. (1978). M.S. Thesis, North Carolina State University, Raleigh.
Izard, M. K. (1981). Ph.D. Thesis, North Carolina State University, Raleigh.
Izard, M. K., and Vandenbergh, J. G. (1982a). *J. Anim. Sci.* **55**, 1160–1168.
Izard, M. K., and Vandenbergh, J. G. (1982b). *J. Reprod. Fertil.* **66**, 189–196.
Jacobs, V. L., Sis, R. F., Chenoweth, P. J., Klemm, W. R., Sherry, C. F., and Coppock, C. E. (1980). *Theriogenology* **13**, 353–356.
Johns, M. A. (1980). *In* "Chemical Signals: Vertebrates and Aquatic Invertebrates" (D. Müller-Schwarze and R. M. Silverstein, eds.), pp. 341–364. Plenum, New York.
Karlson, P., and Butenandt, A. (1959). *Annu. Rev. Entomol.* **4**, 39–58.
Karlson, P., and Luscher, M. (1959). *Nature (London)* **183**, 55–56.
Kelley, R. B. (1937). *Bull.—C.S.I.R.O. (Aust.)* **112**.
Keverne, E. B. (1974). *New Sci.* **63**, 22–24.
Kiddy, C. A., and Mitchell, D. S. (1981). *J. Dairy Sci.* **64**, 267–271.
Kiddy, C. A., Mitchell, D. S., Bolt, D. J. and Hawk, H. W. (1978). *Biol. Reprod.* **19**, 389–395.
Kiddy, C. A., Conley, H. H., and Hawk, H. W. (1980). *J. Dairy Sci.* **63**, Suppl. 1, 91 (abstr.).
Kirkwood, R. N., and Hughes, P. E. (1979). *Anim. Prod.* **29**, 231–238.
Kirkwood, R. N., and Hughes, P. E. (1980). *Anim. Prod.* **31**, 205–207.
Kirkwood, R. N., and Hughes, P. E. (1981). *Anim. Prod.* **32**, 211–213.
Kirkwood, R. N., Forbes, J. M., and Hughes, P. E. (1981). *J. Reprod. Fertil.* **61**, 193–196.
Knight, T. W., and Lynch, P. R. (1980). *Anim. Reprod. Sci.* **3**, 133–136.
Knight, T. W., Peterson, A. J., and Payne, E. (1978). *Theriogenology* **10**, 343–353.
Ladewig, J., and Hart, B. L. (1980). *Physiol. Behav.* **24**, 1067–1071.
Ladewig, J., and Hart, B. L. (1981). *Biol. Reprod.* **24**, 1165–1169.
Ladewig, J., Price, E. O., and Hart, B. L. (1980). *Behav. Neural Biol.* **30**, 312–322.
Lamond, D. R. (1964). *J. Reprod. Fertil.* **8**, 101–114.
Laser, D. B., Smith, G. M., and Gregory, K. E. (1976). *J. Anim. Sci.* **43**, 63–70.
Lauderdale, J. W. (1972). *J. Anim. Sci.* **35**, 246 (abstr.).
Lesmeister, J. L., Burfening, P. J., and Blackwell, R. L. (1973). *J. Anim. Sci.* **36**, 1–16.
Lindsay, D. R. (1965). *Anim. Behav.* **13**, 75–78.
Lindsay, D. R., and Robinson, T. J. (1961). *J. Agric. Sci.* **57**, 141–145.
Lombardi, J. R., Vandenbergh, J. G., and Whitsett, J. M. (1976). *Biol. Reprod.* **15**, 179–186.
Lyle, A. D., and Hunter, G. L. (1967). *S. Afr. J. Agric. Sci.* **10**, 597–608.
MacLeod, N., Reinhardt, W., and Ellendorff, F. (1979). *Brain Res.* **164**, 323–327.
McClintock, M. K. (1978). *Horm. Behav.* **10**, 264–276.
McClintock, M. K. (1981). *Am. Zool.* **21**, 243–256.
McGrath, T. J. (1981). M.S. Thesis, Texas A. & M. University, College Station.
Mavrogenis, A. P., and Robinson, O. W. (1976). *J. Anim. Sci.* **42**, 1251–1255.
Melrose, D. R., Reed, H. C. B., and Patterson, R. L. S. (1971). *Br. Vet. J.* **137**, 497–502.
Milligan, S. R. (1980). *Symp. Zool. Soc. London* **45**, 251–275.
Morgan, P. D., Arnold, G. W., and Lindsay, D. R. (1972). *J. Reprod. Fertil.* **30**, 151–152.
Nalbandov, A. V. (1978). *In* "Novel Aspects of Reproductive Physiology" (C. H. Spilman and J. W. Wilks, eds.), pp. 3–10. Spectrum Publ., New York.
Nancarrow, C. D., Hearnshaw, H., Mattner, P. E., Connell, P. J., and Restall, B. J. (1974). *J. Reprod. Fertil.* **36**, 484 (abstr.).

Nersesjan, S. S. (1959). *Anim. Breed. Abstr.* **30,** 220.

Oldham, C. M., and Martin, G. B. (1979). *Anim. Reprod. Sci.* **1,** 291–295.

Oldham, C. M., Martin, G. B., and Knight, T. W. (1979). *Anim. Reprod. Sci.* **1,** 283–290.

Ott, R. S., Nelson, D. R., and Hixon, J. E. (1980). *Theriogenology* **13,** 183–190.

Paleologou, A. M. (1977). *Vet. Rec.* **100,** 319, 320.

Paterson, A. M., and Lindsay, D. R. (1980). *Anim. Prod.* **31,** 291–297.

Paterson, A. M., and Lindsay, D. R. (1981). *Anim. Prod.* **32,** 51–54.

Patterson, R. L. S. (1966). *Nature (London)* **212,** 744–745.

Patterson, R. L. S. (1968). *J. Sci. Food Agric.* **19,** 38–40.

Perry, G. C., Patterson, R. L. S., MacFie, H. J. H., and Stinson, C. G. (1980). *Anim. Prod.* **31,** 191–199.

Petchey, A. M., and English, P. R. (1980). *Anim. Prod.* **31,** 107–109.

Peters, J. B., First M. L., and Casida, L. E. (1969). *J. Anim. Sci.* **28,** 537–541.

Petherick, D. J., Rowlinson, P., and Bryant, M. J. (1977). *Anim. Prod.* **24,** 155–156 (Abstr.).

Petropavlovskiĭ, V. V., and Rykova, A. I. (1958). *Anim. Breed. Abstr.* **27,** 798.

Radford, H. M., Nancarrow, C. D., and Mattner, P. E. (1978). *J. Reprod. Fertil.* **54,** 49–56.

Rowlinson, P., Boughton, H. G., and Bryant, M. J. (1975). *Anim. Prod.* **21,** 233–241.

Sambraus, H. H., and Waring, G. H. (1975). *Z. Saeugetierkd.* **40,** 49.

Scalia, F., and Winans, S. S. (1975). *J. Comp. Neurol.* **161,** 31–56.

Schinckel, P. G. (1954a). *Aust. J. Agric. Res.* **5,** 465–469.

Schinckel, P. G. (1954b). *Aust. Vet. J.* **30,** 189–195.

Shank, C. C. (1972). *Z. Tierpsychol.* **30,** 488–528.

Shelton, M. (1960). *J. Anim. Sci.* **19,** 368–375.

Shelton, M. (1980). *Int. Goat Sheep Res.* **1,** 156–162.

Shelton, M., and Morrow, T. (1965). *Prog. Rep.—Tex. Agric. Exp. Stn.* **2340,** 20–21.

Shorey, H. H. (1976). "Animal Communication by Pheromones." Academic Press, New York.

Short, R. E., and Bellows, R. A. (1971). *J. Anim. Sci.* **32,** 127–131.

Short, R. E., Bellows, R. A., Carr, J. B., Staigmiller, R. B., and Randel, R. G. (1975). *J. Anim. Sci.* **41,** 379 (abstr.).

Signoret, J. P. (1970). *J. Reprod. Fertil., Suppl.* **11,** 105–117.

Signoret, J. P. (1972). Ph.D. Thesis, University of Paris.

Signoret, J. P. (1974). *Ann. Biol. Anim., Biochim., Biophys.* **14,** 747–755.

Signoret, J. P. (1976). *In* "Mammalian Olfaction, Reproductive Processes, and Behaviour" (R. L. Doty, ed.), pp. 243–256. Academic Press, New York.

Signoret, J. P., and du Mesnil du Buisson, F. (1961). *Congr. Int. Reprod. Anim. Insemin. Artif., 4th, 1961* Vol. 2, pp. 171–175.

Sipilov, V. S. (1965). *Veterinariya* **42,** 81–83.

Skinner, J. D., And Bonsma, J. C. (1964). *Proc. S. Afr. Soc. Anim. Prod.* **3,** 60–62.

Smith, M. C. (1978). *Cornell Vet.* **68,** Suppl. 7, 200–211.

Stinson, C. G., and Patterson, R. L. S. (1972). *Br. Vet. J.* **128,** xli–xlii.

Thompson, L. H., and Savage, J. S. (1978). *J. Anim. Sci.* **47,** 1141–1144.

Thompson, L. H., and Schinckel, P. G. (1952). *Emp. J. Exp. Agric.* **20,** 77–79.

Tomkins, T., and Bryant, M. J. (1974). *J. Reprod. Fertil.* **41,** 121–132.

Underwood, E. J., and Shier, F. L. (1941). *J. Dep. Agric., West Aust.* **18,** 13–21.

Underwood, E. J., Shier, F. L., and Davenport, N. (1944). *J. Dep. Agric., West. Aust.* **21,** 135–143.

Vandenbergh, J. G. (1969). *Endocrinology* **84,** 658–660.

Vandenbergh, J. G. (1973). *J. Reprod. Fertil., Suppl.* **19,** 411–419.

Vandenbergh, J. G. (1975). *In* "Hormonal Correlates of Behavior" (B. E. Elefthériou and R. L. Sprott, eds.), Vol. 1, pp. 551–584. Plenum, New York.

Waring, G. H., Wierzbowski, S., and Hafez, E. S. E. (1975). *In* "The Behaviour of Domestic Animals" (E.S.E. Hafez, ed.), pp. 330–369. Baillière, London.

Watson, R. H., and Radford, H. M. (1960). *Aust. J. Agric. Res.* **11,** 65–71.

Weston, J. S., and Ulberg, L. C. (1976). *J. Dairy Sci.* **59,** 1985–1988.

Whitten, W. K. (1958). *J. Endocrinol.* **13,** 399–404.

Williamson, N. B., Morris, R. S., Blood, D. C., Cannon, C. M., and Wright, P. J. (1972). *Vet. Rec.* **91,** 50–58.

Wilson, E. O., and Bossert, W. H. (1963). *Recent Prog. Horm. Res.* **19,** 673–710.

Wiltbank, J. N. (1967). *In* "Factors Affecting Calf Crop" (T. J. Cunha, A. C. Warnick, and M. Koger, eds.), pp. 44–59. Univ. of Florida Press, Gainesville.

Wiltbank, J. N. (1970). *J. Anim. Sci.* **31,** 755–762.

Wiltbank, J. N., Gregory, K. E., Swiger, L. A., Ingalls, J., Rothlisberger, J. A., and Koch, R. M. (1966). *J. Anim. Sci.* **25,** 744–751.

Wiltbank, J. N., Dasson, C. W., and Ingalls, J. E. (1969). *J. Anim. Sci.* **29,** 602–605.

Wysocki, C. J. (1979). *Neurosci. Bio. Behav. Rev.* **3,** 301–341.

Zimbelman, R. G., Lauderdale, J. W., and Moody, E. L. (1977). *Proc. Conf. Artif. Insemination Beef Cattle, 11th, 1977* pp. 66–75.

Index

BELOIT COLLEGE

Pheromones and reproduction in

000
010101

0 2021 0011306 9